Madness
at the Movies

*Understanding Mental Illness
through Film*

James Charney, MD

JOHNS HOPKINS UNIVERSITY PRESS | Baltimore

Johns Hopkins University Press
2715 North Charles Street
Baltimore, Maryland 21218–4363
www.press.jhu.edu

All quotations from films are the author's own transcriptions made from watching a given film. The quotes are not taken from official versions of the screenplays, which often differ from the final films. Any errors are the author's own.

Library of Congress Cataloging-in-Publication Data is available.

ISBN 978-1-4214-4562-5 (pbk)
ISBN 978-1-4214-4563-2 (ebook)

A catalog record for this book is available from the British Library.

Special discounts are available for bulk purchases of this book.
For more information, please contact Special Sales at specialsales@jh.edu.

For Noah

And for Eleonora and Izabella
from Greppen, with love

CONTENTS

I grew up on Long Island, not far from New York City, loving movies. A child of the 1950s, I went to the movies almost every week, first with my parents and then on my own or with friends. My mother loved musicals and dramas; my dad wasn't interested at all. I took after my mother. I loved the entire experience of going to the movies. Our local cinema was not very special, but it was magical to me. No matter what the feature film, there were cartoons, nature films, newsreels, and coming attractions. Sometimes the coming attractions were the best part of the show—even mediocre movies looked good in a coming attraction short.

I loved the horror films, even though they gave me nightmares. I still get the shivers thinking about *Them!*, a movie about giant radioactive ants created by atom bomb tests (lots of 1950s horror films reflected the anxieties and paranoia of the Cold War, but as a kid I didn't know about any of that—they were just very scary movies, and I loved them). Years later I watched *Them!* again and I was pleased to see how well made it was. So many of those B horror movies were just bad; if I was going to be terrified by a scary movie, at least I had chosen a good one!

I've written elsewhere about why we like horror movies (see Recommended Reading at the end of this chapter). It's still something of a puzzle. As a kid, I would often watch them from behind my hand, fingers spread just enough for me to peek at the screen. One time when I was nine, my mother was delayed picking me up from the theater, so I stayed and watched *The Creature from the Black Lagoon* a second time. Boy, was that a mistake! I had bad dreams for weeks. But still I went back.

Sometimes as a family we would go to roadshow presentations. You bought your ticket in advance for those. They were a luxury: a ticket for a roadshow presentation cost $2.50 when an ordinary double feature cost 35 cents. Unlike most films that ran continuously, these had a firm starting time, and because they were long epics, they even had intermissions, like a live play. Some had glossy programs. We saw *The Ten Commandments*, *Around the World in Eighty Days*, and *This Is Cinerama* with its wraparound screen. We went to fancy movie houses in New York City, like Radio City Music Hall and the Roxy Theater, for some of these shows. They were special outings that remain happy memories.

HOW I LEARNED TO LOVE CLASSIC MOVIES

I went to college at Columbia University, where I was able to take what I believe was the first history of film class at the school. This was years before there was anything like a film studies major, much less a department of film studies. There, I saw silent films for the first time, and black-and-white films from the 1930s and 1940s that blew me away, like the sophisticated comedies of Ernst Lubitsch: *Ninotchka* with Greta Garbo and *The Shop Around the Corner* with Jimmy Stewart and Margaret Sullavan. I loved Howard Hawks's fast-talking screwball comedies, like *Twentieth Century* with John Barrymore and Carole Lombard and *Bringing Up Baby* with Cary Grant and Katharine Hepburn.

I had never seen a Marx Brothers movie until I took that class. I couldn't imagine how they allowed such comic anarchy in the movies, but they did, and it was wonderful. My favorite was *Duck Soup*. I loved Groucho with his leering slouch and quick wit.

Casablanca became my favorite film, a wartime love story for the ages, with a tough and sentimental Humphrey Bogart and a beyond beautiful Ingrid Bergman. I wanted to be Bogart. I had a poster of him in my room and memorized much of his dialogue. "Here's looking at you, kid" and "This could be the start of a beautiful friendship" may not mean anything if you haven't seen the movie (see it!), but if you have, they will instantly transport you.

I also saw films from other countries for the first time. The showing of foreign films was becoming more common during my college years; before that, it was rare to watch a film with subtitles (it's still rare today in the States, though with streaming services it is becoming more popular). My friends and I discovered the films of Ingmar Bergman, such as *The Seventh Seal* and *Persona*, Federico Fellini with his *La Dolce Vita* and *8 1/2*, and Akira Kurosawa's *Rashomon* and *The Seven Samurai*. Later, we reveled in the independent films of Cassavetes and the wonderful weirdness of Buñuel and developed a new appreciation for the work of Orson Welles. His *Citizen Kane* (1941) has been called the greatest film ever made. It remains amazingly fresh and revolutionary even today.

In the late 1960s and early 1970s American filmmakers like Francis Ford Coppola, Steven Spielberg, and Martin Scorsese came into their own, making films of power and creative energy. Many of them were influenced by the freedom and originality of films from abroad. It was a golden time to love the movies.

During my college days, in the mid-1960s, if you didn't get to see an older film in a class, you had only one other option. There were no such things as VHS tapes or DVDs and certainly nothing like the streaming services we have today. The Thalia was a run-down theater on the Upper West Side that showed classic movies, one of a few such theaters in New York. It presented smartly put-together double features, which would be shown for a few days at a time. You were at the mercy of whoever made the choices, but if they were showing a movie you wanted to see and you were an enthusiast like me, you made a beeline there, no matter what. It was at the Thalia that I first saw *Dinner at Eight* and *Grand Hotel*, two MGM extravaganzas with big stars of the 1930s, and many of the other Marx Brothers films I loved.

I had become the very definition of an amateur: a lover and appreciator of movies. One who had begun to learn how to read them, to understand how they worked. I subscribed to *Variety*, the professional journal for plays and films, and imagined I would write for them some day. I loved *Variety*'s slangy style (with headlines like the famous

1935 "Stix Nix Hick Pix"; that is, "Farmers Don't Like Farm Pictures"). I can remember a time I stood outside the *Variety* office in New York and simply couldn't bring myself to enter. I didn't have confidence that I was a good enough writer, and I didn't have the nerve to put it to the test.

My dad was a doctor, a well-known gastroenterologist, and his work was his life. He was committed in a way I couldn't imagine for myself, but he encouraged me to give medicine a try, and I did.

BECOMING A DOCTOR

So, I shifted my life plans. I became a pre-med at Columbia but continued majoring in English; you could do that back then. Today, the demands on pre-meds, with so many required science courses, make it almost impossible. I got into the Medical School at Duke University, in North Carolina, one of the most creative programs in the nation. At Duke we were introduced to patients and clinical work in the second year instead of waiting until our last year, like at most med schools. It made a world of difference, giving us a sense of what the work was like early enough to make good decisions about our future specialty.

Medical school is unlike any other postgraduate education. It is modeled on the guilds from the Middle Ages: students apprentice to practicing physicians and learn from their experience. Though the first years of medical school are traditional classes that focus on the basic sciences like biochemistry and physiology, the initiation into the privilege of being a doctor starts with an introduction to the cadaver. That unnerving first time, standing with a student-partner over a dead person whose body you will be dissecting to learn anatomy, separates you from other people. As physicians, we are privileged to violate the norms of social engagement. We are permitted, invited, to touch another person in private places and ask awkward questions in order to diagnose and treat what is causing them pain or discomfort. A doctor can palpate a belly, put a stethoscope on their chest, look closely into their mouth or ears, ask them about the color of their stool or other bodily discharges.

Duke brought physician-students into the clinical world earlier than other medical schools, introducing us to the learning model described in the catchphrase, "See one, do one, teach one." This is only a slight exaggeration.

Going on rounds with the senior physician could be daunting. He or she would fire questions about the patient who had been assigned to us, and we had better have the answers: what was the result of last night's blood tests, what did you notice when you examined the patient's eyes or palpated her belly, what diagnoses might explain her symptoms, what tests did you think should be done next? This way of teaching (Socratic on steroids!) forced us to be thorough in our examinations, to think on our feet, and to get by on very little sleep.

It also inspired me. These were teachers I wanted to emulate.

I loved working with children and thought initially I would become a pediatrician. But once I was allowed to follow an admired pediatrician around in his office, I realized how hectic the typical practice was. This pediatrician would see each child for only a few minutes before moving on to the next. He was someone who would have wanted to spend more time to get to know his patients, but the demands of seeing mostly well children for checkups didn't allow it. That wasn't for me.

Then I did a wonderful rotation with Drs. Pearce and Easley, two old-time obstetrician-gynecologists (Eleanor Easley was the first female gynecologist in North Carolina). I loved learning from them and I loved delivering babies. What I didn't love were the hours. Babies are delivered when they are good and ready, and that often means in the middle of the night. Also, the gynecologic part of their work was basically surgical, and after working at Dr. Easley's side in the operating room a few times, she gently took me aside and said, "Jim, whatever you do, don't choose a specialty where you work with your hands." Very good advice. She was right; surgery was not for me.

So, I found myself gravitating to psychiatry. It used the skills of analysis I had learned as an English major, and people's stories fascinated me. I wanted to learn how to help. In psychiatry you got to spend time with your patients and really get to know them. This was a specialty that allowed an authentic relationship to develop, especially with children. I liked that a lot.

My love of movies continued while I was in medical school. I wrote a weekly column called *On Film* for the local newspaper, *The Durham Chronicle*. The column allowed me to keep up with the latest films and gave me an outlet to talk about them.

While at Duke I met Diane, the woman who would become my wife. She was working on her PhD in French literature. We both played piano and we met on a blind date to play duets. Two years later, we were married. Fifty years later, we still are.

MOVIES IN SEATTLE

My psychiatric residency after finishing medical school was at the University of Washington in Seattle. I arrived there in 1972, and I stayed not only for the two years of the General Psychiatry program but for the additional two years of a Child Psychiatry Fellowship. We loved the Pacific Northwest, a gardener's paradise. The weather was eccentric, with mild, rainy winters that could feel dreary to someone from the East, and summers that felt like the best of spring. People from Seattle would say, "We have two seasons. Winter and August." That suited us fine.

Another reason we loved it there was the Seattle Film Society. I can't remember how this wonderful group started, but it was in full bloom when we arrived. They would offer curated film programs built around a theme, usually the work of a single director. If memory serves, film showings occurred weekly, so in the fall, attendees might see films by Howard Hawks, like *Only Angels Have Wings*, *His Girl Friday*, and *Red River*. Seeing the films in this way showed, for example, Hawks's range, from a romantic drama about daredevil pilots in South America starring Cary Grant and Jean Arthur, to a fast-talking newspaper comedy, to a John Wayne Western with Montgomery Clift that focused on the conflict between Wayne as a tyrannical father and Clift as his son. Each movie was accompanied by a brilliant biographical handout that included an analysis of the film. This became an important part of my film education. I don't know who wrote those handouts, but I really wish I did because I would want to thank them.

IT'S NOT EASY TO LEARN THERAPY

The UW psychiatry program was excellent, teaching an eclectic mix of therapeutic models. It's where I gravitated away from individual psychodynamic therapy into more active therapies, working not only with individuals but with couples and eventually with families.

Teaching talk therapies is complicated because therapies are supposed to be private. In order to teach them, you must show what happens in them. During the first years of my psychiatric training, the dominance of the psychoanalytic model made that difficult. However, things were changing. New ways of practicing therapy allowed for a co-therapist student to be in the room or for the therapy to be observed from outside. We didn't have video cameras at the ready, though that was coming, but we did have one-way mirror rooms and telephones.

The patients would know they were being observed by students or other doctors positioned behind the mirror in an adjacent room. Sitting there was like watching a movie. The shape of the mirror-window even mimicked the shape of a movie screen. This was wonderful for learning play therapy with young children, or family or couples therapy. It also worked for individual therapies. "See one, do one" operated here too. We would get the chance to watch an experienced therapist engage with a patient, demonstrating a specific way of doing therapy. Then we would do a therapy session with a patient, and other students and the senior doctor would watch from behind the mirror. If a student got stuck, not knowing how to respond to something the patient said (this happens a lot in the beginning), the telephone in the room might ring. It would be the teaching doctor suggesting a response to try; allowing the student to say it and see where it leads. Soon after, the telephone was replaced by a "bug in the ear," a small earpiece that allowed the teacher to coach the next response without the interruption of the telephone. This was very helpful. Watching therapies as though they were movies, but with the added benefit that someone could intervene in what was happening, came back to me years later as I was developing the Yale course that became this book.

I had wonderful mentors at the University of Washington and made lifelong friendships with my teachers and fellow residents. I got to spend several months of my Child Fellowship at a clinic in Maui, Hawaii, part of the WWAMI Program, bringing specialist doctors to underserved areas. As one of only two child psychiatrists on the island, I would often see families in their homes, and taking off your shoes at the door was their custom. I flew every week in a single-engine plane (just me and the pilot) to the island of Lanai, back then called the Pineapple Island for its only crop. I treated the children of the pineapple workers and their parents in a makeshift clinic in the school auditorium. Another day, I would drive with a colleague three hours on a Maui coast road with some 300 curves (with the Pacific Ocean on the left and jungle waterfalls on the right) to the isolated town of Hana for another children's clinic in the only hotel there. Hana is where Charles Lindbergh chose to spend his retirement, and no wonder: this place fulfills every fantasy of paradise. It certainly did mine. I loved my time on Maui, and we considered staying on, but being so far from family weighed on my wife and me, so we decided that after the fellowship I would look for a job back East, which brought me, in 1976, to New Haven, and to Yale.

TEACHING "MADNESS AT THE MOVIES" AT YALE

I loved teaching and Yale University gave me many opportunities. At first, I was full-time at the Medical School, but I soon realized that academic medicine was not for me. I was not interested in research or publishing in journals. I liked to see patients and teach. So, I switched to the Clinical Faculty and opened a private practice office focusing on family therapy with children and adolescents. I also became a consultant to several local public schools, and for some twenty years I was the school psychiatrist to Choate Rosemary Hall, a prestigious boarding school nearby. I thought of these consulting positions as opportunities to teach, and they were.

At Yale I taught regularly in the two departments where I had appointments, the Department of Psychiatry and the Child Study Center. My interest and background in family therapy was unusual at Yale back then. Both departments were still mostly psychoanalytic in their approach to talking therapy. But they did ask me to teach a family therapy seminar, and I was able to encourage interested residents to try their hand at it whenever they could.

A social worker colleague and I put together a group for medical students to talk about the challenges they experienced as they began to assume the role of physician. It can be quite stressful to become someone to whom others turn for life-saving treatments when you are insecure about what you actually know or can do. The Medical School had never considered helping students with this transition, and the students were enthusiastically grateful for the opportunity to explore it with each other.

I also taught diagnosis and interviewing to medical students in their first psychiatric rotations—skills that would serve them well in whatever specialty they chose to pursue. The psychiatric mental status exam is a structured series of questions and behavioral observations that, like the physical examination, needs to be practiced over and over. Just as you must listen to many hearts before you can be confident of what you are hearing and what it might mean, you need to learn how to ask about changes in mood, energy, appetite, thoughts, and worries before you can make a confident psychiatric diagnosis. I taught this in small tutorials, just a few students at a time, on the hospital ward using in-person interviews with patients that the student did not know, so that there would be no prior knowledge of the patients' diagnoses.

I would sit in the room with the students and watch them do an interview, telling them in advance that at some point I would step in and take over, to underline a technique or show how to get a more useful response. We would discuss the interview and determine the likely diagnosis. I would encourage the student to practice as many times as possible in the coming week, then we would meet again to interview a different patient. Even though I am now retired from my private practice, I still teach interviewing and the mental status exam whenever I am in New Haven. It is a delight for me to see how much the students improve in a few short weeks.

In 1993 I discovered the Freshman Seminar program at Yale College. This was revolutionary for Yale University, which was not often open to new ideas: a series of unusual seminars on subjects that did not fit easily into the standard curriculum, taught by experts who were not necessarily on the Yale faculty. These seminars were made available exclusively to entering freshmen. Each seminar had to be sponsored by two of the then twelve colleges of the university. The seminars could only be taught a limited number of years to give other subjects a chance in the rotation.

My first Freshman Seminar course was one I called "The Family in Literature," a cross between psychiatric family theory and comparative literature. We analyzed how families were portrayed in classic works of fiction, from Aeschylus to Shakespeare to James Agee in his remarkable novel, *A Death in the Family.* One of the works I included was a first novel by Judith Guest called *Ordinary People*, which I thought was a good complement to the Agee novel on how families grieve a sudden loss.

Then, one day in 1996, my wife and I went to the movies. The Yale Film Society regularly screened classics, as well as new films. The film that evening was *Ordinary People*, based on the book, and it moved me deeply with its quietly detailed portrait of an adolescent and his family, separate in their grief and unable to help each other. *Ordinary People* also had one of the best examples of good, compassionate therapy I had ever seen in a commercial film.

It gave me an idea. Could I find other movies as effective in their portrayal of mental illness and therapy and make a course of them?

I presented this to the Freshman Seminar boards, and "Madness at the Movies" was born. After three years as a College Seminar, it became a regular seminar in the Blue Book, the Yale College course book, co-sponsored by the departments of Psychology and Film Studies. I taught that course at Yale for more than ten years.

I loved teaching "Madness at the Movies" and it proved very popular. As a seminar, which values exchanges in class between students and the teacher, it was capped at twenty-five students. Each sponsoring department required that I choose one-third of each class from students who were majoring in that department's subject: so, one-third psychology majors, one-third film studies majors. I made a point of choosing the final one-third from as widely varied backgrounds as I could find: students majoring in physics, English, history, economics, art history, computer science, philosophy, music, and more. For that varied one-third, I required no prior formal education in film or psychology, just an interest in film and in human nature.

More than 150 students would apply each year for the 25 spots. During the "shopping period" at the beginning of each term, I would have each student fill out a brief questionnaire asking them to tell me about themselves and why they wanted to take the class. The eclectic mix made for lively discussions that often went in unexpected directions.

Most years there was one session with an invited guest. Often it was Richard Brown, who had created "Movies 101," an adult education class at New York University in New York City. For thirty years his class provided opportunities for movie enthusiasts to have a first look at new movies and to see him interview major film stars and directors. He is a wonderful interviewer, funny and warm, and even the most reluctant actor loosens up when talking to him. He was asked to do interviews with Golden Age film performers such as Jimmy Stewart, Audrey Hepburn, and Robert Mitchum for the Library of Congress. You can see excerpts from many of his interviews online. In my class, he talked about *Psycho*, *Annie Hall*, and *Hannah and Her Sisters*, giving the students a vivid sense of the decisions that go into making a film.

A highlight visit one year was with Joe Greco, the writer and director of a very good film called *Canvas*, which we screened for the university community the day of his visit. It is about the effect of a mother's bipolar illness on her husband and child. A beautiful movie.

Joe Pantoliano came to class that day too. Joey is an actor with a remarkable filmography, including major roles in *Memento, The Matrix, Midnight Run,* and *The Fugitive.* He played Ralph in *The Sopranos,* whose death is one of the most memorable in the series. Joey, who produced *Canvas,* also played the father in a tender and touching performance. In class, he talked about his own problems with depression and how they informed his portrayal. Bringing guests like these to the seminar added a different dimension to our discussions, helping my students better understand how complicated the process of creating a movie can be and how exciting.

A WORD ABOUT WORDS

I call this book *Madness at the Movies* because that is exactly what it's about. It also suggests, I hope, that I will be plain-speaking, avoiding jargon or specialized language. And it suggests that the book might be fun to read. I also like the title because of the alliteration; it's catchy and grabs most people's interest. In the early days of teaching my course, if anyone asked about it and heard the title, they immediately "got it" and started recommending movies and forms of madness I might want to include. That enthusiasm was infectious.

The word "madness" has a long history (dating back to the fourteenth century) and, unlike words like "crazy" or "insane," it's not a put-down or an insult. It has always meant what it means now: a disorder of the mind that causes bizarre, irrational, compulsive, or psychotic behavior, or changes of mood that cause the person emotional distress and affect his or her ability to function.

The term most commonly used for these disorders in psychology texts and medical journals is "mental illness." It means the same thing, but is an attempt to medicalize madness, to put it in the same category as pneumonia or ulcers. It implies a certainty of understanding that we don't yet have.

Is someone suffering from a mental illness because of genetic vulnerability, a physical defect, environmental causes, or problems of living? For many forms of madness, we just don't know. So why insist on using a medical-sounding name? Though occasionally here I will use the term "mental illness," I prefer just calling it "madness."

This became an issue in the naming of my course at Yale. There is a bit more to my origin story.

I was an odd duck to both departments that were co-sponsoring my course. I was a psychiatrist teaching psychology students and an amateur appreciator of movies teaching film students. I must give them credit for supporting me even though I had never taken a film studies or a psychology class and even though I was a psychiatrist (a medical doctor) in a world of psychology PhDs—very different worlds, with very different languages.

After my "Madness at the Movies" class had been running at Yale for several years, I was unexpectedly called into the office of the Department of Psychology. They told me how much the department liked the course and the students' enthusiasm for it. Then they said that the department had a problem. They were bothered by the name of the course. "We don't use the word 'madness' here in the psychology department. We say 'psychopathology.' We want you to change the course title to 'Psychopathology in the Movies.'" I tried to argue my case: that "madness" exactly described my subject. It was a good, solid, Old English word, and it was catchy too. People responded to it. My argument fell on deaf ears. The Yale Course Book required a more formal title. Starting the next term, the title of the course had to change.

A few weeks later, the office of the Film Studies Department, my other sponsor, called me in. You can probably see where this is going. They praised the course but told me that the film studies people had a problem with my course title. They didn't like using the word "movies" in the course catalogue. "We don't teach 'movies' at Yale, we teach 'film.'" The department chair was fine with my keeping "madness" in the title, but "movies" had to go.

Sigh. The next semester, the class was called "Psychopathology in Film" in the Yale Blue Book. Would you be as eager to take that class as you would one called "Madness at the Movies"? I don't think so. That title is airless, has no character, no energy. It doesn't sound like fun. And my class was fun.

Fortunately, it didn't matter. The course was already well known in the college as "Madness at the Movies," students were still eager to take it, and we never referred to it as anything but "Madness at the Movies."

▪1▪

"What do you think you are, for Chrissake, crazy or something?"

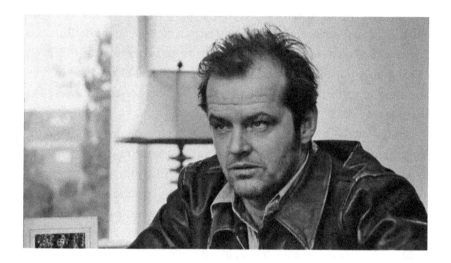

Introduction

Our subject is the experience of madness. What is it like to have your thoughts, perceptions, and feelings—how you see the world and yourself—be shaped and distorted by mental illness?

We will examine this inner world. And we will explore how films work to help us understand it.

To enjoy this book, you do not need to have a background in psychology or in film. What matters is that you are interested, not just in madness or movies but also in how our minds work, in what it means to be human.

Many people get their knowledge of mental illness from what they see in movies or on television. As a cultural force, movies shape our understanding and can even shape our definitions of what madness is, for better or worse. This is why I think it is important to examine how it is represented in movies.

There are many valid approaches in the field of film studies to thinking about movies, with a wide range of theoretical perspectives. These studies help advance our artistic appreciation and cultural understanding of film in many ways.

I do not begin with a theoretical paradigm either from film studies or psychiatry. Mine will be a practicing psychiatrist's view, specifically focused on the clinical question of how mental illness is portrayed. This requires a humble ability to observe and interpret, relying on what I see as well as on the consensus of medical understanding of each illness, to finally discover what diagnosis best fits that portrayal.

Guided by the body of essential research in psychology and psychiatry that constantly informs clinical practice and my many years of experience watching, interpreting, and teaching film, I apply my psychiatric skills to an understanding of human experience and how it is represented in the movies. My goal is to teach not psychiatric diagnosis but how to observe and interpret behaviors that signify madness in films. I will also be talking about film craft—how the film helps us experience the mental illness of the main character.

As a psychiatrist and an autodidact on film, I believe I am particularly well placed to study how madness is portrayed. Treating the characters in fictional films as though they were real, taking them as seriously as they take their fictional selves (and as their creators take them), I can use my clinical skills and experience to examine their history, their behaviors, and what the film allows us to know about how they think, and make considered judgments on the accuracy of these representations.

The conjunction of the medical and the humanities is something I have encouraged and valued for my entire teaching career. These disciplines can learn from each other, but in academia they have too often been kept apart. In *Madness at the Movies*, I bring them together to understand the nature and experience of mental illness.

Movies don't just show the behaviors of madness, they can help us sense what drives them. They are immersive. They touch us emotionally. The best of them can pull us into their reality until it becomes our reality. We don't just watch; we become absorbed as though we are living it too. When that happens—and it does in most of the movies here—it's a remarkable thing.

We will also consider the question of diagnosis: what it means to put a name to a mental illness. The films examined in this book get much right in their portrayals. Exploring what they get wrong (including factors that don't fit with how a particular mental illness is experienced by most people) can open discussion and help us see the real nature of the madness.

Finally, in the last chapter we will look at psychotherapy. Does it help, and if so, how? Can films really show us what therapy is like? I'll save you the suspense. The answer is "no." But they can come pretty close.

WHY USE FILM TO STUDY MADNESS?

When I began to look for films that might work to study the experience of mental illness, I found myself watching them differently. Not just for enjoyment or to entertain, but to see if they were comprehensive enough, with enough detail and example in their portraits of the main character, to give us something to analyze. I wanted to be able to examine a fictional movie character with as much depth as I would a patient who came to my office. But a film could do more, because I would be seeing that character not just in an office but with the people who mattered and the world they lived in. Doctors must intuit so much of this when we see patients in an office or hospital setting.

As I planned the course that is the basis for this book, I decided to also explore how the craft of film is used to convey what the person experiences and suggest what he or she is thinking and feeling. I wanted to help my students see how these films worked. I also wanted to only present films that were considered masterpieces: not just classics, but films whose excellence and ability to move an audience had been proven over time.

As a film aficionado, I had been surprised at how little most Yale students knew about films made before they were born. These were films that defined the history of movies. Many of my students had never seen a black-and-white or silent movie. Many had never heard of the great directors of the twentieth century, such as Ingmar Bergman, Billy Wilder, or Howard Hawks. They didn't know the stars of the so-called first Golden Age of movies (usually considered the 1930–40s), such as Humphrey Bogart, Cary Grant, Jimmy Stewart, James Cagney, Ingrid Bergman, Greta Garbo, or Katharine Hepburn. They had never heard of many of the great international stars, such as Anna Magnani, Marcello Mastroianni, Catherine Deneuve, Simone Signoret, Jean Gabin, or Charles Laughton. Alfred Hitchcock and Marilyn Monroe they knew, but either only by name or for one or two films. To my surprise, this was often true for the film studies majors too.

The students who applied for my seminar often did not recognize all the films on the syllabus. They were interested in the subject (movies and madness). The film titles were not the draw. However, without exception, when the course ended, they thanked me for introducing them to films and filmmakers that were new to them. They would tell me that the course had opened a new world of classic movies for them to explore.

Yale used to have a film society that showed some of these classic older films, but as DVDs and online streaming became more available, the need for scheduled theatrical film showings abated, and they finally stopped. Ironically, the wide availability of these resources has led to fewer classic movies being watched. If you didn't know about them, or if someone didn't present them to you, it wouldn't occur to you to look for them. And besides, there are so many new films to choose from.

I wanted to change that. Not only by choosing movies that showed madness in three dimensions, but also by making sure the movies we discussed were acknowledged masterpieces, no matter how old. I showed different films in class over the years, seeing how each worked to teach about mental illness. I finally settled on the classic movies that I thought were most powerful in their portrayals. These are the films featured in this book. They are all the best I have found to help us understand what living with a mental illness feels like; the best at using the techniques of film to enhance that understanding.

I write in each chapter about aspects of movie history, including how these films were received and what they tell us about prevalent assumptions about mental illness and treatment at the time they first came out. If you understand something of the world and times the movies portray, it will add to your appreciation. I also talk about why these films are considered masterpieces.

Films have a unique ability to draw the watcher into their world using images, action, story, atmosphere (a sense of place and time), sound and music, and, of course, great acting. They can convey action and states of mind (thinking, imagining, feelings) through camera and editing techniques, such as cuts, juxtapositions, focus, the placement of the camera, close-ups of faces and objects, point of view, and montage (putting together fragments of film to make a continuous whole, conveying the passage of time or of events). Movies are particularly good at conveying sensory experiences. We can get inside the head of someone suffering from a madness, seeing the world through his or her eyes.

A film can draw the viewer deeply into its world, especially the world of its central characters. I will talk about how films heighten our identification with a particular character, how they shape our reactions to both events and people, how they can make objects develop an emotional valence. It's not just the screenplay or cinema magic that engages us; the quality of the acting makes a big difference too.

The overall structure of a movie can prove instructive. For instance, most films are in three acts, like a play. This is not always obvious, but if you look for it, you will see it. The first act introduces the characters and the situation, often pointing to a conflict. The second act shows how the conflict affects the main players and may introduce additional complications to the story. The third act brings the story to a conclusion, not always resolving things but usually pointing to where they will lead. These acts are often indicated by a fade-out of one scene into another, or a change of pace or tone. Sometimes, there will simply be text on the screen reading, "Six Months Later." The acts give a rhythm to the movie that keeps the audience engaged and interested in what will happen next. And in the films here they often expose the worsening of madness symptoms and how they affect family and friends—until things get better, or don't.

WHAT IS A CLASSIC MOVIE?

To be considered a classic film, a movie must be at least a generation (twenty-five years) old. And it must have something about it that makes it stand out: originality, brilliance of execution, a story that speaks over the years to the human condition. To call a new movie a "classic" is making a prediction that it is special and will be remembered years from now. These predictions can be notoriously bad. Some films that were touted as unusually important were quickly forgotten. Other films received bad reviews or were unappreciated when they were first released (for instance, *The Night of the Hunter* and *Peeping Tom*), but were rediscovered years later and are now seen as worthy of the designation "classic."

Not every classic film is a masterpiece. Many are classics because of their role in film history: the first to deal with a particular subject, or define a genre, or use a film technique. For instance, *King Kong* is a classic because it was the first popular monster picture with stop-motion animation, which was state-of-the-art in 1933, and it used it to portray King Kong, the dinosaurs, and other prehistoric creatures. It set the standard for all the monster films that followed. However, it shows its age, with stiff acting, a slow pace, and obviously artificial sets. Despite that, it is entertaining, and the set pieces (Kong fighting a Stegosaurus, the battle on top of the Empire State Building) are iconic and gripping. It works.

The movie *Frankenstein* (1931) is a classic for much the same reason. The image of the Monster is part of our culture. The Monster's encounters with a blind man and with a child, neither of whom is frightened of him, respecting his humanity (the blind man can't see, and the child accepts him as he is) are touching and real and have inspired similar scenes in many movies since. The scene in

Dr. Frankenstein's laboratory when he captures lightning and wakes the Monster to the cry of "It's alive!" still brings chills, despite the wooden, declamatory acting. The movie isn't great, but it has great moments, some of them historic because they were the first of their kind. That makes it a classic too.

The movies of Fred Astaire and Ginger Rogers from the 1930s have by-the-numbers plots and unremarkable direction, but the dance numbers are sublime, some of the best ever filmed, defining the developing romance between Fred and Ginger with incredibly graceful and romantic ballroom dancing and energetic and often funny tap dances. The movies are classics because the dances are classics, inspiring every dance style since, from ballet to tap to hip-hop.

Many not-great movies can count as classics because they have embedded themselves in popular culture with images, situations, lines of dialogue, or moments of brilliance that not only reflect their times, but also speak to us today. On the other hand, there are classics that are indeed masterpieces: films that are great, that work, that show the creativity and signature styles of the controlling artists—the director, the writer, the actors, or the composer. In the best films, it is all of them, working together to create something wonderful.

You can make a case for calling a movie a classic by pointing to its place in film history or in popular culture. To consider a movie a masterpiece is more an opinion than a statement of fact. You can argue for it, but one person's masterpiece is another person's snooze. There are many people who think Andrei Tarkovsky is one of the greatest film directors of all time. I find most of his films pretentious and boring. As my mother, an occasional font of wisdom, used to say, "That's what makes horse races!"

In my opinion, all the featured movies in these essays qualify as both classics and masterpieces.

One of the questions I ask prospective students of my class is to name their favorite movie. I'm looking for unexpected choices, which can give me an insight into their interests and their personality—sort of a movie Rorschach test. So, in a gesture toward full transparency, and so you can get to know me better, here are a few of the films that I love, films I would be happy seeing again and again (but which, because they aren't about madness, are not in the book): Buster Keaton's *The General*, *Bringing Up Baby*, *The Wizard of Oz*, *Swing Time*, *The Big Sleep*, *Notorious*, *The Third Man*, *Casablanca*, *Yankee Doodle Dandy*, *The Best Years of Our Lives*, *Singin' in the Rain*, *Some Like It Hot*, *8 1/2*, *The Seven Samurai*, *Wild Strawberries*, *Les Enfants du Paradis*, *Chinatown*, *Lawrence of Arabia*, *Annie Hall*, *Moonstruck*, *Close Encounters of the Third Kind*, and *The Godfather, Parts 1 and 2*.

What about the "Other Vision" movies discussed at the end of each chapter? I think they are all excellent films worth seeking out and watching. They are usually not as completely focused on portraying madness as the featured movie, and there may be aspects of the films that just don't work or are simply wrong, which I point out. Though some are classics, many are not. I include them because of particular moments in each that explore different aspects of the mental illness discussed in the chapter. They give us another viewpoint, either through telling a different story or by using different techniques to convey the madness experience. I see them as complements to the featured film.

HOW I CHOSE THE MOVIES

The essays here are meant to be casual and personal and clinically rigorous when addressing the question of diagnosis. I chose films that speak to me, that I find interesting and engage me each time I see them, and that illustrate madness categories that play to my strengths as a psychiatrist. I make no attempt to be encyclopedic or comprehensive. Other movies might serve, but these are the ones I like.

I don't write about every form of mental illness: about anorexia, drug or alcohol addiction, attention deficit disorder, autism, borderline or histrionic or narcissistic personality disorders, post-traumatic stress disorder (except maybe a glancing mention), or gender dysphoria. These are all worth study. But I had to make choices, and I chose the forms of madness that most intrigued me, and that I hope will most interest you.

I narrowed my movie choices to make it a bit easier to decide what to include. The first decision I've already explained: to choose films that I (and others more expert than I) consider masterpieces, great films. I also decided to limit myself to standard-length films that were originally shown in theaters.

Long-form television movies hardly existed when I first began teaching my course. They are not only common now, but many are very good. They might be worth including in a book like this. But, for now, I think the book is rich enough without them, focusing as it does on classic films. It's also too soon to know which current series will have staying power. However, I could see myself writing a follow-up to this book focusing on limited series: for instance, *The Sopranos*, *In Treatment*, *Homeland*, *Girls*, *Crazy Ex-Girlfriend*, and *Mare of Easttown*. These are very well done and deserve to be appreciated.

There are no films here that give supernatural explanations for any form of madness (such as *The Exorcist*), no films based on fantasy (*Lord of the Rings*, *The Shape of Water*), and only one film based on the Marvel or DC Universes (*Joker*, as one of the most successful films of the last decade, demanded attention; my discussion of the film, however, shows why I usually avoid this genre). We are trying to stay in the world of the real: real madness and real people. Superheroes, fantastic creatures, and the supernatural have their place, but not here.

Periodically, I will refer to the important issues of how women are portrayed in a film. Movies reflect the attitudes of their time, and some of the portrayals in these and other films are quite dated. Too often women are portrayed as victims, as helpless, as having no agency, or as sexual objects inviting violence. The film noir "femme fatale" may powerfully control men with her sexuality, but that is a stereotype too. These issues and those of the portrayal of race, class, and gender identity are subjects that deserve recognition. I will refer to them if they highlight something about madness. But, as a psychiatrist, I think it best to keep my focus on what I know: the clinical study of mental illness, and how films influence popular understanding.

The walk-through descriptions of the films are quite detailed because these films are dense with incidents and behaviors that well illustrate the featured madness. They give us a lot to consider—a reason I chose them.

One important thing to point out: even though these films are best of breed, none of them is perfect. They will sometimes get some aspect of an illness wrong because of the needs of the story or because the creative artists simply didn't know any better. But those mistakes can be instructive and provide us with something more to discuss. What they get wrong can actually increase our understanding of what the madness really is.

THE REASON FOR THE SEQUENCE OF THE MOVIES

When psychiatrists begin training, they are usually put on a hospital ward with the most dramatically ill patients, those with psychotic illnesses such as schizophrenia. One reason for this is that the symptoms of these illnesses are so different from common experience that they are easier to discern, easier to see as different. The more extreme, the clearer it is that this is not "normal." This makes it easier for a young trainee to learn to keep a professional distance and yet balance that with compassion and empathy. As the trainee moves out of the hospital and begins to see people whose mental illness, however disabling it may be, allows them to function, they may recognize themselves and their own, perhaps milder version of the illness. That can make them a better therapist ("I feel your pain"), but it also may make it more difficult for them to be objective ("How can I help you when I have the same problems you have?"). Maintaining that balance is central to psychiatric training, and in fact to the training of anyone learning to be a healer.

We will follow that path here for the same reasons. As we progress through the book, we move from severe psychosis, illnesses involving a loss of reality, with hallucinations and delusions (*Through a Glass Darkly* and *Repulsion*), to paranoid delusion (*Taxi Driver*), to the personality diagnosis of the psychopath (*The Night of the Hunter*, *Strangers on a Train*), someone who on the surface may look more like us, who is not obviously responding to things that are not there (such as hallucinations or illusions), but who we still understand to be mentally ill. Then we move to dissociative states such as multiple personality (*Psycho*), to obsessions (*Peeping Tom*), and, finally, to the anxiety disorders and symptoms of obsessive-compulsive disorder, OCD (*As Good as It Gets*). By this time, we are looking at more common forms of madness, ones that we may have experienced ourselves, what I call "garden-variety" disorders.

HOW TO USE AND ENJOY THE BOOK

Each chapter focuses on one particular mental illness, examining a film that features it, then, in the Other Visions section, I explore examples of other films that portray the illness differently.

For each chapter I start with an introduction to the featured film and to the artists who made it. I talk about how the movie was made, how it reflects its time, and how it was received by the public and by critics. Then my walk-through of the film describes what happens moment by moment, accompanied by commentary about important aspects of the characters' madness and about film craft, how the movie works.

You will likely have the best experience with this book if you can watch each movie before reading the chapter that discusses it. Most of these films are easily found on streaming services, in your university or public library, or for rent or purchase online. I particularly recommend The Criterion Channel (https://www.criterionchannel .com) and Mubi (https://mubi.com), streaming services that offer well-curated selections of great films, old and new.

Of course, the best way to see any movie is on a large screen, in a darkened theater with an audience. If you have the opportunity to see any of these movies that way, grab it. Watching in a theater is immersive; you have few distractions, the darkness helps you stay focused, the big screen pulls you in, and the audience reaction can enhance your own. Laughing by yourself at a comedy is nowhere near as satisfying as laughing with others. The gasp of surprise while watching a thriller or finding tears in your eyes during a tender moment in a drama are all the better when shared with an audience: strangers in the dark, together.

No written description of a movie can possibly fully convey all that is there. I can only describe what I see, what I think matters in that moment. When you watch the film, though the broad outlines of what you see will be the same as what I describe, you might well notice different things: a look on another character's face, something meaningful that you notice on a table, or someone's tone of voice. My walk-through will, I think, convey what is most important for my discussion. If you have seen the film before, reading about it here can refresh your memory and suggest other ways of understanding what you have seen. This is the beginning of a silent dialogue with me, which I encourage.

If your first experience of any one of these movies is to read my moment-by-moment description, I think it will be more than enough to understand why I chose it to represent the featured madness. I don't think you need worry that it will somehow "spoil" the movie for you when you finally get to watch it. I have lived with these films for more than twenty years and have seen every one many times. They stay fresh even when I know exactly what will happen in the story. I would say *Psycho* is the one exception. In that film the surprise is uniquely powerful; see that movie first, if you can.

My discussion of each madness will give you some idea of how psychiatrists make a diagnosis, how we observe behavior and use what the person says about his or her experience to begin to define the illness (or determine if there is one). I hope this will help develop your skills of observation and analysis. I also hope it will help you understand how very complex this process of understanding really is.

Diagnosis, both medical and psychiatric, is an opinion. It is a knowledgeable one, based on scholarship and experience. But, especially with film when the information is often incomplete and there is much we can't know because we can't ask, there is room for uncertainty and disagreement. The purpose of trying to form a diagnosis is to figure out what you are dealing with when patients come to you distressed by how they are feeling or functioning (or when someone is brought to you because others are concerned about them). Once you have determined a diagnosis you can then plan a treatment. Every diagnosis (whether it's cancer, pneumonia, the flu, depression, or paranoia) has a history of therapies that have been tried with varying degrees of success. You will choose among those and offer them to the patient. Observing behavior is an important part of the diagnostic process and studying the films in this book can help you be a better observer.

I will be frequently complaining about the *DSM-5*, the *Diagnostic and Statistical Manual of Mental Disorders*, which codifies diagnoses for research and insurance billing purposes. If you study abnormal psychology or if you become a therapist, you will see it referred to a lot. There is a reductionistic quality to this manual, an implied certainty, that I object to. People are more complex than a code can ever convey. Our movies here will underline that.

Since this is a personal selection of movies I like, I do not attempt to cover everything in the world of abnormal psychology. If you want more information about a particular madness (for instance, to learn about the research that has been done to understand the etiology of the illness) or want to find out about illnesses that I don't discuss, I suggest you refer to an abnormal psychology textbook. You will find that their brief case studies tell us little about the experience of each madness. But the other subjects they do cover, the best of them do well. I would recommend the textbook *Abnormal Psychology*, written by my Yale colleague Susan Nolen-Hoeksema, sadly deceased, published by McGraw-Hill. Her book, in its 8th edition, is a model of clarity and compassion. Another good textbook is *Abnormal Psychology: The Science and Treatment of Psychological Disorders*, 14th edition, by Ann M. Kring and Sheri L. Johnson, published by Wiley.

ANOTHER WORD ABOUT WORDS

There is a worthwhile movement to stop using words such as "schizophrenic" to describe someone with schizophrenia (and rather to call them "a person with schizophrenia"). This is laudable, a way of saying that people are not defined by their illness.

I don't think such discretion works with the category of madness called the personality disorders, including the psychopath, the narcissist, and others. When this diagnosis fits, though it may not describe the totality of their character, it does speak to the essence of their nature, who they are and how they interact with the world. Here, their madness is not a disturbance from the normal, it is their "normal," and it does define them. So, when speaking of psychopaths, I call them psychopaths.

THE ELEPHANT IN THE ROOM

You may wonder why I am including Roman Polanski's *Repulsion* and Woody Allen's *Hannah and Her Sisters* in this book, when their creators are so controversial.

There is no better film to show a woman's gradual but rapid descent into psychosis than *Repulsion*. The story, the acting, and the brilliant but measured special effects all not only contribute to an immersive and disturbing experience, but show accurately what it's like to be Carol, dramatically losing touch with reality. Similarly, the Mickey subplot in *Hannah and Her Sisters* defines generalized anxiety and hypochondria better than any other film I know.

That these movies are the works of people whose personal lives are controversial and even sordid seems to me beside the point. We are exploring the work, not condoning what the artist does behind closed doors.

As Walt Whitman wrote, we contain multitudes. We all at times have behaved badly. Should we be judged only by the bad? If so, many other artists would be dismissed, ignored, and vilified: Caravaggio, who was a low life and a murderer; Wagner, a virulent anti-Semite; Picasso, who was a misogynist and a thief; Hitchcock, with his fetish for blondes and a history of bullying performances out of them. The list could go on. Should we really close the door on their best works because of their worst behavior?

In a recent lecture, author Tobias Wolff was discussing his love for the work of Ernest Hemingway. He was asked how he could love the work when the man is the exemplar of a toxic version of manhood. Hemingway was seen that way while he was alive. With the cultural changes of recent decades, his persona seems even more to be despised. Wolff's reply was that though he would likely not want to ever meet or spend time with Hemingway for those very reasons, he still admired the work. He pointed to several of Hemingway's stories as evidence that he understood women, however badly he might have treated them in life.

Wolff said (I paraphrase), "I like to think of a masterwork as having arrived sealed in a glass bottle, floating on the ocean. Isolated from whoever wrote it. So, I can appreciate it for just how very good it is." He also said, "I like to think that Hemingway's stories are the best of him; that writing them he left the worst of himself behind."

I am not advocating for the personal lives of any of the artists represented in the films here. It is not my role to judge them. I will leave that to others who are better placed, and to history. It is the films that matter; and what they can teach us here about madness and about the craft of moviemaking.

BRIEF WORDS OF CAUTION AND ENCOURAGEMENT

This is a book about mental illness. Some of these films can be distressing to watch. Ironically, it's not the violent movies, nor the ones about psychosis, but the films about families and relationships that are often the most troubling. We will talk about why.

Every year that I taught the "Madness at the Movies" course, I would give this warning to my students during the first class. I would invite any students who thought they might be disturbed by one of the films, or were upset by a film they had watched for class, to come and talk to me. I'm sure that if you are reading this for a class, your teacher will be equally open to your concerns. Many of my students would talk in class about moments in a film that they found challenging to watch, and they were able to use that difficulty to explore the issues in the film that troubled them.

DIVERSITY

I wish there was more diversity among the creators of the films here. Though the behind-the-scenes artists who made them come from very diverse backgrounds and from many countries, they are mostly white males. Until recently, the culture of Hollywood and the movie industry in general limited opportunities for women and people of color. What is lost, besides work and creative expression, is the experience of a broader world, of people and cultures too often unseen and unknown. Especially in the exploration of issues in mental health, this is regrettable.

Things seem to be changing, a change that promises to make movies not only more inclusive but more interesting. But change happens slowly, in fits and starts, and though things are better, there is much more to do.

I would have liked to have been able to include films by women, by artists of color, by LGBTQ+ artists, and by other underrepresented groups. I have not yet found time-tested films by these artists with the specific focus on madness that is my subject. I am sure they will come, and I will be excited to see what new insights and perspectives they bring.

If you know of a film that you think I should consider for future editions, please tell me. I can be reached at james.charney@yale.edu.

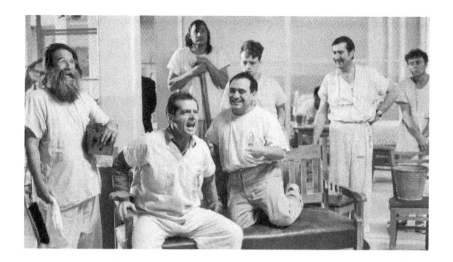

One Flew Over the Cuckoo's Nest (1975)

Jack Nicholson, Louise Fletcher, Danny DeVito,
Christopher Lloyd, Will Sampson
Director: Miloš Forman

The movie *One Flew Over the Cuckoo's Nest* can help us ease into the more detailed examinations of the individual madness categories in the other chapters. It gives us a broad overview of what mental illness looks like in a story that is more political than clinical.

When I tell people about the subject of my course and of this book, *One Flew Over the Cuckoo's Nest* is on most people's list of films they suggest I include. After all, it takes place in a mental hospital and most of the characters are considered mad. However, the story it tells never looks closely enough at any specific mental illness for it to be instructive. It isn't really about madness, but about nonconformity and challenging authority. For that reason, my discussion here will be brief, looking at the glimpses we get at the appearance of madness.

One Flew Over the Cuckoo's Nest is based on the 1962 novel by Ken Kesey, which was turned into a play the following year starring Kirk Douglas as R. P. McMurphy, the role played in the movie by Jack Nicholson. The novel and play were both successes, and Douglas was determined to make them into a movie. But he couldn't figure out how to make it work and eventually abandoned the project.

The problem was that both the novel and the play are narrated by Chief Bromden, a Native American incarcerated in the psychiatric hospital with McMurphy. His thoughts are psychedelic and imagistic. Bromden is psychotic, obsessed with the paranoid conviction that the hospital is run by a mysterious "Combine" as a place to house nonconformists, especially Native Americans. How do you make a movie out of this?

Time passed, movies changed, what was acceptable and what could be talked about changed. And especially ideas about psychiatry changed. The novel was inspired in part by the work of R. D. Laing (notice the similarity to R. P. McMurphy's name), a Scottish psychiatrist who wrote extensively in the early, 1960s about how psychiatry was a political force, labeling as ill those who simply "broke the rules." He saw psychiatry as conservative, repressing individual differences, and saw madness as an enlightened state. He said, "Madness need not be all breakdown. It can also be Breakthrough. It is potentially liberation and renewal—as well as enslavement and existential death." He encouraged the mad to "journey" through their experience (not illness) and claimed that distinctions between patient and therapist were a conspiracy to confuse and control.

You can see how this fits with Chief Bromden's paranoia. These ideas took hold and led to the deinstitutionalization movement, which got patients out of the hospitals many of them had lived in for years. Unfortunately, discharging these patients into the community was not coupled in the United States with an increase of outpatient services, and it led to dramatic increases in the number of people living on the streets.

In the early 1970s, hospitals were being repopulated, and though there was a push to make them more humane, in reaction to Laing there was an insistence that the mad were still mad and needed to be "cured." Nurse Ratched is what happens when there is an abuse of authority in such a system. The ultimate exercise of that authority was the use of electroconvulsive (or shock) therapy, ECT, which is portrayed as a horror in the film. In reality, when used judiciously in people who have not responded to other treatments, it can be lifesaving.

In the 1960s, Kirk Douglas's son Michael was beginning what would become a very successful career in the movies (*The China Syndrome*, *Romancing the Stone*, *Fatal Attraction*, *Basic Instinct*, and recently, *The Kominsky Method*). He tried repeatedly to get *Cuckoo's Nest* made for his father, but the problem of how to tell the story eluded him. In 1971, it began to come together with a new screenplay by Bo Goldman that reflected the changing times, and with Miloš Forman on board as director. But by then, Kirk Douglas was too old to play McMurphy.

Cuckoo's Nest was the breakout role for Jack Nicholson. It defined his persona and made him a star. Louise Fletcher's performance as Nurse Ratched won her an Oscar for Best Actress. The film won Best Picture and Best Adapted Screenplay. The Best Director award went to Miloš Forman. Nicholson won Best Actor.

The film was no longer tied to the paranoid thoughts of Chief Bromden. In fact, for fully half the film you don't know whether the Chief can talk, much less what he thinks. *Cuckoo's Nest* became the story of McMurphy who, Christ-like, must die to resurrect the mad and set them free, helping them realize that they are the sane ones, hiding from an insane world.

The cast and crew of this movie took over two floors in the Oregon State Hospital and lived there while filming. They observed and mingled with the psychiatric patients on the other floors, encouraged by the head of the hospital, Dean R. Brooks, a nonactor who plays Dr. Spivey in the movie. Many of the patients were given roles as extras, filling the background with glimpses of real mad behavior. Others got to work with the crew.

In the story, R. P. McMurphy is transferred from a prison farm, where he was serving time for having sex with a minor, to the hospital. He outsmarts himself, thinking that serving his sentence in the psychiatric hospital will be a walk in the park compared to prison. He is a born troublemaker, someone who loves breaking the rules and challenging authority. He is high on life and is dismayed when he sees the inmates of the hospital; they seem defeated, passively accepting whatever rules the dictatorial Nurse Ratched imposes in the guise of "helping them." He begins by entertaining himself, encouraging small rebellions, but soon takes up a cause to break Nurse Ratched's hold on them, and to encourage an enthusiasm and spontaneity that matches his own.

Most of the patients with speaking parts have eccentricities of behavior that would not put them in the hospital today. The movie tells us little of their prior lives, except for Chief Bromden and Billy Bibbit. Once the Chief allows McMurphy in on the secret that he can both hear and talk, he tells him how he watched his father become diminished by drink, leaving the Chief to feel small, even though, physically, he is a giant. He has remained silent in the hopes that he might not be seen (in the novel we understand his silence differently: he is avoiding the mysterious "Combine"). Billy, who stutters badly, is overwhelmed by his controlling mother, a friend of Nurse Ratched; his suicide attempts brought him to the hospital. Both of them are inspired by McMurphy. It ends badly for Billy, but for the Chief, meeting McMurphy helps him to recognize his strength and become free.

+ + +

To prepare you for the closer readings of the movies and madness in the rest of the book, I would like to propose an experiment.

If you have not seen *One Flew Over the Cuckoo's Nest* before, please watch it just to enjoy. Allow yourself to become immersed in the characters and the situations. I expect that you will really like the movie and put it on your list of favorites.

But then I would like you to watch it again. This time, don't just *watch*, but *observe*. Look for behaviors that seem bizarre or irrational, especially in the patients you glimpse in the background—behaviors that you would consider evidence of mental illness. Don't try to put a label on what you think might be wrong with them, just note the behaviors that draw your attention. Consider what questions you might ask, if you could, to help you understand why the patients are acting that way.

There is the white-haired gentleman perpetually dancing; Bancini, who keeps moaning "I'm tired"; the bearded fellow in a wheelchair, muttering to himself; the bald man standing against the cage wall, arms outstretched. What behaviors distinguish Martini, Cheswick, Billy, or Taber? For that matter, do you see anything of madness in how McMurphy acts, or Nurse Ratched?

The discussions in the coming chapters will help you understand these unusual behaviors.

Miloš Forman, the director, likes to show us reaction shots: people, especially McMurphy, registering what is happening around them. It's a signature move. Their reactions inform ours in the audience; they guide how we feel about what's happening in the story.

Context matters when you look at behaviors. Midway through the film, during a group therapy session, Taber, who looks paranoid and intense, suddenly jumps up and down hysterically. That might look like irrational behavior, but we have seen that he accidentally dropped a lit cigarette in his pants cuff—he's screaming because he has burned himself. Often his reactions tell us what we too should feel (for instance, his reaction when McMurphy throttles Nurse Ratched). But not this time.

What about when McMurphy starts talking excitedly as though he is watching the World Series game and there is nothing on the television? Is that mad behavior? It sure looks like it. If not, how do you understand it?

These are the kinds of questions a psychiatrist would ask and that we will examine in greater detail in later chapters.

At the end of the film, when the Chief finds the strength to break a window and escape, we see a different Taber reaction. This time he is exhilarated. And we in the audience are too. This is one terrific movie.

RECOMMENDED READING

Bogdanovich, Peter. *Who the Devil Made It?: Conversations with Legendary Film Directors*. New York: Ballantine Books; 2012.

The author, director of *The Last Picture Show*, talks with directors from the first Golden Age of film (1930–1950) about their work; lots of film craft and film lore.

Charney, James, and Noah Charney. What's to Like about Horror? *Versopolis Arts and Letters Review* [Web site]. May 2016. Available at: https://www.versopolis.com/arts/to-see/94/what-s-to-like-about-horror.

Callard, Felicity: Psychiatric Diagnosis: the indispensability of ambivalence. *Journal of Medical Ethics.* 2014 Aug; 40(8): 526–530. Available at: https://www.ncbi.nlm.nih.gov/pmc/articles/PMC4112451/.

Ebert, Roger. *The Great Movies.* New York: Crown Publishing Group; 2003.

A personal selection with smart and thoughtful observations on each film.

Katz, Ephraim, and Ronald D. Nolen. *The Film Encyclopedia*, 7th edition. New York: Collins Reference; 2012.

A good basic reference to film

Kesey, Ken. *One Flew Over the Cuckoo's Nest.* New York: Berkley Press; 1963.

Laing, R.D. *The Politics of Experience.* Pantheon Books; 1969.

Laing's indictment of conformity and insistence that madness is a social construct not an illness.

Monaco, James. *How to Read a Film: Movies, Media, and Beyond*, 4th edition. New York: Oxford University Press; 2009.

An essential text.

Nolen-Hoeksema, Susan. *Abnormal Psychology*, 8th edition. New York: McGraw-Hill Education; 2020.

Pickersgill, Martyn D. Debating DSM-5: diagnosis and the sociology of critique. *Journal of Medical Ethics.* 2014 Aug; 40(8): 521–525. Available at: https://www.ncbi.nlm.nih.gov/pmc/articles/PMC4112449/.

Thomson, David. *The New Biographical Dictionary of Film*, 6th edition. New York: Knopf; 2014.

Comprehensive and opinionated

Wasserman, Dale. *One Flew Over the Cuckoo's Nest.* From the novel by Ken Kesey. New York: Samuel French, Inc.; 2010.

Contrasting the novel, the play, and the film shows how what one field of the arts does well is often difficult for another to manage effectively, and how the creators adjusted from novel, to play, to film.

∎2∎

"I have seen God. . . . I saw his face. . . . It was a terrible, stony face."

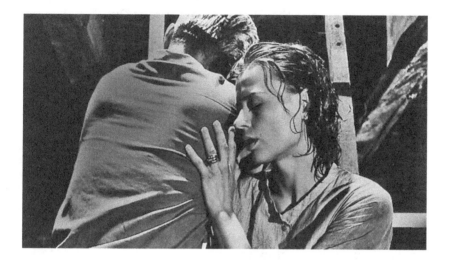

Hallucinations and Delusions

SCHIZOPHRENIA

Through a Glass Darkly (1961)

Harriet Andersson, Max von Sydow, Gunnar Björnstrand
Writer and Director: Ingmar Bergman

Under the credits a mournful cello, the Bach Suite in D minor, sets the mood. The film opens to an impressionistic image of water mingling with clouds, and then we see from a distance four people in the water, talking happily. The moment is elemental, almost primordial. It could be any time, any place. They are chatting back and forth, planning the day. We realize they are a family. On an island, alone together.

That will be the story.

Karin and Minus go to fetch milk, and Martin, Karin's husband, and David, her father, take in the nets. We learn that Martin is a doctor, that David was away in Switzerland, and that there is news about Karin. Something concerning.

This is a quiet, even distancing film. More like chamber music, a string quartet, than the symphonic expanse of *One Flew Over the Cuckoo's Nest*. Instead of a dozen featured characters (with an equal number in the background), here we have only four. Much will happen offstage, and not a lot seems to happen as we watch. But actually there is much going on—relationships tested, misunderstood. Confessions and promises. And the strain of a loved one with a returning madness.

Ingmar Bergman, the writer and director, is one of the towering figures in twentieth-century film, alongside Kurosawa and Fellini. For a long period in the late 1950s and 1960s, his work defined the foreign film: exotic, difficult, thought-provoking, more emotionally and sexually honest than American films were allowed to be. They defined the "art film" too, for better or for worse.

Bergman's father was a Lutheran minister and became religious advisor to the King of Sweden. His parenting was strict and punishing. Bergman says he lost religion when he was eight years old. In this film, and the other two films in what became a trilogy (*Winter Light* and *The Silence*), Bergman examines man's relationship to god (not usually capitalized in the subtitles or on the page). Is there a god? If there is, how do we know and what does he want from us? It sounds pretty heavy, perhaps overly philosophical, and seems to confirm the stereotype of Scandinavian dour austerity; however, the stories are often compelling and moving, with strong emotions under the surface.

Bergman lived a full and interesting life, directing over fifty films in addition to the many plays he both wrote and directed. Married five times, he had affairs with several of his leading actresses: Harriet Andersson, Bibi Andersson, and Liv Ullmann.

Scouting locations for *Through a Glass Darkly*, he discovered the island Fårö, off the Swedish coast. He made this and other films there. It became a much-loved home, and it is where he is buried.

Bergman was a man of the theater. He had his own company in Sweden, and the actors there were the ones he used each summer in his movies. They were a tight-knit group, and many had major careers outside of their work with Bergman.

In *Through a Glass Darkly*, Harriet Andersson is Karin. I think she is a marvel. She had started her career with Bergman in the early 1950s. Introduced in *Summer with Monika*, she was wildly sexy. She made *Smiles of a Summer Night* with Bergman and, after *Glass Darkly*, *Cries and Whispers* and *Fanny and Alexander*—wonderful films, and she is so very different in each. At one point in her career Andersson gave up acting to marry a goat farmer. Bergman coaxed her back to acting with *Glass Darkly*, which was written for her.

Martin is played by Max von Sydow, another member of Bergman's company. He starred in early Bergman films that had international impact—*Wild Strawberries*, *The Virgin Spring*, and *The Seventh Seal*, where, as a knight in the Middle Ages, he famously played chess with Death. He had a long career in commercial films as well: for instance, *The Exorcist*, *The Greatest Story Ever Told* (as Jesus), *Never Say Never*

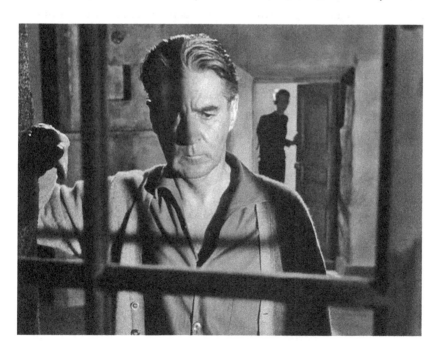

Again (as James Bond's nemesis Ernst Stavro Blofeld), *Hannah and Her Sisters*, and, most recently, in the HBO series *Game of Thrones* (as the Three-Eyed Raven). He was nominated twice for an Academy Award.

The cast is rounded out by Gunnar Björnstrand as David and Lars Passgård as Minus. Björnstrand later played a minister in *Winter Light* and was an important part of the Bergman repertory company. This was Passgård's first film. He would later become a television teen idol in Sweden, but he was dedicated to theater and won serious recognition for his performance as Hamlet.

The cinematographer for *Through a Glass Darkly* was Sven Nykvist. He made several films with Bergman, including *Persona*, *Cries and Whispers* (Bergman's first film in color), and *Fanny and Alexander*. He specialized in using natural light with dramatic effect. I think his camera work here contributes a lot to the mood of the film. We often see the characters in close-up, emphasizing their isolation from each other, or through a doorway, as though we are spying on emotions they would not want us to see. The camera often lingers on a room even when it's empty. Though it is likely Bergman who made these choices, it is Nykvist's use of light, framing, and focus that make them work.

This was the second Bergman film to win the Oscar for Best Foreign Film. The first was for *The Virgin Spring*, the year before.

Bergman's style influenced a world of filmmakers, such as Andrei Tarkovsky, Stanley Kubrick, Guillermo del Toro, Steven Spielberg, and Woody Allen. You see it in Tarkovsky's and Kubrick's measured pace and long takes, and in the shots that hold a place even when there is no one there (defining a mood). *Nostalghia* and *The Shining* are good examples. Allen doesn't mimic his camera work but often wrestles with the same questions of man's relationship to god and religion. Allen does it "funny," for instance in *Sleeper*, *Love and Death*, *Annie Hall*, and *Stardust Memories*. His film *Interiors* was the one time he most directly copied Bergman, and it was a failure. In trying to be "serious" like Bergman, he forgot his strength was in humor. When Allen figured this out, his films gained depth and meaning (*Hannah and Her Sisters*, *Crimes and Misdemeanors*). Allen always acknowledged his admiration for Bergman, even copying the style of his credits: white letters on a plain black background.

The Movie

Karin and Minus are going to fetch milk. She stops—"Do you hear that?" (he doesn't)—she hears a bird, a cuckoo. "Strange," she says, "since my illness my hearing has become so acute. Maybe it's the shock therapy." She has just returned from the hospital after a psychiatric illness. She teases Minus about his growth spurt and his seriousness; he is an adolescent, uncomfortable with girls, trying to be grown up. He appears childish, moody, intense. Karin's teasing, her hugging him and giving him a kiss, upsets Minus. It's too sexual for comfort.

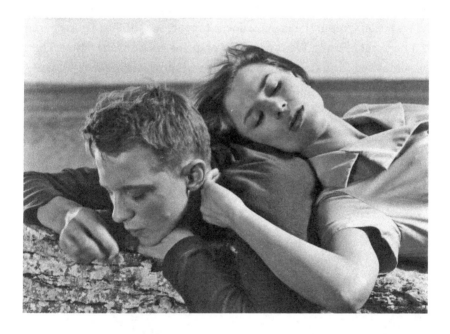

Martin confides in David that Karin's doctor cannot assure him that Karin will stay well. Right now "she is having difficulty sleeping, and her hearing is acute," but otherwise she seems OK. "She knows all about her illness, but not that it may be incurable."

In a funny way Minus seems more disturbed than Karin, but his are the ordinary confusions of adolescence. We don't know yet what is wrong with Karin, but these conversations tell us it is serious.

A foghorn sounds in the distance. No one comments on it. It is a sound anyone can hear. Karin will comment later that the light feels too strong: another unusual sensitivity.

We get more of a sense of the family over dinner. David announces his time on the island will be short—he must go on another book tour. The others are disappointed but not surprised. He has disappointed them before. In fact, he is rarely around. He gives them each a gift, but the gifts are all wrong: he doesn't know his own children. David registers their mood and excuses himself to get tobacco. We follow him into the house: he is pacing, crying—we watch him through an open door (as though we are spying; a Bergman image we will see often) and he walks offscreen; the camera doesn't move, we still hear him crying but he is out of sight. We can feel the emptiness, the desperation. Then he comes back and stands in front of the window, arms outstretched— an image of crucifixion. Composing himself he returns to the family to watch a play written by Minus for his father.

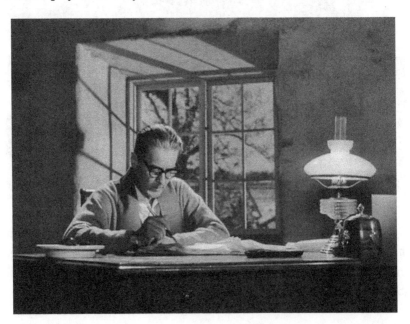

After the play we follow Martin and Karin as they prepare for bed. She talks of wolves and owls in the night and he tries to reassure her, treating her a bit like a child who has had a nightmare. "You are so kind, and I am so horrid," she says, and turns away from his gentle sexual advances. She has lost her sexual interest, at least with her husband. Does this say something about their marriage or about her illness? Maybe both.

The camera moves to the curtained window, looking out to the sea.

Then we are in David's room. He is pacing, looking pained. He sits down, and another window emphasizes a sense of isolation and separateness. He begins to proofread his novel; it sounds like a mediocre romance. Then there is a fade back to the window of Karin and Martin's room. It's later that night. We see her eye caught in the light, and Karin wakens to the sound of birds. She covers her head, then stops short at the sound of a foghorn, gets out of bed and goes upstairs, cautiously entering the attic room.

We have been watching her from the outside: We don't know what she is thinking or reacting to, but she presses herself against the wall and the look in her eyes is strange. She looks out the window and then at a large crack in the wallpaper. The flickering light from the window reflecting the ocean outside makes the wallpaper seem to be moving. The camera moves closer, but what is she seeing? She moves to the center of the room, seems at first to pray but then kneels and begins to moan and touch herself sexually, working her way to orgasm.

Meanwhile we hear the foghorn in the distance.

Bergman seems to be making an effort to keep us out of Karin's head. But that will change.

Next, she is watching her father from his door as he works on his novel. She tells him she is having trouble sleeping and sits on his lap, like a child. "The birds made frightening noises and I didn't dare go back to sleep." He puts her to bed and tucks her in, with Karin saying, "Just like when I was little."

When David leaves, we see a brief moment with him and Minus. Minus, after trying a headstand, asks his father: "Tell me what you really thought of the play?" David says, "It was good." Minus says, "I

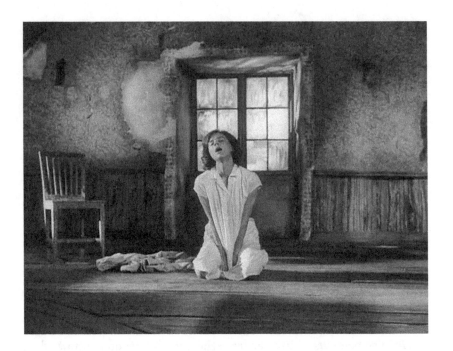

thought it was crap," and runs off. Minus is trying on the role of writer to feel closer to his father. David seems very much aware of his lack of connection, of how little he knows his family.

Karin wakes up, walks to David's desk, checks to be sure no one is looking, and begins to go through his pages. She opens a drawer, finds his journal, and reads it. He writes (and we hear it in her voice), "she is incurable, with periods of temporary improvement. The certainty is almost unbearable. I'm horrified by my curiosity, by my urge to record its course . . . to make an accurate record of her disintegration . . . to use her."

The Bach cello returns. The first time since the opening scene. Music is used sparingly here, as Karin reacts to what she has just read.

When she wakes up Martin, she seems energized and ready to face the day, but then she begins to cry. "I have a confession." She tells Martin what she saw in her father's diary. "Is it true it is incurable?" He tries to reassure her.

That is the end of Act One. As we will see in other films, there are often clear moments, like in a play, that divide the beginning of the film from the rest. Films are usually in three acts: the first act sets up the situation, and the others bring it to a conclusion.

Act Two begins with Martin and David leaving the island for supplies. Minus and Karin are alone. Minus is looking at a girlie magazine instead of his Latin, and Karin catches him, grabs it, and teases him, asking, "Which are your favorites?" Then it's back to Latin study. Minus, whose name to our surprise is short for Dominus, is acting like a normally confused teenager.

Karin talks to Minus about how Martin doesn't understand what is happening to her. She wants to confide in Minus—"I don't think the others would mind"—and for the first time we get a glimpse of her thoughts. Just who are the "others"?

Karin takes him to the upstairs room. This will be our second visit. Finally, we will have a glimpse of what goes on in Karin's mind. Minus watches her press against the wallpaper; we see another close-up of the

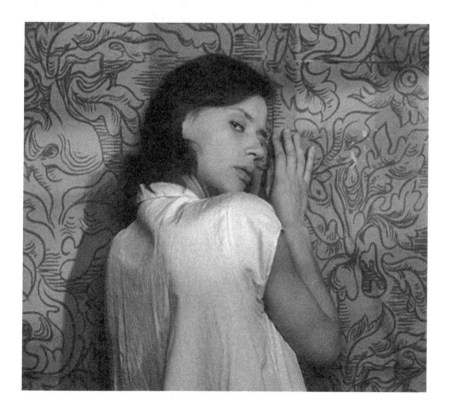

crack in the wallpaper, but this time we hear indistinct murmuring. We are hearing what Karin is hearing, sharing her hallucination. "I walk through the wall you see," she says quietly, "each morning I am awakened by someone calling me . . . someone called me from behind the wallpaper . . . I pressed against the wall and it gave way like foliage and I was inside." Minus doesn't know what to say or do. "I enter a large room, people talk, they understand me. It's so nice and safe . . . everyone is waiting for him to come but no one is anxious . . . I think it is god who will reveal himself." She confides to Minus that "I turn away from Martin . . . I must choose between him and the others . . . I've sacrificed Martin." "Is this real?" asks Minus, and Karin tells him she doesn't know, and though it feels like a dream, "it must be real." Minus says a powerful thing: "It doesn't seem real to me"—exactly the right thing to say. He's more grown-up than he looks.

But what can he do? She angrily tells him to go and he leaves her lying on the floor in a fetal position; but when he turns back, suddenly she is poised and asks him about his Latin. Then she demands he not tell Martin. Her volatile mood and what he has witnessed scare him.

On the boat, Martin asks David what he wrote that so upset Karin, then tells him off: "You haven't written a word of truth in your life."

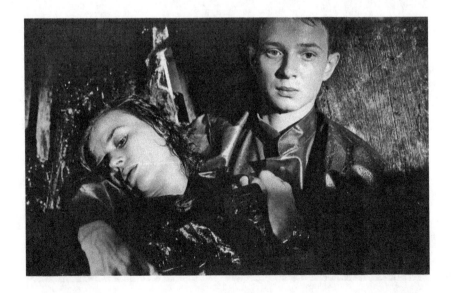

David tells Martin that while he was away he tried to kill himself. He hired a car and planned to drive off a cliff. The car stalled with the wheels over the edge. He is empty and feels without hope except for his love of his family.

Back on the island, rain is threatening, and the foghorn sounds. Karin runs off, and Minus finds her inside an old boat wrecked on the beach. She is lying in the hold. He leans over her, calling her name. She reaches up and pulls him toward her. Fade to a downpour of rain; they are both in the hold, soaking wet. "I'm not well, you have to help me," she says. What just happened? End of Act Two.

The third and final act finds Minus running to the house, then back to the boat with a blanket. He sits with Karin, waiting, until he hears the boat with Martin and David returning. As the grown-ups run to help Karin, Minus collapses on the beach, overwhelmed.

Karin tells Martin, "I must talk to Papa before it starts again," and Martin goes to call an ambulance. Karin tells David she wants no more treatments and wants to stay in the hospital. "I can't continue to live in two worlds. I must choose." She then refers to reading his diary: "I didn't do it of my own free will—a voice told me to do it." Karen adds, "I've done worse than that—much worse. Just now with poor Minus. . . . The voices start and I have to do what they say—is it really my illness?"

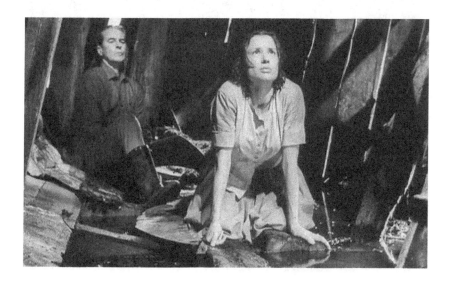

David apologizes to Karin for turning away from her, allowing his books to be more important than his family. When Karin first became ill, he left for Switzerland. He tells her that her mother had the same illness and died from it. "Poor little Papa—forced to live in reality," she says.

Minus hides, unable to face his family.

Karin is packing for the hospital and sends Martin on a false errand to get headache pills. When he returns, she is gone. He searches for her and then hears her talking quietly in the upstairs room. David opens the attic door but does not come in. He is so often on the wrong side of the door. Once again, we see that to know each other they each have had to watch unobserved. "I understand," she says again and again. When Martin arrives, he does come in the room. Karin says, "Martin be still, they say he'll be here any moment now. We must be ready." "Nothing is happening," he says, "No god is coming here!"

Martin sits helplessly. Karin kneels and prays, and when she asks Martin to pray with her, he crouches down, declaring his love. We hear the increasingly loud sound of a motor. Is this a sound in the real world,

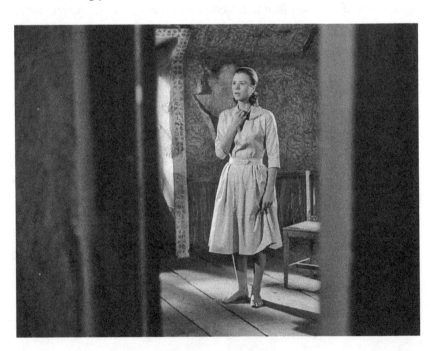

or is it just what Karin hears? Bergman is playing with these confusions, letting the audience experience them as Karin might. The room begins to vibrate. Karin sees the closet door swing open, wider and wider . . . is someone coming? Then through the window we see a helicopter landing—the source of the noise and the vibration that opened the closet door. The sounds and vibration are real; how she understands them is not. The helicopter is a shadow, with the look of a spider.

Suddenly Karin runs to the corner and screams; then, at the window, still screaming, she struggles, pushes Martin away, runs out of the room, and finds Minus at the bottom of the stairs. For a moment they stare at each other. David grabs her, and Martin administers a sedative (remember, he is a doctor). She screams again, struggles, and then settles down.

She is surrounded by her family, holding her. "I was frightened," she says quietly. "When the door opened, the god that came out was a spider. . . . I saw his face. It was a terrible, stony face. He crawled up and tried to force himself inside me. . . . I defended myself. I saw his eyes. They were cold and calm. When he couldn't penetrate me,

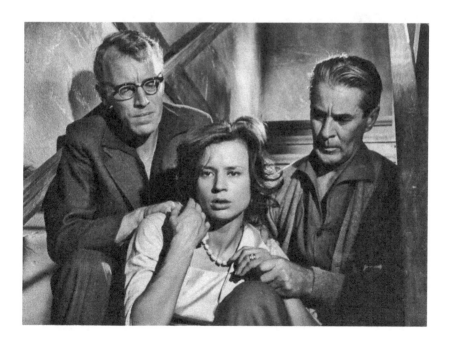

he continued up my chest onto my face, and on up the wall. I have seen god."

We now understand Karin's struggle as she was screaming at the window. If you can, watch this moment again. In a master class of acting, Harriet Andersson shows us Karin trying to push away the stony spider as it first tries to penetrate her, then as it moves up her body and over her face. We see her look of terror and disgust. Bergman has her describe it, but Andersson has already shown it.

There is a knock at the front door: it's someone from the ambulance whom we don't see. (This is a chamber piece—four players; we won't be shown anyone else.)

They are ready for Karin.

Martin and David leave the house. Minus stands in the doorway, watching. The camera is at a distance in the hallway; it doesn't move as he returns inside, crouches behind a stove, and cries.

The Bach theme returns as Minus watches the helicopter take Karin away.

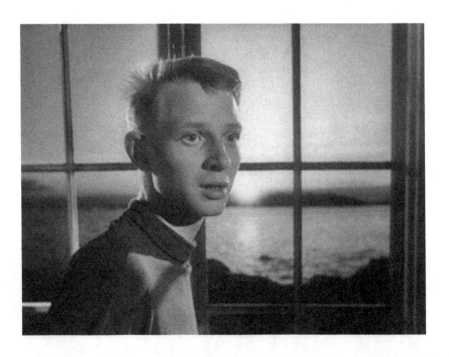

We have a sort of epilogue later that night when Minus comes to talk to his father. He asks for proof of god—something to hold onto when the world seems too much. David tells him that human love is the proof of god, or maybe, it is god. "Karin must be surrounded by god since we love her," says Minus, "will that help her?" "I believe so," says his father. David then leaves to make dinner and Minus whispers, with feeling, "Papa spoke to me."

Fade to black.

The Madness

While I do want to focus on Karin and her experience, I think the film is really about her family and how her illness affects all of them. We will be talking about several films where that is of central importance, such as *Ordinary People* and *A Woman Under the Influence*. Here, because there is only the family, we experience it undiluted.

But let's look at Karin first, and her particular madness.

What do we see that suggests that there is something wrong, besides that we are told she is just out of the hospital and has had shock therapy? Initially there are few clues in her behavior. As they are first walking on the beach, she hears bird calls, a cuckoo, that Minus doesn't hear. Was it really there? We see changes in her mood, sometimes teasing, sometimes serious. But these could well be the normal way a big sister treats her little brother. Her teasing about his looking at naked women in a magazine is perhaps a bit too much for an adolescent sorting out his sexual feelings; but again, there is nothing there that says she is ill.

It's not until we see her wake in the night that we see evidence of her madness. She walks into the attic room, touches the wall, and stares at the crack in the wallpaper; the camera moves closer, staring with her. She steps back to the center of the room and begins to writhe sensually, caressing herself, falling to her knees, and putting her hands between her legs. She groans in what certainly sounds like an orgasm and falls forward, spent. It has the look of religious sexual ecstasy; the image of the Saint Teresa statue by Bernini in the Santa Maria della Vittoria church in Rome comes to mind. We have no idea then what she is reacting to, but we know it is something she is seeing or hearing that we can't see or hear. She is hallucinating.

We are still outside her perceptions. Other films we shall see attempt to depict hallucinations, but these often fall flat, very much like trying to convey the essence of a dream. Bergman leaves us outside her experience but has us watch and wonder. The attic room, and later the shipwreck, become metaphors for Karin's mind, leaving us outside her immediate experience, watching.

In interviews Bergman said he considered showing her walking into the wall and showing what she finds there. I think that would have been a disaster, and obviously he did too. Instead, he relied on the most minimal of special effects.

What else do we learn? In her father's room, when she wakes up alone, Karin begins to prowl through his desk and finds his diary. There she reads that he can't restrain himself from observing her deterioration from a cold distance, as though he is studying a specimen under a microscope. Why? To use in his next novel. She is understandably upset, not just by what he wrote but also, she tells Martin, by the fact that voices told her to find and read the diary, and she felt compelled to do what they said.

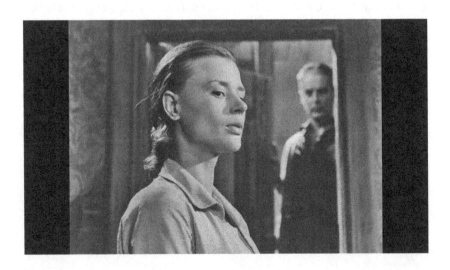

This is called a "command hallucination" and is quite common in the psychotic disorder of schizophrenia.

The second time she visits the attic with Minus, she confides in him about what she is experiencing. For the only time in the movie the first-person camera lets us into her experience; the camera moves closer and closer to the crack in the wallpaper, and we hear the murmur of voices, indistinct but definitely there. But only there for Karin and, very briefly, for us.

The nature of her madness becomes more clear in the final dramatic scene in the attic, when we hear her saying over and over, "I understand," responding to someone talking to her, and reassuring her. It's then that we see the minimal special effects used to convey the intensity of her experience: the motor sounds and vibrations from the helicopter cause the closet door to seemingly open on its own, as though someone or something is coming. But Karin screams, acting as if she is being attacked. On the stairs, after she has been sedated, she tells us what she saw—the stone-cold face of god, a spider who tried to enter her and then crawled up her body and disappeared.

Here we have clear evidence of her seeing things and hearing things that aren't there. These auditory and visual hallucinations are a hallmark of schizophrenia too. More than that, she describes what I would call a paranoid delusion: that she is being invited to walk through the wall and join the "others" waiting for god, and that when god comes, he is an unfeeling spider who tries to possess her sexually. More, that she must make a choice: go with the "others" waiting for this god or stay with the ordinary reality as represented by Martin.

A word about paranoid delusions. The word *paranoia* implies a sense that "they are out to get me, to do me harm," and certainly it can present that way. But more often it simply means that the world is paying special attention, whether for harm or good. When things happen that most of us would consider either coincidence or about something else, the person with paranoia is convinced it is all about them, is meant for them, or has a special meaning only for them. This can be grandiose: for instance, "the FBI is after me because of the antigravity machine I have invented that will change the world"; or "those black invisible helicopters overhead (that no one can see, but that I know are there) are watching out for me, to make sure no harm comes to me because I am so very important." Obviously, paranoia can go the other way too: "that look they gave me when I walked into the room means they hate me, that they want to shun me, even worse, that they want to kill me." Take your pick: these are different levels of paranoia that will generate very different reactions. The milder version—"they don't like me"—may simply mean a person feels ostracized and leaves the room. The more extreme preoccupation, "that they want to kill me," may lead a person to run away in panic or try to attack the perceived persecutors.

Karin's paranoia is not so much grandiose as comforting. She is not alone, she is understood, and she is special enough to be invited to meet god.

All these ideas, and the hallucinations that go with them, fit the diagnosis of schizophrenia, a psychotic illness (meaning out of touch with reality) of distorted thought and perception. Depending on the type, it can first show itself in adolescence (chronic undifferentiated schizophrenia) or in early adulthood (paranoid schizophrenia). Karin seems to have had her first episode recently, in her mid-twenties, which fits best with the paranoid category. Her mother suffered from the same illness and died from it; most likely a suicide, though some people with this illness will die not because they want to but because their delusions drive them to do something dangerous.

I had a patient once, a young man, who had done well with treatment until he decided to stop the medications that were controlling his delusions and hallucinations. The medications often have unpleasant side effects, like constipation, weight gain, and tremors, so it's understandable that patients would not want to take them. But what happens too often is they forget how much the medications have helped in controlling their psychotic episodes, and they think that since they are doing well right now, there's no harm in stopping. But there is, because it's the meds that are keeping them well.

Once my patient stopped taking his medications, within days the scary images and ideas returned. He became convinced that he was being chased by undercover agents, and to escape them, when he felt backed into a corner by these invisible (to us) assailants, he jumped from the fourteenth-floor terrace of his hotel. Amazingly—he landed on a car, which broke his fall (as well as his pelvis and both legs)—he survived. Others are not so lucky.

So, what is this schizophrenia? It's a psychotic illness that has existed forever. It was first carefully described by Emil Kraepelin in 1898. He called it "dementia praecox" and the diagnosis was made if the patient had hallucinations and delusions and showed ongoing mental deterioration.

Kraepelin thought of it as a form of dementia; we now know it is not. Dementia implies a loss of cognitive function, loss of memory leading finally to a loss of self (you forget who you are as well as who those around you are and what they mean to you). This devastating illness is a very different thing from schizophrenia. One can suffer from schizophrenia and be highly intelligent, with no loss of memory. There is a category of schizophrenia (chronic undifferentiated) that does show a gradual deterioration of function, but that is because the illness interferes more and more with the ability to deal with the world, not because it has an impact on memory.

When Paul Eugen Bleuler clarified the work of Kraepelin in 1908 and renamed the illness "schizophrenia," he emphasized that in addition to hallucinations and delusions, the diagnosis required disturbances of the "four A's": affect, association, ambivalence, and autism (another word he coined). As we shall see, this too was not quite right, mostly because the meaning of some of these terms has changed.

By the way, the word "schizophrenia" does not mean "split personality." It means, in Greek, "shattered mind," which is perhaps a bit poetic but is a closer description of what the illness does. There is nothing "split" about someone with schizophrenia. We are not talking about multiple personality, or even about a mood disorder. This is an illness of thought and perception—devastating enough.

Though there is certainly evidence for hallucinations and delusions with Karin, the four A's are less evident. The disturbance of affect that Bleuler covers is more a flattening, a lack of range of expressed feeling, than the mood swings of bipolar illness. We don't see that in *Through a Glass Darkly*. Karin sometimes breaks down in tears and seems somewhat ecstatic when she is anticipating the appearance of god, but these expressions are muted. Perhaps it's the Swedish way, but more likely it's just her.

There is no evidence in the film of Karin having disturbed associations—disconnected thoughts or overly concrete expressions of thought (an inability to read between the lines, to understand what is implied, or suggested, as in a metaphor or a joke). In fact, her descriptions of her hallucinations are remarkably straightforward— as though she is reporting something that happened to someone else. There is no confusion or thoughts that are hard to follow, both quite common in people with a psychotic disorder. What we see here is quite unlike what an acute psychotic episode would look like. Typically, there would be more of a sense of disorganization and excitement; it would be unlikely to see such a calm report of what just happened. On the other hand, we do witness a good example of what was meant by autism: becoming isolated in your own non-real world. (This is not referring to the quite separate illness of autism; the word is here used to describe a symptom.)

Karin's ambivalence shows in the uncertainty about whether to believe her delusions or not. These are articulated thoughts—decisions she tells us she is weighing. More typically ambivalence is behavioral: indecision to the extent that a person gets stuck and is unable to choose whether or how to move. This sort of ambivalence is an extreme symptom, seen more often in those with catatonic schizophrenia. We saw behaviors like this in the background patients in *Cuckoo's Nest*.

When Karin describes her dilemma, that she feels she must essentially choose whether to be crazy or sane, she is expressing something real. Very often, early in a gradual descent into psychosis, the patient knows that their ideas are strange or extreme and can consider the possibility that they aren't real. But as the psychosis progresses (this can change in a matter of hours) they no longer have that sense of distance about what is happening to them and become fully convinced of the reality of their delusions. There are fancy words for this transition: the ideas move from being *dystonic*, meaning that they feel foreign and strange, to being *syntonic*, meaning they now fit comfortably with how the person sees herself and seem convincingly true.

For Karin, though she thinks she is making a choice, the illness is making the choice for her. And it has chosen madness. When she talks about having to decide whether to "sacrifice" Martin to join the voices, she is expressing a part of her delusion. It is a delusion that she is able to choose. The developing psychotic episode is choosing for her. It is a conceit of the movie that she might really have a choice to make, and she certainly believes it.

Why is this sort of diagnostic categorizing necessary? Well, different medical or psychiatric diagnoses will point to a different natural history for an illness and will also suggest how to treat it. For instance, many forms of schizophrenia are indeed chronic and deteriorating. Contrarily, a manic psychotic episode is likely to be self-limiting. It runs its course and fades, though it is also likely to return, and the second stage is likely to be a profound depression with its own serious consequences. So, knowing what you are dealing with can help you better help the patient.

There have been modifications of the Bleuler concept of schizophrenia over the years. The *DSM-5*, the diagnostic manual that is now used to help psychiatric researchers communicate more clearly with each other—to be sure they are talking about the same illness when they look for treatments—has expanded the symptom list to five: delusions, hallucinations, disorganized speech, disorganized or catatonic behavior, and negative symptoms (avolition and diminished emotional expression). We have talked about most of those. It requires only two out of the five symptoms to be present to make the diagnosis (in addition to specifics about how long the illness has lasted, at what age it began, and whether there are complicating symptoms like depression or manic episodes—which of course would point to a different diagnosis).

There is no laboratory test for this mental illness. In fact, there is no such test for any psychiatric illness at the present time. There is no imaging of the brain that is definitive either. These severe forms of madness remain black boxes: we don't know what causes them, we don't know why they present when they do in someone's life. We do know more and more about the natural course of these illnesses if they are not treated, what sort of stresses can make them worse, and for many we have good if not perfect treatments to alleviate the most damaging symptoms. For instance, there are effective antipsychotic medications for schizophrenia that will help dull delusions and can even make hallucinations disappear. These medications don't cure the illness: if a patient stops taking the medications many of the symptoms are likely to return. But they do allow a person to live a sort of normal, functional life.

There are some patients who don't want their delusions and hallucinations taken away. Think of Karin—how special and protected she felt at first, that a group of "others" behind the wallpaper wanted to include her in their wait for god. If the god who finally arrived had been less terrifying and threatening, she might have very much cherished that delusion and been reluctant to have any treatment to diminish it.

In the film she tells her father, "I don't want any more treatments." The treatment she was receiving at the hospital was shock therapy: a standard "last hope" treatment at the time. Properly performed electroconvulsive therapy (ECT) does not look like the scary experience shown in *Cuckoo's Nest*. Though shock treatment works by generating a seizure, there are medications that are administered now (and I think were available then) to control the physical violence of the seizure, yet allow the treatment to be effective. But there is a price to pay: most patients who have undergone shock treatment have gaps in recent memory, which can be very disconcerting. I don't think Karin said she didn't want treatments anymore because she wanted to continue her delusion, or because of the concerns about the shock therapy, but because she had lost hope of ever getting better.

We can't know that, of course. This is one of those times that I as a psychiatrist wish I could have sat down with the fictional character and asked her a few (okay, many) questions. Since the viewer can't do that, we have to surmise, and accept the limitations of our understanding.

This is something physicians often have to do with patients in real life too. It is very hard to really know what makes people tick, what they are really thinking and feeling—in part because it can be hard to gain their trust, and because they often don't know themselves. As psychiatrists, we do the best we can, hoping to establish a relationship of trust and safety. This takes time and effort. We will talk about therapy—what actually happens in therapy, what makes it work and why it sometimes doesn't—in the last chapter.

Let's talk about the family. This is where the *Diagnostic Manual* scheme lets us down. It very much focuses on the individual, which fits its mandate to be specific about a person's mental illness but does not leave room to assess how the people around that person affect the illness and are affected by it. It ignores the family.

Let's not do that.

We've certainly spent time with Karin. When someone is ill, she is likely to be babied, treated like a child, given chicken soup and extra TLC, until she is better. This is how families take care of each other; it is only a problem if it continues after the person is no longer ill. Karin is not all better. She is just out of the hospital, and no one in the family is sure of her recovery. In fact, we find out they have been told she is likely to have a relapse and that it might be permanent. So, they do baby her and walk on eggshells around her. She is so involved in her own world that she can't take the measure of how her behavior affects others. For instance, she is sexually inappropriate with Minus because she is preoccupied and overwhelmed with her own feelings, and perhaps because he seems to be the only family member with whom she can be open. That openness translates into the sexual. The line between her religious and sexual feelings is a fine one. She turns away from her husband sexually, telling him her illness has taken away her feelings. But the feelings are there: They are part of her delusional system. She is sexually excited by her conviction that she is about to experience god.

Let's look at the rest of the family.

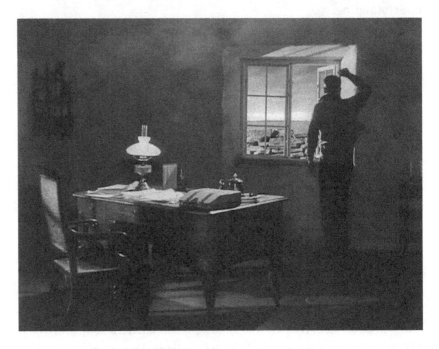

David is a rather unsympathetic character. It is particularly interesting to note that Bergman said that he felt closest to David, that David was most like him. The issue of using the people around you for creative inspiration is something often on the minds of writers, actors, and other artists. Not just using them as muses, but cannibalizing their lives, extracting character traits and experiences and molding them to a story. Bergman admitted that he often did that, and he does that here, about himself, with David. Not only does David find he is unable to stop himself from treating his daughter's illness as a fascinating "car crash" to watch and use in one of his novels, he also divulges a failed suicide attempt in Switzerland. This mirrors an actual suicide experience of Bergman's earlier in his life.

David knows his books are mediocre, but they sell and that brings some small satisfaction. This doesn't fit with how Bergman saw himself. Quite the opposite: he had great confidence in the quality of his work. Clearly David is not a clone of the writer-director, but he does share aspects of his life and personality. At least Bergman thought so.

David knows he has failed his daughter by avoiding her when she began to show signs of a madness very much like the one that eventually killed his wife. It's understandable that he might be overwhelmed with fear and anxiety for her, and perhaps feel an unearned guilt about his wife's illness. He could have no responsibility for his wife getting sick—that was in her genes, in her biochemistry—but did he abandon her as he did Karin? We don't know.

Any suggestion that the family might have prevented Karin or her mother from becoming mad is not valid. The ideas that Karin might never have fallen ill if they had been more in touch with their feelings, or better able to express them to love her better, all border on blaming the family for her illness. There is no evidence that the love of a family can prevent mental afflictions. These are genetically determined illnesses. A patient can be protected from some of the symptoms and protected from causing harm to herself or someone else if carefully watched, but love and caring can't make the illness not happen.

David, however, has good reasons to blame himself; not for her madness, but for running away when she became ill. For not being there. He left the country when Karin was hospitalized, and since then has kept away from her, Martin, and Minus. He sees their disappointment at dinner when he tells them he will be leaving soon, and then again, realizing how inappropriate his gifts to them were, that he has no idea of their interests; if Karin's too-small gloves say anything, it is that he doesn't even know quite how old his children are. His reaction (he cannot bring himself to talk about it directly) is to excuse himself and begin sobbing alone in his room. The emptiness of the room speaks volumes, especially when the camera holds as David leaves the frame, keeping an aloof distance and yet listening, and underlining the distance David feels from his family. Then, still crying, David stands in front of the window, arms outstretched, an image of the crucifixion.

But who is being crucified? Does he feel somehow sacrificed by their quiet chastisement? It's hard to say, but for me, even hearing the depth of his tears, I feel little sympathy. He has brought this on himself. He can't seem to speak from the heart; not a good thing in a writer.

Later, Minus asks his father what he thought of the play he wrote and performed for him. His father just tells him he liked it. Minus's reaction is to chatter away about how he has written dozens of plays this summer, they just "flow" out of him; then turns on a dime as teenagers do, and says they are all "crap." The two are talking past each other, there is no connection, though Minus is trying to make one ("I'm an author just like you, papa"); we see the look on David's face as Minus runs off—he knows there is no connection and doesn't know what to do.

Later, when Martin berates him as someone with no feeling who avoids reality (dismayed as he is at hearing what David has written in his diary about Karin), David agrees and then tells him of his suicide attempt. Yet, the lost hope that he says inspired this moment of desperation sounds too intellectual and self-pitying. Is there any possibility for David to redeem himself?

Perhaps redemption lies in the fact that his children still love him. And they still turn to him. Karin, after the incident in the shipwreck, by telling him she wants no more treatment and calling him "papa," is asking to lean on him as one should be able to do with a loving parent. He stays and gently begins to apologize for letting her down, telling her how his wife's madness scared him into running away. "Poor papa," she says. There is a tender moment of connection.

This does not stop her from showing the extent of her madness just a few minutes later in the attic. Too little, too late. But, it's a start. This is something that David acknowledges to Minus when he comes to talk to him at the end of the movie. If "god is love" means anything

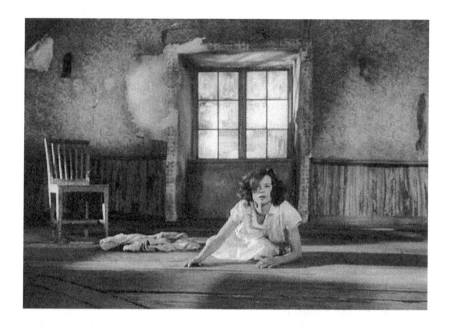

(it seems such a cliché), it means that you don't need to search for a supreme being to see something miraculous; the powerful feelings of connectedness, support, and love in a family are miracle enough. They might be enough to have hope for Karin. And for Minus too, who is so sweetly grateful that "Papa talked with me."

Did David's absence, his inability to speak about feelings, cause Karin's madness? Of course not. But his not being there spoke volumes and increased her vulnerability, making that psychotic delusion so much easier to embrace. Remember, one of the attractions of what was happening behind the wallpaper was a feeling of acceptance and belonging. This is something she was not able to get in front of the wallpaper, in the real world.

Which brings us to Martin. He is a doctor and yet he feels impotent, unable to help her stay sane. He is smart enough to know he cannot be her doctor, that he must be her husband, and he frequently tells her how much he loves her (unlike David), but he treats her like a child and she chastises him for it: "You always say and do the very right thing—and it's always wrong." She is infantilized, but she invites it, talking in a childish way, asking to be taken care of. Relationships are a dance; it indeed "takes two to tango." It is never one person doing something to the other; there is always the other's reaction and reply. Karin blames her illness for her lack of interest in being intimate with Martin, but perhaps it's also that she has invited him to treat her like a child, not like a grown woman.

Martin's reaction to being told by Karin's psychiatrist that she is likely to relapse is to become more protective, more caring, in a way that puts walls between him and Karin. She is not sure she wants to be protected from her delusions. "I'm her strength, she needs me," says Martin to David. But she is willing to "sacrifice" him to her madness. His helplessness is palpable, especially in the scene in the attic. She tells him to sit; he does. She asks him to kneel with her; he does. All he can do is watch her leaving him for a world of delusion, and there is nothing he can do to stop it.

Yes, on the stairs he can give her a shot, a sedative, to calm her down, to stop her screaming. This allows her to be held for the first time by all the family—they are all there: David, Martin, and Minus— as she tells them of a god with the stony face of a spider. This is a pietà of another order: a family confronting a sad reality, but confronting it together, maybe for the first time. And maybe for the last time, as Karin is led away to the helicopter ambulance, and we see it fly away.

By this time we are watching with Minus. Bergman frequently shows us Minus watching his sister become overwhelmed by her illness and expressing a sympathy with her that the others can't manage. He is a pubescent teenager, dealing with a growth spurt, embarrassed by the fact of girls, wanting to impress his father with the twenty-seven plays he wrote that summer, wanting to solve the problems of the world, but sometimes just standing on his head like a kid. He has the spark of life: was his father as enthusiastic about writing when he was Minus's age? Minus is less tightly wrapped emotionally than the other members of the family, and as a result he becomes our emotional barometer. When Karin confides to him what she is seeing in the attic room, you can see the pain and fear in Minus's eyes. And the helpless love he feels for his sister. Unlike the others, he knows the right thing to say. It is a version of "I know you believe what you are saying, but it does not make sense to me. I don't see it, and I don't think it's real." This is what a good psychiatrist or a very good friend would say. It speaks to whatever part of Karin's mind still wonders if this is real, and to the extent that it supports reality, it is helpful. Here it shows his sympathy and tenderness. It also shows he is an adolescent who has no idea what else to do in such an emergency.

When he finds her in the shipwreck, they embrace and the image fades to rain. It certainly looks more sexual than fraternal, that embrace. And Minus's reaction of embarrassment and avoidance afterward confirms that something happened that crossed a line. Just an overly passionate kiss, or something more? We don't know. But we know that Karin is also ashamed and tells David she "couldn't help herself." Minus gets her a blanket and they sit, huddled together in the dripping hull of the ship—a primal scene—until they hear the sound of the motorboat returning. Once Minus has told the grown-ups that Karin needs help, he collapses on the beach. And for the rest of the movie he is hiding, unable to face what has happened.

Minus may well be the healthiest member of this family, emotionally. He allows himself to cry—not like David, with self-pity, but for Karin. He approaches his father for comfort, for hope—and for once, his father delivers. Whatever we make of David's declaration that god is love, it means something important to Minus. His father is someone he can go to for support, and for love. And perhaps they can face this crisis in the family together. That is its own miracle.

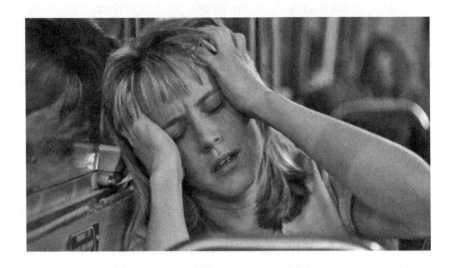

Benny and Joon (1993)

Mary Stuart Masterson, Johnny Depp, Aidan Quinn
Director: Jeremiah S. Chechik

Benny (Aidan Quinn) is Joon's (Mary Stuart Masterson's) brother and he takes care of her. She needs his care because she has a diagnosis of schizophrenia, though the film never actually says it. When Joon takes her medications she is fine, but without them she is prone to rages.

Sam, a relative of a friend, comes to their home to stay: it's Johnny Depp in an early role, and though he is not mad, he is certainly eccentric. He is obsessed with the silent movie clown Buster Keaton and seems to go through life channeling moments from his films, as well as those of Charlie Chaplin. Depp is a marvel at managing this without it becoming precious or unconvincing. There are moments of real grace as he charms Joon with his antics.

He and Joon fall in love. Benny is angry and worried that Joon can't be okay outside his care, and he is probably right. The film wants us to believe that Sam's love can cure Joon, which is wishful thinking, but almost works in this sweet and touching movie. It is at its most convincing and most powerful, however, in the short scene that is the reason I'm including it in this chapter.

Joon has stopped her meds. She and Sam are on a city bus, and she begins to respond to voices only she can hear. She becomes agitated, drumming on the seat in front of her, subvocalizing (in other words, as we saw with Karin in the attic room and as we will see in *Spider*, another portrait of schizophrenia, muttering intently but quietly so that you can't make out what she is saying). Then she holds her head and begins crying out, "I am not, I am not"; the voices are calling her names or accusing her. We never see or hear her hallucinations; we only see how she reacts to them. Sam tries to comfort her, but she is too upset. Each sound of the brakes of the bus seems to startle and upset her more and she begins to bang her head on the seat. Sam asks the driver to stop the bus and call for help.

They let all the other passengers off while waiting for the ambulance. Joon is alone, pacing the length of the bus, shouting, shaking her head. When the medics come on the bus, she confronts them "Think I don't know who you are, I know just who you are . . . leave!" She sounds paranoid (and probably is), but she also has experience with hospitals so she recognizes what's happening. When they try to restrain her to take her to the ambulance, she kicks the window of the bus and shatters it.

Benny arrives moments later just in time to watch helplessly as Joon is strapped onto a stretcher in the ambulance, with Sam sitting beside her as it drives off to the hospital.

This scene, with parallels to what we see with Karin, is real and convincing. It shows the intensity of an auditory hallucination, and how disturbing it can be not only to the person experiencing it but to the people who love her. Joon goes from sitting quietly to becoming agitated in moments—then to hitting her head, pacing, shouting, and wrestling with aides trying to help. We don't get to know what the voices are saying or whether she is also seeing something that isn't there, but we do see how it affects her. This is acute psychotic decompensation; as with Karin, only seen from the outside. We are witnessing the behaviors even though we can't see the world through the character's eyes, and from these we must imagine what she is experiencing.

This is a decision of the filmmakers. It is very hard to convey the inner experience of a hallucination without it looking ridiculous. Think how hard it is to tell someone about a dream you had, particularly one with fantastical elements, without it losing its power for you, or its meaning. Some films can pull it off (like *Repulsion* in the next chapter) but most can't; so a solution is not to try, and just count on the actor's performance to convey what is happening.

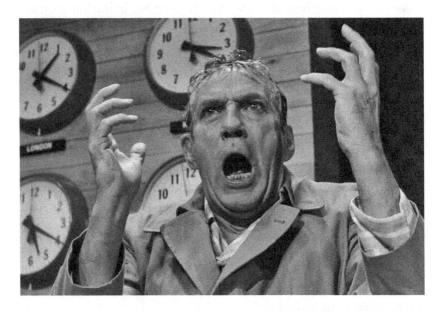

Network (1976)

Peter Finch, Faye Dunaway, William Holden
Director: Sidney Lumet

Written by Paddy Chayefsky, who got his start writing dramas for television (*Marty*, 1953), this is a wonderfully talky drama that was really quite prescient. It's a very good example of seeing acute psychosis from the outside.

Peter Finch is Howard Beale, a highly respected news anchorman, in the days when there were few channels, no cable, and news anchors could sign off each night saying, as Walter Cronkite of CBS News famously did, "And that's the way it is . . . " and be believed.

Beale is experiencing a psychotic decompensation, which feels to him like a holy rapture (not every psychosis is terrifying; sometimes the delusions are grandiose, as here, and make the subject feel important, that their life has meaning).

One evening he announces during a broadcast that he is going to commit suicide. He is told by his boss that he needs to take some time off and rest. That night he wakes, responding to voices we can't hear; they are command hallucinations, telling him what to do. Muttering "I must make my witness," he shows up in the studio in pajamas and a raincoat and is allowed to go on his newscast. He declares: "I don't have to tell you things are bad . . . worse than bad, they are crazy. We sit in the house and our world gets smaller, and all we say is 'please leave us alone in our living rooms.' Well, I'm not going to leave you alone. I want you to get mad! . . . You've got to say 'I'm a human being, my life is worth something!' So I want you to get up, go to the window, stick your head out and yell: 'I'm mad as hell, and I'm not going to take it anymore!'"

The people do, yelling all over the country, in one of those film moments that have become iconic. Beale becomes the "Mad Prophet" of the airwaves, and soon he is the star of a reality show preaching anger at the status quo. This is before such a thing as "reality shows" existed on television. Things do not go well . . . but I'll leave that for you to see when you watch the film. *Network* is quite brilliant, and Finch is wonderful in it (he died shortly after the movie was released, and posthumously won an Academy Award for his performance). This film is a critique of television, popular culture, and politics. But central to the story is this man, a man of honor, whose madness is perverted by television to make sure that "getting mad" doesn't change a thing.

There is a great punchline. He tells us it was God talking to him that night, telling him to give witness. He said to God, "Why me?" And God said, "Because you are on television, dummy!"

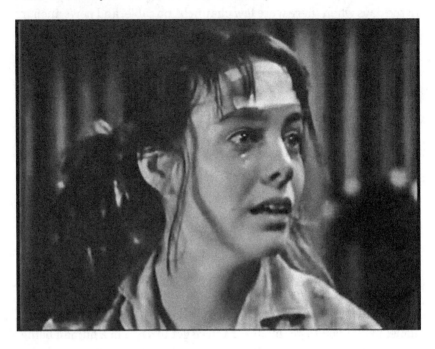

I Never Promised You a Rose Garden (1977)

Bibi Andersson, Kathleen Quinlan
Director: Anthony Page

This is an earnest, well-intentioned film based on the popular novel by Joanne Greenberg. There is much to recommend it, especially the acting of Kathleen Quinlan as Deborah, the young girl hospitalized with a diagnosis of schizophrenia, and Bibi Andersson as Dr. Fried, who is wonderfully sympathetic as her therapist.

Deborah is in a mental institution after attempting to kill herself. She has an elaborate delusional system, a seductive primitive world that intrudes and dominates when reality challenges. A very effective moment occurs in an early therapy session when Deborah is talking about believing she has a tumor. She says, "Uparu punishes us all," and when Dr. Fried asks what that means, suddenly we see prison-like bars slam down between Deborah and Dr. Fried, the therapist's voice drowned out by drums and angry chanting. This hallucination works, because the only image is the bars: a powerful and unexpected vision. We hear the drums and voices, but they are incoherent, and more unnerving because of it.

Later we see Deborah in the hospital hallway, upset and gesturing bizarrely. She rounds a corner, and suddenly there is a man, face painted, dressed in animal skins, threatening her with a spear; she turns to run, and behind her is an army of men with drums and spears and painted faces, chasing her back down the hall. We cut from what Deborah is seeing to a view of her chaotically running down the empty hallway and into the bathroom; crouching in fear, banging her head against the floor until it bleeds, then scrawling some letters in blood on the wall.

This is a powerful moment, undone I think, by how her hallucinations are conveyed. What the film shows us—a cliché of primitive native warriors—borders on the silly. What we might imagine she sees to cause her to so desperately run away, what might scare us, becomes cartoonish. On the other hand, when we see what things look like from outside (the running, the odd gestures, the self-harm) we understand how difficult it might be for a therapist to understand what is driving Deborah. The balance is challenging. We will see in the next chapter that Polanski, in *Repulsion,* is much more subtle in showing us what Carol sees—the distortions of the rooms, the softened walls, the cracks, even the hands groping in the hallway—all are more suggestive than literal, and more powerful for it.

Other moments in the film are more successful, showing how Deborah's therapy and her relationships with the other patients help draw her away from this delusional world into a reality she can handle. For instance, when she burns herself with a cigarette, unexpectedly feels the pain, and realizes that she can be in the real even if it hurts. Or when, encouraged by Dr. Fried, she first allows herself to cry in sympathy with her father, whom she had thought of as uncaring, tears that her delusional world would never have permitted. There are many such moments in this film, both touching and convincing.

RECOMMENDED READING

Bergman, Ingmar. *The Magic Lantern: An Autobiography.* Chicago: University of Chicago Press; 2007.

Greenberg, Joanne. *I Never Promised You a Rose Garden.* London: Penguin Classics; 2022.

An autobiographical novel describing the author's experience as a patient with psychosis and her complicated delusional world.

Kaysen, Susanna. *Girl, Interrupted.* New York: Vintage Press; 1994.

Kaysen calls this a memoir, but said in an interview in the *Paris Review* that "it's not about me." Susanna is likely showing symptoms of borderline personality disorder. However, the descriptions of her time in the hospital and her psychotic episodes ring true to the experience of schizophrenia.

Wang, Esmé Weijun. *The Collected Schizophrenias.* Minneapolis: Graywolf Press; 2019.

The author uses her own experience with schizoaffective disorder to explore what it is like to live with such a debilitating illness.

∎3∎

"I must get this crack mended."

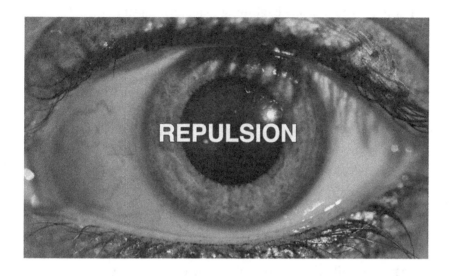

The Experience
of Acute Psychosis

SCHIZOPHRENIA

Repulsion (1965)

Catherine Deneuve
Director: Roman Polanski

A woman leans into a wall, and the wall melts, leaving an impression of her hand. This image is indelible, disturbing, and frightening. And it's just the beginning. The story of a woman repulsed and driven crazy by sex, *Repulsion* may be the world's worst date movie.

Roman Polanski's first English-language film, *Repulsion*, was initially released more than fifty years ago. He has had a remarkable career, as well as personal scandals and tragedy, with films like *Rosemary's Baby*, *Chinatown*, *The Tenant*, and *The Pianist* confirming his importance as a director.

But in 1965 he was just beginning to make himself known. His first feature, *Knife in the Water*, had gotten him into trouble with the Polish authorities even though (or maybe because) it was the first Polish film to get an Oscar nomination for best foreign film. Arriving in London, speaking no English, he was seen as exotic and brilliant, and managed to quickly become a part of the arts scene.

He had been working on the script for *Repulsion*, which he had started earlier in Paris. After being turned down by mainstream producers, he found a backer in Compton Films, which distributed foreign films notable only for how much nudity they featured, including low-budget films with titles like *Naked as Nature Intended*. These films were made on the quick, with cheap sets, inexperienced actors, and barely a script. Polanski was a different animal; if he was going to make a low-budget horror film, it was going to be one with his stamp on it.

He demanded the best, managing to persuade Gilbert Taylor to be his cinematographer. Taylor was impressed with the spare brilliance of *Knife in the Water*. Made in Poland on a small budget, it was an intense and sexy thriller. Taylor had recently made Kubrick's *Dr. Strangelove* and the Beatles movie *A Hard Day's Night*; he liked challenging projects.

Polanski recruited Catherine Deneuve, at the time the most famous actress in France, who was just as well known for her sex life, having just given birth to the child of her lover, director Roger Vadim. She was eager to make a film in English to widen her audience, and she and Vadim had been charmed and impressed by Polanski during his time in Paris.

What Polanski achieved with *Repulsion* was not just scary or psychologically convincing—it was art.

It's hard to recapture the effect this film had on audiences when it was first released. Much like Hitchcock's *Psycho*, *Repulsion* was unlike anything anyone had seen before: a powerfully effective and convincing portrait of someone gradually going mad.

The Movie

It opens with a close-up of an open eye, unblinking, and a slow, threatening drumbeat. The credits roll, the title *Repulsion* moves across the screen, followed by the actors' names and other credits at odd angles, and, finally, the name of the director, Roman Polanski, cutting across the eye, a seeming violation. It is a reminder, whether intended by the filmmaker or not, of the iconic image from Buñuel's surrealistic classic *Un Chien Andalou*, of a razor blade in close-up cutting open an eyeball.

With that image, we are in a world of implied violence, and, the eye tells us, a world we will see in close intimacy through the main character, Carol (Catherine Deneuve). It is her eye we see as the camera pulls back to her beautiful, impassive face. She sits staring, not moving until someone asks, "Have you fallen asleep? You must be in love or something." We soon learn that Carol is a manicurist, a young woman from Brussels living with her sister in South Kensington, London.

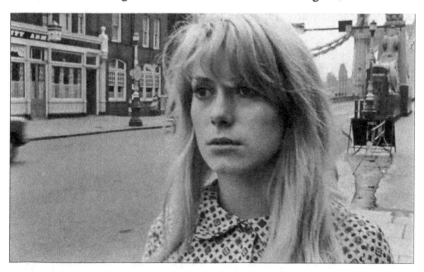

The camera follows her closely as she walks home, oblivious to the life around her. Later, we see her staring at her food, awkwardly unaware as Colin, a pleasant fellow, tries to ask her out on a date. She seems withdrawn, child-like, a bit spacey, with no sense of humor. She bites her nails, and very early in the film comments on a crack in the apartment wall (which Polanski cleverly doesn't show us; we will wonder later, was it really there?). She is increasingly disturbed by the evidence of her sister's lover in the apartment: his straight razor and toothbrush in her glass, his undershirt in the hamper. We begin to see the world through Carol's eyes. Sitting alone after her sister leaves to go out to dinner with her boyfriend, Carol stares at her reflection in a tea kettle, distorted like a fun-house mirror. We hear the bells of a convent play yard, and the camera pans across the objects on a mantle to focus on a family picture featuring a very young Carol, separate and staring. Fade to Carol in bed and sounds of a ticking clock and her sister making love in the room next door.

Startled by seeing the boyfriend shaving the next morning, she sits in her room, brushing away something unseen. We hear the sound of someone playing scales on the piano, over and over. There is a pervasive uneasiness in the ordinary. Carol stares at her sister's bed; the sheets indicate the lovemaking of the night before. She picks up the boyfriend's undershirt from the floor, trying not to touch it, and gags in disgust.

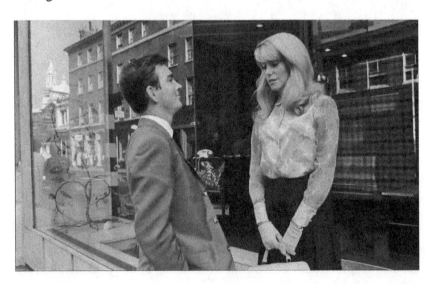

When Colin finds her sitting on a bench staring at the cracks in the sidewalk, he offers to drive her home. They have nothing to say to each other: she is in her own world, and when he hesitantly kisses her, she stares unresponsive and then runs off, back to the safety of the apartment, where she frantically brushes her teeth and tosses her sister's boyfriend's razor into the trash.

Her sister is going on holiday with her lover, Michael—she will be away ten days. This is going to push Carol over the edge. We have already seen her isolation, her trance-like preoccupation with and avoidance of men, and her moments of disgust. Michael's flippant "Don't do anything I wouldn't do" as he and Carol's sister leave doesn't bode well. Carol watches them pack up the car and go. She is now alone. End of Act One.

We cut to the beauty parlor and Carol's view of a woman customer seen upside down—looking quite grotesque—as she holds forth on the subject of men: "There's only one thing they want, and they love begging for it. . . . They are all the same, just like children." Carol's staring disconnection gets her sent home, and we begin to see images of decay and loss of control. She absentmindedly leaves an uncooked rabbit on the kitchen counter (it will convey the passage of time as it rots and draws flies). She sees Michael's razor—recovered from the trash by her sister—and she opens it, fascinated. She gets a glass of water, and we hear the drip-drip of the faucet, then a cracking sound. We see a close up of her glance at a crack in the wall—did this just happen?

She wanders into her sister's bedroom, and as she closes the armoire door, she sees reflected in the mirror a man in the room. We are as startled as she is: the quiet slowness of the film up until now has lulled us into her world. The music underlines the shock and certainly gets our attention. But there is no one there. Then she is back in her own bedroom, hearing someone in the hall, the clock ticking. Next morning, she starts to run water into the bath but is transfixed by Michael's undershirt for who knows how long—except we see that the bathwater has overflowed onto the floor.

The scene shifts to her walking outside; jazz music announces a world beyond her apartment, and we see her looking more and more disheveled, wiping something only she can see from the side of her nose, from her shoulder. Then she is back in the apartment, again in her nightgown, and for the first time we see her hallucination—until now only implied—when the wall of her apartment cracks open with a crash. She retreats to her bedroom, locks the door. We hear someone in the hall, we see him pushing open the door, a man rapes her. She screams silently; we only hear the ticking of the clock. The sharply ringing phone finds her on the floor the next morning: it's Colin calling.

Back at work we find she has missed three days. As she works on a customer's nails, she cuts her and blood drips onto the floor. Carol cowers in the corner and is sent home. Her friend at work, Bridget, asks what's wrong: "Is it a man?" End of Act Two.

As Carol walks home, she doesn't even notice a car accident nearby. Back at the apartment, which is becoming increasingly sexualized but is also her only haven, the potatoes on the counter and the rabbit are rotting unnoticed; the walls crack open and become soft, melting under her touch.

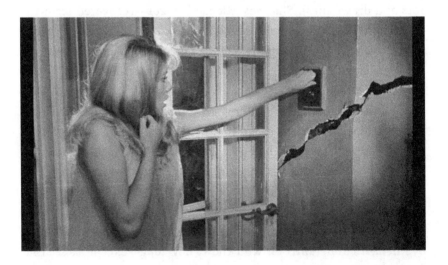

Colin, who is worried about her, makes the mistake of forcing his way into the apartment. When he does, she hits him with a heavy candlestick, showing no emotion, almost robotic as she hits him again and again and then drags his body into the water-filled bathtub. Blood leaks into the water. The images are horrifying, but made worse by her worsening hallucinations.

There is another silent rape which leaves her lying naked on the floor.

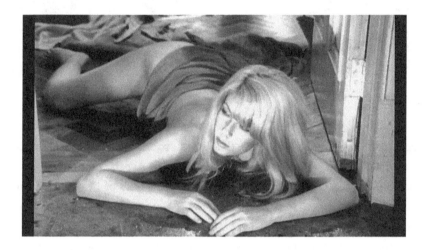

In the hallway hands reach out from the walls to grab and caress her. The rooms become distorted, larger, empty.

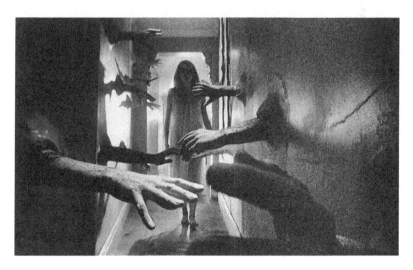

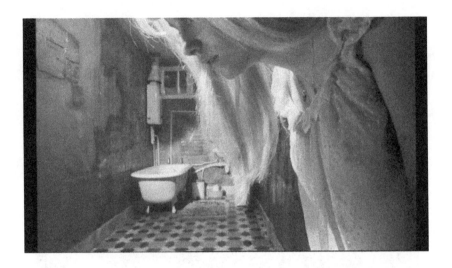

There is another murder, this one again a seemingly impassive reaction to a sexual intrusion. The landlord clumsily tries to seduce Carol and she takes Michael's razor to him. Again, her face shows no feeling, but there is no mistaking the intensity of her attack; she cuts him again and again, just as she hit Colin again and again. The apartment seems to close in on her.

When Michael and her sister return, the sister goes into the apartment first and we hear her scream. Her screams sound very much like the lovemaking sounds Carol overheard earlier, under-lining the sexual implications of what has happened. They find Carol under her sister's bed. Michael carries Carol out of the apartment. We again hear the clock ticking and the camera pans to the family photo we saw earlier, zooming into a close-up of the young Carol. Only now the picture looks different. We see her isolation, the strange emptiness in her look. Just what does she see as she stares, looking where?

I find this film fascinating. It is an intense portrait of a young woman's disgust at things sexual (well, disgust and attraction), which leads her to kill. Not exactly a turn-on. The film is so well done, the details so right, that it has a powerful impact. It is one of my favorites for the study of madness in film.

Repulsion, Taxi Driver, Peeping Tom: all these films start with a close-up view of an eye, telling us that we are in for a voyage into the psyche. And so often that voyage turns horrific, or at least thrillingly intense.

We in the audience are always watchers. After all, watching movies is a voyeuristic pleasure. We sit in the dark with a group of strangers and get to see the secret and not-so-secret lives of other strangers. We get to see them in ways no one else would see them: when they are alone, when they are having sex, when they are doing their work. And we get to watch (as Peter Sellers as Chauncey Gardiner in *Being There* says, "I like to watch," and he does, and we do too). So, when we see an eye, we know we are going to see the world as someone else experiences it, or at least as the artists who made the film think that someone experiences it. When we are lucky enough to be in the hands of an acute observer like Polanski, we are in for a treat and a very interesting ride.

A comment about the cinematography and sound design in *Repulsion*: The black-and-white photography by Gilbert Taylor is extraordinary. He uses light and shadow to highlight both what Carol sees and the emotion (or lack of it) in her face. Encouraged by Polanski, he gives us such extreme close-ups that her face is often distorted—not made ugly, but pulling us into her world even more completely.

The apartment becomes a character, sometimes comforting, more often mysterious and alienating. Notice the light on Carol's face as she begins her walk down the hallway in Act Three; she moves out of the shadow, her face half-lit as the camera follows her, and we see her silhouette, occasionally highlighted by her blonde hair. The apartment is changing shape. The hallway becomes longer, the bathroom with Colin's body, enormous. The spooky repetitive music is coupled with the sound of a dripping faucet, then there is a musical startle and hands reach out to grab her again.

Often, we only hear the sounds that she hears (we don't see what is causing them): the interval bell from the convent outside, the clatter of spoons from the buskers on the street, the obsessive scales played on the piano in another apartment, the ringing of the telephone or the doorbell. There are long moments of complete silence. But also the ticking of a clock at night, the faucet dripping, the flies buzzing on the decaying rabbit, the dull thud of the candlestick as she hits Colin in the head. When there is music, it is often another sound effect; the rat-tat-tat drumbeat outside, the see-sawing mumble as the apartment comes to life, the odd theme for Carol when she is in repose. All this adds to our sense of unease and greatly adds to the effectiveness of the film.

Catherine Deneuve's performance is remarkable. Of course, she is very beautiful. In fact, she later became the new face of the image of France.

There is a tradition in France of choosing a beauty every generation as the model for statues of "Marianne," who is to France what the Statue of Liberty is to the United States (perhaps not coincidentally, Liberty was a gift from France to the United States to honor its one-hundredth birthday). Deneuve was that face for a decade.

Her dewy beauty and her look of innocence are perfect for this role. Especially since so often all she needs to do is look distracted as though she is daydreaming, disconnected from the real world or, later, absorbed in another, hallucinated world. This is not easy for an actor to do. She is totally convincing.

We must credit Polanski for this since it's reported that he walked her through every moment of her performance, talking in French only to her, often taunting her to provoke the necessary anger for her homicidal moments. But the details are hers. Polanski may tell her that she needs a "tic," a compulsive gesture to show she feels somehow dirtied by any association with the masculine (Michael's razor, his toothbrush, his undershirt), but she convinces us with how she brushes the side of her nose, her shoulder, her skirt, seeming to want to rub away anything that touched a man.

The Madness

The film is in two parts. The first, relatively slow opening section lasts a bit over forty-five minutes, and we learn much about Carol's world, but watching over her shoulder, not through her eyes. When she sees a crack in the wall early on, we don't see it. She walks the streets of South Kensington, London, but mostly we just see that she is withdrawn, and how oblivious she is to her surroundings. And yet, something penetrates. During that first walk, a workman crudely flirts with her; there is a close-up of him (she is seeing him), and it will turn out that he is the man of her rape-hallucinations. That she has registered his presence is emphasized on another walk a while later, when the little work tent he was standing near is now empty and she looks for him there.

She doesn't respond to Colin's pathetic attempts to engage her. She almost doesn't seem to realize what he wants: a date, some attention. Early on we begin to wonder about her. Something is wrong with this girl; so passive, so vacant, so childlike in her unawareness, but we don't know what.

What are we reacting to? She seems oblivious, to have no appetite, and she certainly has no sense of humor; she just doesn't "get it." Is it because she is a foreigner? After all, she is from Brussels. Her sister seems to have adjusted; she's even found herself a married lover in Michael. So, what could it be? We don't know, and we actually never know for sure. Early on, the camera closes in on a family photo that we will see again at the end. We see Carol separate from the rest of her family, standing behind them, seemingly isolated and staring into the distance. Does this tell us there was something wrong with her way back then? We don't know, but the image seems to carry more meaning when we see it again.

Carol is preoccupied and bothered that her sister's boyfriend is staying at their apartment. She sees his toothbrush and razor and moves them away, holding them with the tips of her fingers as though to touch them is to pollute. Of course, it is uncomfortable for her to hear the sounds of lovemaking from the next room. This would be disturbing to anyone, though it might just make you feel more sexy and perhaps frustrated that you didn't have a lover there for yourself. Is this how she feels? Perhaps, but clearly the repulsion she shows indicates that she is confused. She throws away Michael's undershirt, but then we see she is holding it almost as a fetish object that transfixes her so much that she loses track of time and lets the bathtub overflow.

When she is alone and finds his straight razor again, she opens it with great delicate curiosity. We can't help noticing how it looks like an erection (whether or not Polanski intended the association, it's there, as it is when the postcard that her sister sends her features the Leaning Tower of Pisa). At work, she often seems to be daydreaming. Here in a beauty salon, a world of women, the talk centers around how coarse and problematic men are, and how much the women want them. This is the first place that Carol draws blood, accidentally stabbing a client with her manicure scissors.

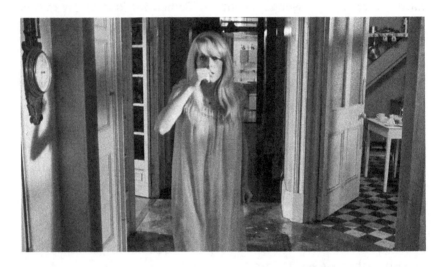

Polanski likes his little jokes amid the horror. When Colin breaks into the sanctum of Carol's apartment (a sort of violation, though with the best of intentions), the door is left open. He pleads with her, and as she stands there with the heavy candlestick at her side, we see the old lady next door with her silly little dog waiting for the elevator. As long as that bit of the outside world is there, nothing bad can happen. Polanski seems to relish the irony that something so ordinary could delay or protect from violence. But the old lady gets on the elevator, Colin goes to close the door, and Carol begins to bludgeon him with the candlestick.

We don't actually see her hit him, but we see blood spurting onto the door, and we hear the thud again and again as she bashes his head just out of the frame. Her face remains impassive, oddly calm. It is only after she stops (and the music signals a moment of panicked realization) that we see her become upset and try to cover up what she has done. She nails a board to the door to keep it shut, she rubs it down to remove the blood, and she drags his body into the bathroom. Improbably, she lifts him into the water-filled tub, where his blood mingles with the water. Shades of the bathtub scene in the classic French thriller *Diabolique*.

In the next shot, she is quietly crocheting, the familiar rhythm calming and normalizing her world. But soon she hallucinates being raped, and the apartment begins to change. It is here that the film shifts.

Now we fully see the world as Carol sees it: we are not just watching her walk through the world but seeing it with her eyes. We witness the bedroom door being pushed open, the man standing there, then coming to the bed to rape her. We see the apartment hallway become longer and darker, and the bathroom seems to become this abattoir— enormous, distorted, with the loud ominous sound of dripping water. We don't need to see Colin lying in that tub to know he is there.

Then, as Carol backs away from the bathroom, hands reach out from the hallway walls and grope her. The apartment is now violating her too.

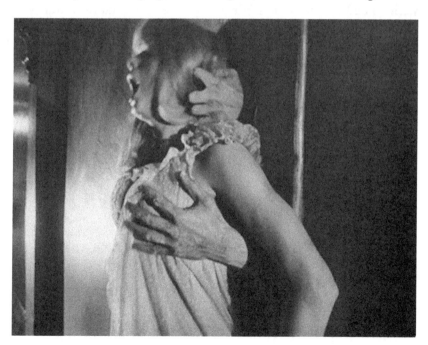

The apartment cracks open with the sound of thunder, the walls are soft and yielding, sensually holding the imprint of her hands, and she begins to behave more and more bizarrely. After the second hallucinated rape we see her garishly putting on makeup, writing invisible words on the glass doors of the living room, ironing with an unplugged iron, humming distractedly. And finally, the ceiling of her bedroom seems to lower itself to crush her.

Then there is a shift away from this subjective view as the sister and boyfriend return. Now we are again watching from the outside. As the sister goes from room to room in the apartment, seeing the furniture upended, the rotten rabbit carcass, and finally the body in the bathroom, she screams hysterically. We hear her scream and, as I pointed out earlier, it sounds just like the sexual screams that Carol heard before in the loneliness of her room. Even her sister's panting and whimpering sound sexual, and only stop when Michael slaps her (which audiences today react to viscerally, but I think was hardly noticed when the film came out). He then finds Carol, catatonic under the bed, and carries her out with an odd sympathetic smile on his face. The camera wanders to the family photo, and this time we see the picture again, closing in on the image of Carol in isolation, gazing blankly, until once again only her eye fills the screen.

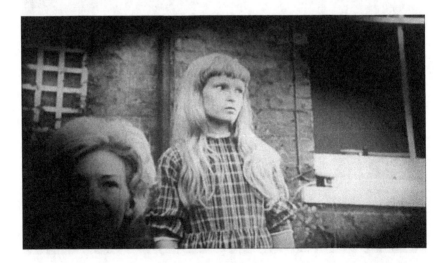

Do we have enough here for a psychiatric diagnosis? I think we have more than enough.

Usually a film will only give us the positive symptoms of a mental illness; the more passive, negative symptoms—the absence of normal behaviors—are harder to show, or simply less interesting for the audience. Here we have both. Let's work backward, because if we start at the beginning, the symptoms are too nonspecific to be useful. But we know how it turns out. She hallucinates vividly, hallucinations that have a specific theme. They are paranoid and sexual, hallucinated experiences of being stalked in her own apartment, of being raped repeatedly, of the apartment become a sexual creature that cracks open, grabs her, and responds softly to her touch.

We know she sees things. Does she hear things as well? In other words, does she have auditory hallucinations? This is not so clear. We notice many things she hears the bells from the convent, the clattering busker spoons, the ticking clock, the sexual moans of her sister, the sharp ring of the telephone. But these all seem to be real sounds that you or I would hear, as well. What makes them special is how they affect Carol, how she is drawn to them or responds to them.

Does she hear anything we don't hear? Well, yes, she hears the thunderous cracking of the walls (which she also sees), which we are allowed to hear, too, but only late in the film when we are well into her head, her perceptions. She certainly doesn't seem to hear voices.

The most likely diagnosis for this sort of psychosis is schizophrenia, but though many of her symptoms fit, it is unusual with this diagnosis to experience auditory hallucinations and not hear voices too.

Would we say she was delusional, another symptom of schizophrenia? It seems so. Her disgust at the ordinary presence of a male in her home conveys a delusional preoccupation with men and sex. We see her brushing herself with increasing frequency, as though she had been dirtied. Is this a delusion or a hallucination? Is she just feeling dirty, or actually seeing dirt that isn't there? We have already noted her flattened affect; that distracted, disconnected look, her flat, quiet way of speaking, her lack of eye contact with any male and with most females.

She seems to show concrete thinking. This is also called "literal thinking." It means a person understands most things based on the physical world, what she can see and hear. But the person will have a hard time thinking abstractly, being able to infer meaning or generalize, to understand when someone is joking, or be able to read a person's tone or body language. It is another symptom of schizophrenia. Carol shows this in her lack of a sense of humor and her frequent misunderstanding of what is said to her by Colin, though you could also attribute that to English not being her first language. Let's not over-read our symptoms.

She doesn't eat and doesn't seem to take pleasure in anything. It's a shock in the one scene when she laughs to see her react with energy to her workplace friend Bridget's description of the scene where Charlie Chaplin thinks his roommate is a chicken (*The Gold Rush*). But is she really finding it funny, or just briefly sharing in her friend's delight? It's hard to tell. Either way, it is sadly the only moment when she really seems to connect with another person. She never seems to have this connection with her sister, who barely sees how disturbed Carol is, so involved is she in her affair with Michael.

The episodes of violence are not typical of schizophrenia, though the nature of her psychotic process makes the violence here seem inevitable. She is repulsed by men's sexuality just as she is attracted to it, and when that sexuality gets stirred up, she must defend against it. Unfortunately, two men got too close, pushed too hard in very different ways, and impulsively she strikes out to "protect" herself.

What's missing from the diagnosis? We don't see any organized delusion, such as that she has special powers, or that someone is giving her special messages from the television or radio. She doesn't seem to feel controlled by another's thoughts, though she is controlled by her reaction to her own sexual feelings.

She doesn't seem obviously depressed, though you could make a case for that: she stays in her apartment for days at a time just wearing her nightgown, doesn't groom herself (her boss at the salon tells her to wash her hair), she can't concentrate or do her job properly. Her sleep is problematic, though it looks like she sleeps well after the imagined rapes. Most of these possibly depressed symptoms can be explained by her paranoid delusions and hallucinations. She certainly never looks clinically sad or tearful; quite the opposite, we only see her looking blank or in a very brief frenzy. She doesn't show much anxiety, even when in a fraught situation. As she sits on the couch talking to the landlord, oblivious to the effect her bare leg and her disheveled night-gown are having on him, she seems quite calm and in control. Even as she reaches for the razor and holds it in readiness, she remains calm. It is only when he clumsily pounces on her (it would have been easy for her to push him away without violence) that she becomes animated and puts the razor to use.

Psychosis can be difficult to portray in films, which rely on behavior and the visual. The internal experience, what the person sees and imagines, how he or she thinks, which is the essence of the illness, can be very hard to show. *Repulsion* is more successful than most. We begin by observing Carol's mannerisms, her facial expressions which convey an inwardness, a social awkwardness, and a seemingly blank, empty look. All this suggests that there is a lot going on inside her head which we are not privy to at first. As the film progresses, we begin to experience what she is experiencing, and the outward appearance, though it doesn't much change, becomes more understandable.

The world in her head is full of danger: sexual menace confus-ingly mixed with sexual excitement. As her hallucinations become more vivid, she pulls back from the real world. Where before she could manage the minimal responsibilities of her job as a manicurist, which often allowed her to retreat into daydream, now her world is circumscribed by the apartment that both protects her (womblike) and assaults her.

Schizophrenia, the most likely diagnosis for Carol, is a disorder of thinking and of perception. Delusions are not visual. They are distortions of thought: someone is "after" you, they are spying on you, they are putting thoughts into your head that aren't yours, someone is trying to control your thoughts, they are trying to hurt or kill you,

there are conspiracies that center on you. Common to all these delusional thoughts is the idea that "I am important," otherwise why
would they be spying on you or trying to hurt you? Why else would
the TV or radio or website send messages meant just for you? There is a
special mission you must perform, you must act.

Of course, the delusions may not be just grandiose. Often, they are
the opposite: thoughts like, "I have a disease that is rotting my insides
and will kill me," or, "because I am evil, there are devils who will send
me to Hell." How can this be conveyed in a film? We'll see good and
bad examples in the films we discuss. *Repulsion* doesn't even try to put
words to the delusions. Polanski only shows Carol reacting to those
thoughts. We have to imagine them.

He is particularly successful at showing the persuasive vividness
of visual and auditory hallucinations. Carol hears the man in the hall
before she sees him breaking into her room. She hears thunderous
cracking sounds, that eventually we hear as well, as she hallucinates
cracks widening in the walls. What Polanski doesn't try to do is focus
on the "voices," which are the most common psychotic experience of
someone with schizophrenia.

Carol shows most of the symptoms of schizophrenia outlined in the
DSM-5, which we talked about in relation to Karin in *Through a Glass
Darkly*. Because in this film we are watching Carol's first psychotic
decompensation, an acute deterioration, the symptoms are more
clear-cut and dramatic. Karin, you remember, has just returned from
the hospital and was supposedly better. We never saw her first psychotic break, which is often the most dramatic.

It is interesting to see how different the Bergman film is from
Polanski's in the portrayal of this illness. One tells us the delusions, the
other shows us the hallucinations. In *Repulsion* we experience Carol's
hallucinations firsthand: we see and hear walls cracking, hands in the
hallway groping her, a man forcing himself on her, and rooms changing their appearance. In the Bergman film hallucinations are only
seen from the outside and then described. In contrast, Polanski is never
explicit about the delusions associated with Carol's hallucinations. They
are clearly focused on men and sex, but we have to intuit their meaning

from her actions. She never puts them into words. But, Karin, in *Through a Glass Darkly*, tells us what she believes (the delusion) and what she experiences (the hallucination): her delusion of being invited to meet god and the hallucinated encounter with a spider-god. She tells us, but we never see that spider, or the people inviting her into the wall.

At the end of the film, Carol is found under her sister's bed, seemingly unresponsive. The neighbors at first think she is dead. This is catatonia: an extreme and final decompensation. Note that a tendency toward violence is not part of the diagnosis. This is actually quite rare with this illness. If there is violence, it is more often toward the self.

One feature of this film that fascinates many, especially in the last few years, is the repeated focus on the family photograph. We see it early in the film, and it is the last image of the movie, as the camera closes in on the picture until all we see is Carol's eye. We see that Carol is separate from her family and seems to have the same blank look, but also seems to be staring at something. Many have imagined that she is staring at her father who sits in the foreground, and they have wondered if this implies that she experienced sexual abuse as a child. We can't know, of course. The movie doesn't tell us. In interviews, Polanski says that thought never occurred to him. He wasn't interested in how she got that way. The photo does seem to say to us that she was always a bit odd, that there was something wrong with her even as a child. But could abuse or any similar trauma cause her madness?

Our current understanding of schizophrenia does not allow for childhood experience causing the illness. There is probably a genetic vulnerability from birth; it does run in families. However, it is likely that one's family experiences can either protect that person from the worst of the illness, delay the onset of symptoms, or define the themes of their delusions and hallucinations when they finally manifest. Schizophrenia, by the way, usually first shows itself in adolescence (for the most debilitating types) or in the late twenties (for primarily paranoid types of schizophrenia), but it is thought that the vulnerability is there from birth, just as a tendency to high blood pressure, colitis, or migraine headaches is probably something you are born with but does not show until you are older.

Repulsion is a quietly unsettling movie, with several moments that shock and images that endure. The first time Carol puts her hand on the wall and it softens to show her handprint is really creepy. The distortions of the apartment space and the shock of the hands grabbing her in the hallway are the stuff of nightmares. Both murders are profound in their violence, even though the actual blows happen unseen, just out of frame. Much like the shower scene in *Psycho*, which actually never shows the knife piercing flesh, the thudding sound of the heavy candlestick hitting Colin's skull tells us all we need to know.

This is one of the best films I've found to show the deterioration into psychosis and the experience of both auditory and visual hallucinations. The brilliance of the portrayal of Carol before she completely falls apart and as it happens is remarkably convincing. This is a film that, fifty years on, holds up remarkably well: as a shocker, as art, and also as a perceptive psychological study of a vulnerable young woman.

▌ OTHER VISIONS ▌

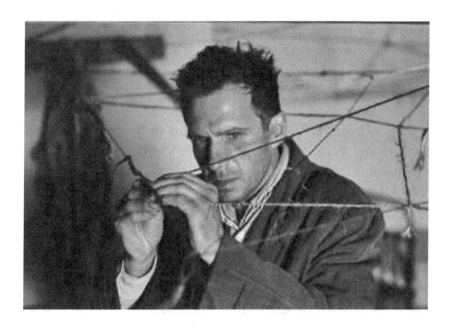

Spider (2002)

Ralph Fiennes, Miranda Richardson, Gabriel Byrne
Director: David Cronenberg

More focused than *Repulsion* in conveying the thoughts of someone with paranoid ideation, 2002's *Spider* features Ralph Fiennes's brilliant portrayal of Dennis "Spider" Cleg, a man with chronic schizophrenia recently released from the hospital to a halfway house.

A train pulls into the station in London. People rush onto the platform, until the crowd disperses and we see someone, alone, slowly climb down from the train. He is thin, almost emaciated (we will learn he doesn't eat), awkward, and socially stiff. He mumbles and subvocalizes, talking to himself and responding to voices only he can hear.

He finds his way to the halfway house, barely able to make his needs known, not making eye contact with anyone. His notebook, which we see is filled with incoherent ramblings that make sense only to him, provides a way of showing his thoughts. He is anxious and fearful, disconnected like Carol, but much less okay on the surface. Carol can go to work and behave appropriately, at least until she is left alone and begins to fall apart. The everyday oddness of Spider, who wears layers of unwashed clothes for paranoid reasons only he knows, prevents him from passing in the normal world.

There is a telling bit of dialogue:

Mrs. Wilkinson: Mr. Cleg. . . . How many shirts are you wearing? One, two, three . . . four! Now really, is this absolutely necessary?

Dennis: Oh indeed it is, Madam. Clothes maketh the man; and the less there is of the man, the more the need for the clothes.

Dennis demonstrates something we don't see in *Repulsion*: hallucinations of smell. He becomes convinced he smells gas in his room. Even when reassured there is nothing there, panicked, he uses newspaper stuffed inside his clothes to protect himself. He comes across as so outwardly "strange" that if you saw him walking toward you, you would likely want to cross the road to avoid him.

The film shows us his visual hallucinations: faces from his past appear on people in the present. We don't realize until the end of the movie how dramatically those hallucinations affect his ability to know who is in front of him or to remember his past without distortion.

The film takes the bold step of showing the adult Dennis watching his parents when he was young (is it memory or does he think it is happening now?) and then seeing his mother's face in the women he meets in the present. It's a clever game that the writer and director play with us. We are as convinced of the reality of his visions as Dennis is and are shocked when we discover the truth.

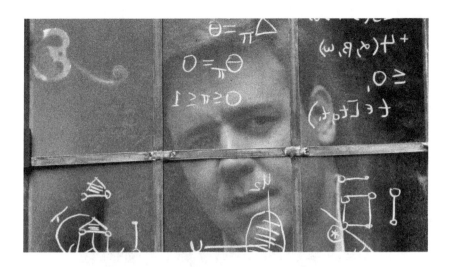

A Beautiful Mind (2001)

Russell Crowe, Jennifer Connelly
Director: Ron Howard

This Academy Award winner for Best Picture is based on the real life of John Nash, a Princeton professor, brilliant mathematician, and Nobel Prize winner who developed the field known as game theory that helps explain how opposing participants make decisions. He also suffered from paranoid schizophrenia.

Nash, portrayed by Russell Crowe, is recruited by a man in the Defense Department to look for coded messages in magazines and newspapers.

He often meets with his former roommate, Charles, and Charles's young daughter, Marcee. Nash becomes convinced he is being followed by foreign agents and flees a lecture at Harvard, fearing for his life.

When he is taken to the psychiatric hospital (which he thinks is a Soviet prison) he is diagnosed with schizophrenia. It is discovered that there never was a defense project and the man who recruited

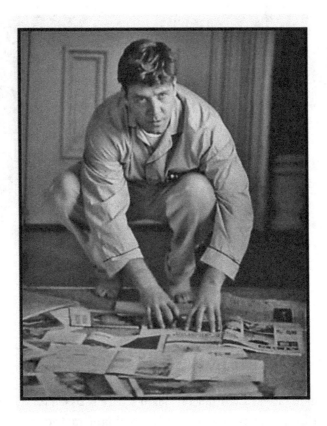

him doesn't exist. Nash is put on medications, which help control his delusions and hallucinations. But he dislikes the side effects (which many psychiatric patients do), especially because they dull his ability to think, so he stops taking his meds. And his preoccupations return.

This is a very common problem when treating someone with a psychotic illness. The medications we have now to help treat schizophrenia also have problematic side effects (they can make patients feel tired and slow and can often cause weight gain). Once medications begin working and the delusional ideas and disturbing hallucinations go away, the patient is eager to stop taking them. But with schizophrenia, meds only control the symptoms, they don't cure the illness. If you stop treatment, the illness is likely to return.

The climax of the film occurs when Nash forgets to mind his infant daughter, leaving her alone in the bath, and telling his wife she is being watched by Charles. It's then that he realizes that Charles doesn't exist. And that Charles's daughter Marcee doesn't either: "Marcee never gets old! She doesn't get old!"

Supposedly, this rational "Eureka!" moment of understanding begins his cure. That, and the love and support of his wife.

This, unfortunately, is Hollywood hogwash. You can't rationalize your way out of paranoid thinking. In fact, one of the dilemmas of paranoia is that, if you accept the premise of your delusion, it all looks very logical. Nash's premise is that he is a genius (which was true) and that he was hired by the government to trap spies (which was not true). His paranoid world was built from there, including hallucinating people who didn't exist.

This film is beautifully made and does a persuasive job of conveying the powerful immediacy of Nash's delusions, as well as how real hallucinations can seem. It's a shock (and I'm afraid a spoiler) to discover late in the movie that none of it was real. Unlike with Spider, whom we know right away is ill, Nash appears brilliant and difficult, not a nice man, but there is no reason to think he is "mad." The viewer just credits his social eccentricities to genius. The writing and direction do a wonderful job of convincing us of the reality of his experience. Then we realize it was all a con. However, it's a trick we are glad was played on us because we have had the opportunity to really feel what it might be like to live with the paranoid delusions of schizophrenia.

The part of the con that is not worth celebrating is the suggestion that it is possible to cure this chronic illness with logic and love. One might wish it were so, but it's not.

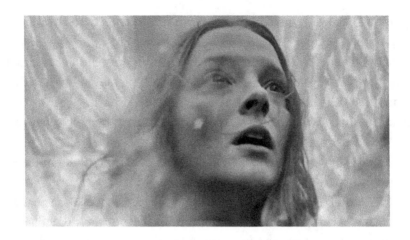

Saint Maud (2019)

Morfydd Clark, Jennifer Ehle
Writer and Director: Rose Glass

This first feature film by writer-director Glass is a powerful and effective low-key horror film, more a psychological drama than really scary. But it quietly manages a creepy sense of dread (greatly helped by a spare, chilling score) as we watch Maud, a nurse and a recently converted religious fanatic, who, convinced that God has a plan for her, decides that she must be the "savior" of Amanda, the woman in her care, a once-famous dancer and choreographer who is dying of cancer.

The entire film is seen through Maud's eyes, with a voice-over that conveys her piety and chatty relationship with God. What works here is that, as she begins to react to moments she takes as proof of her relationship with God—like a crucifix falling from a table just as she asks for a "sign," an ecstatic trembling-choking not unlike an orgasm after moments of high religious feeling, or a churning vortex appearing in her glass of beer—there is never a cut-away suggesting that these things aren't happening. When God finally speaks to her, he speaks Welsh, translated on screen. (I think we can credit that choice to Morfydd Clark's background; I understand that God's voice is hers, digitally lowered into a masculine growl.)

We only see and hear what Maud does, which not only fosters the ambiguity that perhaps these religious visions are really happening, but also, more usefully, like with *Repulsion*, lets us feel the power and immediacy of these experiences which we will come to understand as madness.

Maud begins to mortify herself, putting nails in her sneakers, and walking painfully through the town, her feet bleeding. Then we see her in her room, rising from the floor and floating gently, back arched, in mid-air. Later we pull away from a close-up and see that she now has giant angel wings, white and glowing. When Amanda tells Maud that she is "the loneliest person she has ever met" and that she was not inspired by her religious convictions but was pretending in order to entertain herself because "dying is so boring," Maud begins to cry. Suddenly Amanda is transformed into the Devil and Maud is thrown across the room (shades of *The Exorcist*). She grabs scissors and frantically stabs Amanda, leaving the scissors in her neck. Blood is everywhere.

Back in her room, Maud calmly washes away the blood, wraps a sheet around herself, looking every bit like her Saint, Mary Magdalene, and walks to a nearby beach. She opens a large canister, which we had previously seen her fill with acetone, and pours it over her head. Looking up, she sees an opening in the clouds: heaven is waiting. As the people on the beach cry out for her to stop, she sets herself on fire. We see her standing there, burning, with angel wings again, and people dropping to their knees in awe and worship. Then there is a slam-cut, a real shocker that shows the horrible reality, and confirms that this is madness; it was always madness.

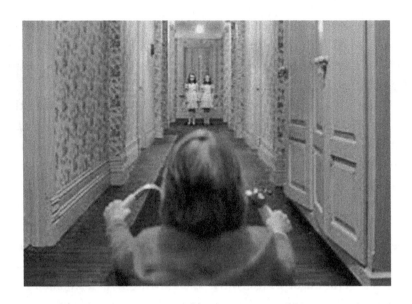

The Shining (1980)

Jack Nicholson, Shelley Duvall
Director: Stanley Kubrick

Movies of the supernatural are not welcome here. Except when one is as good as this one at showing the experience of horrific hallucinations.

There are ghosts and supernatural events in this story of a family intentionally marooned as caretakers in a grand hotel that is snowbound in winter. Jack Torrance plans to use the time to write.

We learn that the previous caretaker went crazy and killed his family and himself. Soon the young boy, Danny, begins to have visions, seeing strange twin girls, one drenched in blood, chanting together "Come play with us, Danny," and the word "REDRUM" scrawled in blood on a wall ("murder" spelled backward). Jack wakes from terrifying dreams of killing his family and has violent outbursts. Soon, he is hallucinating talking to a bartender in the great hall, with the hotel full of guests from fifty years before.

Jack's wife discovers that the pile of pages he has supposedly been writing are filled with nothing but the phrase "All work and no play makes Jack a dull boy," typed obsessively, again and again and again.

The film is filled with images of terror, famously one of the elevators opening silently to a tidal wave of blood. But even the less dramatic moments can bring shivers: that lone bartender telling Jack that he needs to "correct" his wife. This leads Jack to chase her through the looming halls of the hotel, finally taking an axe to the door behind which she and Danny are hiding. "Here's Johnny," he shouts, as only Jack Nicholson can.

One could make the case that Jack's mental deterioration comes from the stress of being isolated and his insincere sobriety, but we see that deterioration happen too soon after they arrive for that to be convincing. Essentially the madness here is a construct, a frame for the ghost story, which is the main event. What matters for our purposes, though, is how convincing the hallucinatory moments are; how scary, how real, how powerful. Attributing them to supernatural forces doesn't take away from how close they are to real psychotic hallucinations and delusions.

RECOMMENDED READING

Carr, Jeremy. *Repulsion* (Devil's Advocates). Liverpool: Auteur Publishing; 2021.

> A close examination of *Repulsion* as a horror film, emblematic of many of Polanski's themes.

Greenberg, James. Roman, Polanski "Foreword." *Roman Polanski: A Retrospective.* New York: Harry N. Abrams; 2013.

Kiernan, Thomas. *Repulsion: The Life and Times of Roman Polanski.* London: New English Library; 1981.

Saks, Elyn R. *The Center Cannot Hold: My Journey Through Madness.* New York: Hachette Books; 2008.

> A memoir of living with schizophrenia by a highly regarded professor, lawyer, and psychiatrist.

Sacks, Oliver. *Hallucinations.* New York: Alfred A. Knopf; 2012.

> Sacks is a humanist and a scientist. He writes with empathy and curiosity about the varieties of hallucination, both psychotic and neurologic.

▪4▪

"Listen you fuckers, you screw-heads. Here is a man who would not take it anymore. Who would not let . . . A man who stood up to the scum . . . Here is a man who stood up."

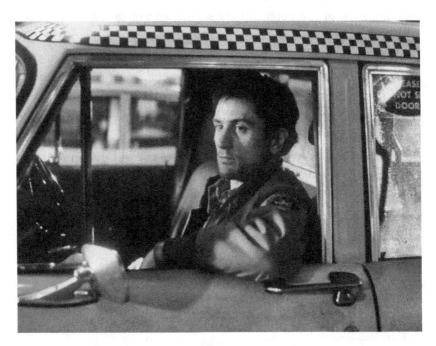

Paranoia and Delusion

Taxi Driver (1976)

Robert De Niro, Jodie Foster, Cybill Shepherd
Director: Martin Scorsese

The first image is of steam rising into the street from the subways below. A taxicab appears, cutting through the steam in slow motion. There is suspenseful, growling percussive music. Is this a vision of

Hell? We see eyes, bathed in a neon red glow, looking left and right; the music is suddenly lush with a sexy saxophone; then we see impressionistic blurred images of the city, New York City, and the eyes again.

We have seen in *Repulsion* a film opening with the close-up of eyes, but these eyes are different. Not empty and staring like Carol's, but searching, watching. We are in a different world and will be seeing that world through very different eyes.

Taxi Driver is regarded as one of the greatest films of the twentieth century. *Sight and Sound* magazine rated it the fifth-greatest film of all time in a 2012 directors' poll. It was directed by Martin Scorsese, with a remarkable performance by Robert De Niro as Travis, the taxi driver of the title, and an original screenplay by Paul Schrader. De Niro was nominated as Best Actor for *Taxi Driver* but lost to Peter Finch for *Network*. He later won Best Actor for *Raging Bull*.

De Niro is considered one of the greatest film actors of all time. In addition to this film, which made his reputation, he starred in *Mean Streets*; *Bang the Drum Slowly*; *The Deer Hunter*; *Midnight Run*; *The Godfather, Part II*; *Cape Fear*; *Casino*; and *The Irishman*. In later years, he has been featured in comedies such as *Analyze This* and *Meet the Parents*.

Paul Schrader's use of voice-overs for Travis was inspired by the diary of Arthur Bremer, who tried to assassinate Governor George Wallace, a segregationist who was running for president, in 1972. The idea for Iris's story (the child prostitute played by Jodie Foster in *Taxi Driver*), and the images of Travis as a cowboy and Sport with his Indian headband, came from the John Ford film *The Searchers*, a classic Western from 1956 that starred John Wayne as a Civil War veteran who obsessively searches for his niece, captured years earlier as a child by Comanches. When he finds her, she has married an Indian, has little memory of her childhood, and has no desire to return to "civilization."

Schrader was brought up in a strict Calvinist home and was not allowed to see a film until he was eighteen. Once he discovered the movies he made up for lost time. His influences were austere European and Japanese directors such as Carl Dreyer and Yasujiro Ozu. There is a strong moral backbone underpinning all his films, including this one. He and Scorsese, with his strict Catholic upbringing, make a powerful pair. Their films together are often violent, but they are resonant with judgment and mercy. Schrader has been a prolific screenwriter and director, with a large catalogue of films frequently nominated for awards, including *Mishima: A Life in Four Chapters*; *The Yakuza*; *Cat People*; *Bringing Out the Dead* (with Nicolas Cage); *Affliction*; and *First Reformed* (with Ethan Hawke).

Martin Scorsese's direction of *Taxi Driver* is a master work. His cinematic flourishes always add to the intensity of the moment, whether it is exploring the tawdriness of the city, Travis's first view of Betsy as an angel in white, the expressions of Travis's isolation and loneliness, or Travis's transformation into a killing machine. There is a propulsive energy to this film that is unmistakable. Starting with *Mean Streets*, his films include *Goodfellas*, *Raging Bull*, and *Casino* (with De Niro and Joe Pesci); *The King of Comedy* and *Cape Fear* (with De Niro); *The Age of Innocence* (based on an Edith Wharton novel, starring Daniel Day-Lewis); *Gangs of New York* (with Day-Lewis and Leonardo DiCaprio); *The Aviator* (with DiCaprio); *The Departed* (with DiCaprio, Matt Damon, and Jack Nicholson); *The Irishman* (with De Niro, Pesci, Al Pacino, and Harvey Keitel); and *The Last Temptation of Christ* (screenplay by Schrader). As you can tell from this list, people who have worked with Scorsese tend to want to keep working with him.

Finally, I must comment on the remarkable music of Bernard Herrmann for this movie. Many of the images and scenes here are grim, though the gorgeous cinematography (by Michael Chapman, who also did *Raging Bull* with Scorsese)—the use of rich color and soft focus and slow motion—tempers the ugliness. But what really makes a difference, what actually makes the movie work, is the music. Herrmann, who also wrote the music for *Citizen Kane*, *Vertigo*, and *Psycho*, created a sophisticated, lush sound for *Taxi Driver*, with a romantic saxophone solo that is often in direct contrast to what we are seeing: the ugly racism, the hookers and hangers-on, the violence. Then he couples that with throbbing bass notes and percussive beats that tell us something is very wrong—with both the city and Travis.

Put all this together and you have a film that fires on all cylinders.

Older films often seem slow to today's audiences, and because they were not allowed to be as explicit, the violence and sex can seem tame. But the 1970s was a decade of transformation in the movies, with the studios allowing a freer expression in language, violence, and sexuality. *Taxi Driver* moved the needle and set a standard for raw toughness and sensitivity that has been a reference point for every ambitious film since. Though there have been more violent films over the years, I don't think any has more power, more ability to shock, than this portrait of a desperately lonely man and the climactic carnage in *Taxi Driver*. Though over forty years old, this film still packs a punch.

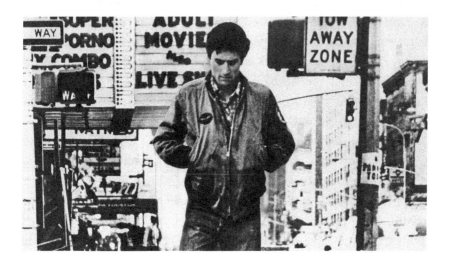

The Movie

Unlike *Through a Glass Darkly* or *Repulsion,* both of which take place in a condensed period of time (*Glass Darkly* in just a few days, *Repulsion* in a couple of weeks), this film is episodic. Except for the day of the shootout, we are witness to moments in Travis's life over several months, punctuated by montages of him driving his cab at night, angrily preoccupied with the sad people of the sidewalks. The moments create a pattern and tell his story, but they are as isolated as he is.

After the title credits, we open on a taxi garage office where we meet Travis Bickle. He is interviewing for a job driving a cab at night. This interview is as close to a mental status examination as we will get, and it is quite revealing. We learn that Travis can't sleep; he wanders the city at night, so "I might as well get paid for it." He will work "anytime, anywhere," implying that he will even go into the roughest Black neighborhoods. (This film is not at all politically correct by today's standards. The language is raw, racist, and frequently obscene. I will respect the language of the film and of its time in describing it here.)

Asked about his work history, he says, "It's clean, like my conscience," an attempt at a joke that fails. Travis is awkward, socially uncomfortable. He is guarded about his lack of education ("some here, some there") but in mentioning that he is recently honorably discharged from the Marines and that he served in Vietnam, he bonds with the interviewer. Asked if he would be "moonlighting," he doesn't know what that means. We will see this again: he is unfamiliar with everyday language and with popular culture.

Another thing we will see several times in this film is the so-called God's-eye view camera shot. It's a Scorsese signature in his films. A view from high above, as though looking down from the heavens. We see the interview room this way. The shot is usually at a moment of stillness or contemplation, or to give a sense of perspective, or, with Travis, to emphasize his isolation. There are many examples in this film, small and large.

Travis gets the job, and we hear his first voice-over, the words in his diary. These voice-overs are worth quoting at some length because they say so much about how Travis sees himself and sees the world: "I'm working long hours. . . . The rain washes the garbage and the trash. All the animals come out at night. . . . Someday a real rain will come and wash all this scum off the streets." We hear this over images of his yellow taxi driving past "whores, skunk-pussies, buggers, queens, fairies, dopers, and junkies." "Venal" he calls them—

a word you wouldn't expect someone with his lack of education to know. Does it point to a Catholic upbringing? We don't know, but it's one of many questions we wish we could ask.

After work we see him go into a porno movie house, which in the 1970s were common in the Times Square area, and try to chat with the girl selling tickets and candy, asking her name. The camera watches from above as he uses his candy purchases to prolong the moment. He is awkward and insistent, and the girl threatens to call the manager.

He still can't sleep. But the next day he sees Betsy. We see her revealed in the crowded sidewalk, in slow motion, all in white. Travis observes her, seemingly pure and special, and says, in voice-over, "They cannot touch her."

A brief scene introduces us to Betsy: she works for the "Palantine for President" campaign with Tom, played by Albert Brooks. Tom is taken with Betsy, and she enjoys his humor but otherwise is not interested in him. This is one of the very few scenes in the movie that does not directly involve Travis, but it's important that we see how very different Betsy's world is from his.

That night he is sitting with some other cab drivers; he is part of them but somehow separate. "How's it hangin'?" asks one; Travis doesn't understand. There is a mention of driving to "fuckin' Mau Mau Land" and Travis's attention shifts to the other tables, staring at fancily dressed Black men, pimps and gangsters, and he is so preoccupied that he doesn't hear his friends asking him a question. Travis puts a pill in a glass of water and watches it dissolve. The camera looks straight down on the glass (a God shot) and slowly zooms in, the water fizzing—an image of his isolation, his preoccupation, his disconnection from those around him. End of Act One.

Travis, wearing a sport coat, is walking toward Palantine headquarters. He goes in and volunteers to help, but he only wants to talk to Betsy. He makes it obvious he has no interest or knowledge of Palantine ("I don't know exactly what his policies are") but tells her she is beautiful and that "I saw in your eyes you are not a happy person, you need something, maybe you call it a friend." She is intrigued and agrees to meet him for coffee and pie.

He tells us in another voice-over (reading from his diary again) that he chose apple pie with yellow cheese and that she had a salad. These details seem to matter to him; he is trying to learn to be a "person." Their conversation is friendly enough, though he often doesn't understand her references—"organiz-ized" and "thimk"—and the Kris Kristofferson song about a "prophet" and a "pusher." "I'm no pusher," says Travis, taking it as an accusation, and Betsy says, "Yes, but the part about the walking contradiction, you are that." After the date, Travis realizes he doesn't know her last name: "I gotta remember stuff like that." Navigating in the world of other people simply doesn't come naturally to this lonely man.

Later, Palantine himself is a passenger in Travis's cab. We see Travis recognize him in the rearview mirror—much of his world is lived in that mirror. Ever the politician, Palantine asks Travis (looking carefully at his taxi license to get his name) what "bugs you the most, Travis?" Wrong question—Travis starts hesitantly, then warms up, "I don't know, I don't follow things closely. They need to clean up this city, it's like an open sewer, it's full of filth and scum. I smell it, I get headaches it's so bad. They should just flush it down the fuckin' toilet!" Palantine is startled, but calmly tells him "I think I know what you mean" (he doesn't), and gets out, shaking his hand.

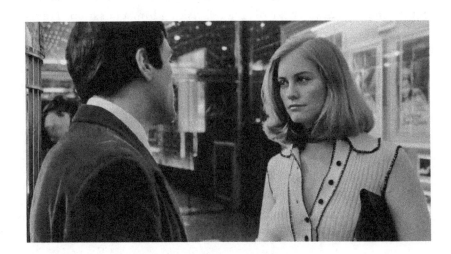

When we first see Iris, she is running away from someone and jumps into Travis's cab. He watches in his rearview mirror as she is pulled out by Sport, who throws some money at Travis and tells him to forget what he saw. The crumpled bill sits there on the seat. We will meet Iris and Sport again.

Afterwards, some kids throw eggs at Travis's windshield. It really does seem like an ugly, dangerous city.

Travis's idea of a date is to take Betsy to a porno film. After all, it's where he goes. She is hesitant but he insists lots of couples come there. As soon as the film starts, she leaves, telling him "taking me to this is about as exciting to me as saying, 'let's fuck'" (this angel can talk dirty too). She returns the record album he bought her and climbs into another cab.

The next scene is poignant but predictable. Travis is on the telephone in a hallway, trying to get Betsy to talk with him, to consider going out with him again. He apologizes for his poor judgment. As he pleads, the camera drifts away and focuses on the empty hall leading out. It's a touching image of loneliness. The film is full of these unexpected embellishments—often a movement of the camera, or a change of focus tells us more than any dialogue.

Travis has sent her flowers, which have been refused. He tells us that "the smell of the flowers made me sicker, the headaches are worse. I think I got stomach cancer."

When he tries to see Betsy at the headquarters and is told to leave, he suddenly assumes a martial arts stance, ready to fight—a reflex from his military past. He has been rebuffed, and he screams at her, "You are in Hell and you are going to die in Hell like the rest of them!" Then he tells his diary, "I realize now that she is just like the others—cold and distant—like all women."

Back in his cab, his new passenger is played by Martin Scorsese. He insists that Travis sit in his cab with him as he watches the apartment where his wife is being unfaithful. "Do you know who lives there? A nigger lives there. I'm going to kill her. With a .44 Magnum. Do you know what that gun can do to a woman's face? Or to her pussy? That you should see. You must think I'm pretty sick . . . you don't have to answer. I'm paying for the ride." This man is acting crazier than anything we have seen Travis do so far. But it puts an idea into Travis's head: a gun, a .44 Magnum.

Later Travis tries to get some help. He asks a senior cab driver, Wizard, for advice. "They got me real down, I want to go out and do something. I have some bad ideas in my head." Wizard doesn't know what he is talking about, and Travis can't bring himself to say more. Wizard throws some clichés at him about life and work and then dismisses them with, "What do I know, I'm a cabbie. But relax, Killer, you are going to be all right."

That's the end of Act Two.

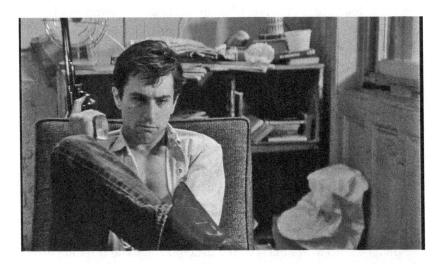

Now things change. We see Travis watching Palantine on TV. As he writes in his diary (and we hear in his voice-over) that he is going to stop taking pills and eat better, we see what he is eating: a bowl of bread, milk, whiskey, and sugar. Not the Breakfast of Champions. He reflects that "loneliness has followed me my whole life everywhere, there is no escape. I'm God's Lonely Man."

Then he meets "Easy Andy," a gun and anything-else-illegal salesman: "I could sell to some jungle bunnies in Harlem, but I just sell quality goods to the right people." The casual racism is telling. In another God shot, the camera caresses the gun barrels as he describes each one. Travis asks for a .44 Magnum, which Eddy says could stop an elephant. He recommends something smaller, a .38 snub nose, which Travis tests pointing it out the window at possible victims. Travis buys four guns and a special holster, and Andy offers him drugs, even a Cadillac. But Travis has what he needs.

Now he is exercising, again seen from above. "Too much abuse has gone on too long," he says, and we see him at a shooting range, trying out each gun. The jump cuts convey his intensity and restlessness, the sound of each shot loud and unsettling. At the porno movie, he mimes shooting at the screen. "The idea has been growing in my brain for some time—all the King's horses can't put it back together again." There is a montage of him practicing with each gun and holding his hand over a flame, testing his resistance to pain. We see him creating an automatic slide to hide a gun in his sleeve (would he really know how to make something like this?); he splits the nose of each bullet to make it more deadly and tapes a knife to his cowboy boot.

Another God shot shows Travis lying in bed, military jacket on. He is preparing for battle, and he still can't sleep.

At a Palantine rally, he talks with a Secret Service man, trying to be clever but just raising suspicion. They try to get his picture but can't.

Back at his room, we come to the most famous moment in the movie. He is bare-chested but with holsters at his side. Then, looking

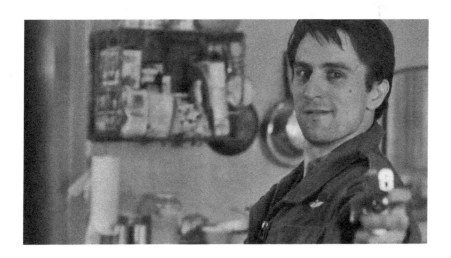

in the mirror, wearing his military jacket, pretending conversation. "I saw you coming you shitheel. I'm standing here, you make a move. You talkin' to me? You talkin' to me!? Well, I'm the only one here. Oh yeah . . ." and he draws his gun. Getting ready.

Then, again in voice-over: "Listen you fuckers, you screwheads. Here is a man who would not take it anymore. Who would not let . . . ? A man who stood up to the scum the cunts the dogs the filth the shit. Here is a man who stood up . . . you're dead!" He is pumping himself up to do something big—and violent.

At an all-night market he overhears a robber, comes from behind, and shoots him. He is primed to kill. The market owner is only too glad to hide Travis's gun and beat the dying robber with a tire iron: "He's the fifth motherfucker this year."

Then we see Travis watching a dance program on the TV. His loneliness is palpable as he watches the couples together, dancing. We see how focused he is on Blacks. He holds a gun in his lap.

He writes a pathetic letter to his parents, lying to them that he works for the government so he can't send them his address, that he has a girlfriend named Betsy, who they would really like, and that he has lots of money and is fine. He can't remember their birthdays but hopes this card will suffice. "I hope you are well and no one has died. One day there will be a knock on your door and it will be me."

Next, he is watching TV again, this time a soap opera, a girl is breaking up with her boyfriend; Travis pushes slowly with his foot until the TV crashes to the ground. Later he is doubled over with a headache.

Now he reaches out to Iris, the hooker who was dragged from his cab earlier. She is twelve years old.

He has his first encounter with her pimp, Matthew (known as Sport), played by Harvey Keitel, a Scorsese regular. It's Sport who notices Travis's boots and calls him "cowboy," first thinking that he is a cop wanting to entrap him. Travis pays for Iris's time and they go upstairs. He doesn't want to have sex with her; he wants to rescue her. But she doesn't think she needs to be rescued; she is just fine as she is. "I got no place else to go—they protect me from myself."

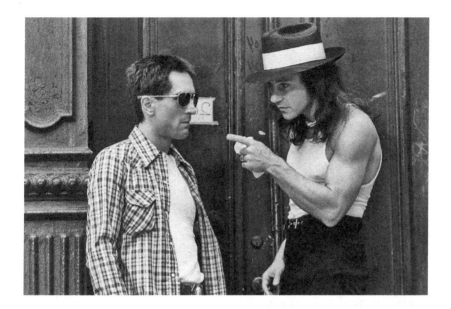

She is touched by his concern and agrees to meet him next day at a coffee shop.

Jodie Foster, who plays Iris, was the same age as her character when the movie was made. Foster was an old hand by then, having starred in Walt Disney kids' movies for years. This was her first role outside of that world, and it was quite a change. She would not have been able to see this movie at a regular theater, she was too young. Foster says she was taken in hand by De Niro, who rehearsed with her repeatedly. She brought her own intelligent observation to the role, spending time with a young prostitute to learn her habits. Her scene with De Niro at the coffee shop was mostly improvised and is completely convincing. She has had a long and very successful career since *Taxi Driver*. She won an Oscar playing a rape victim in *The Accused* and another as a fledging FBI agent in *The Silence of the Lambs*. She has moved into directing, with *Little Man Tate*, about a child prodigy, an episode of *Orange Is the New Black*, and an episode in the Netflix anthology series *Black Mirror*.

Over coffee and her breakfast, which is toast with jam and lots of extra sugar, Travis tries to persuade Iris to leave Sport, calling him a killer. They talk about her going to a commune in Vermont, but it's not

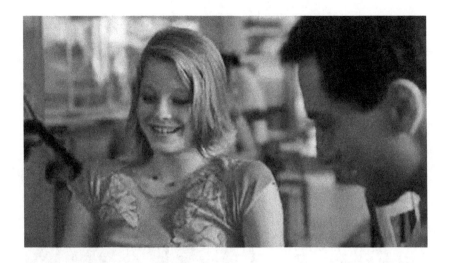

clear that Travis knows what a commune is. He tells her he will give her money so she can go away.

The next scene is one of the only other scenes in the film without Travis. We see Sport romancing Iris, who tells him she doesn't like being a hooker. Travis has gotten into her head. Sport tells her he is glad she doesn't like it, and that she is his support, that he depends on her. It's exactly what she needs to hear. They dance in a close embrace, to the same lush music that we so often hear under the tawdry images of the city throughout the movie.

Meanwhile, Travis is getting ready. He puts money in a letter for Iris, telling her that when she gets the letter, he will be dead. In voice-over he says, "Now I see clearly my whole life pointed in one direction—there has never been any choice for me."

Cut to Travis getting out of his cab at a Palantine rally. We see him from the knees down. The camera tracks to where he is standing, and as he raises his arm to put a pill in his mouth, we see him revealed: wearing his military jacket, head shaved into a mohawk. He looks fierce, and in no way will he blend into a crowd. So, when he works his way toward Palantine, he is spotted by the Secret Service agents and they give chase—his plan to assassinate the candidate foiled. He has worked himself up into doing a killing, and if this one doesn't happen another one must. So, he heads toward Iris, to rescue her.

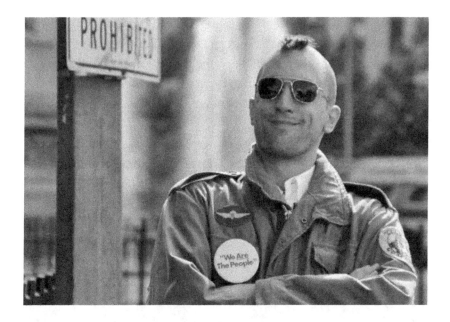

Now follows one of the most brutal killing sprees in film. At the time, nothing came close. In order to get this scene approved by the bosses at Columbia Pictures, who wanted Scorsese to totally eliminate it, the colors are de-saturated. The blood is less red. Do we notice? Does it really make a difference? Does it make the violence any less disturbing? It's hard to know, but I doubt it. But it did allow Scorsese to keep the scene as he and the screenwriter envisaged it.

First Travis confronts Sport, standing at his spot on the street. "How's everything in the pimp business? How's Iris?" says Travis. "I don't know nobody named Iris. Get back to your fuckin' tribe!" Travis pulls out one of his guns and shoots Sport in the belly.

He sits down in front of Iris's building. We don't know what he is thinking, but he seems calm. Readying himself to "rescue" her, and possibly for his own death. Then he walks into the building. In the hallway, he shoots the fingers off one hand of the pimp's timekeeper. Then Sport appears. How he got there is hard to imagine, but there he is. He shoots Travis in the neck. Travis shoots back—there is blood everywhere. Sport is down, and Travis shoots him a couple more times to make it stick. Then he climbs the stairs, with the timekeeper grabbing him and yelling "I'll kill you" over and over. A mafioso comes out of Iris's room and shoots Travis in the shoulder; Travis shoots him, then stabs the timekeeper's other hand through with a knife. When that doesn't stop him, Travis shoots him in the head. There are dead bodies everywhere. Iris has seen the mayhem, and she is screaming.

Travis is holding his bleeding neck, blood all over him. He puts a gun under his chin and pulls the trigger. Nothing. A second gun is empty too. He sits down and his head falls back. Is he dead?

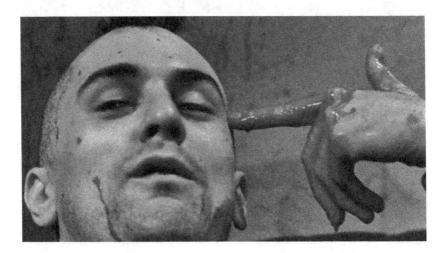

A policeman peers into the room, gun drawn, then another. Travis lifts his head, looks at the cops, puts his finger to his head and mimes pulling the trigger. Then falls back.

Then we have a final, iconic God shot. From high overhead the camera looks down on the carnage, the police frozen in position, and slowly, to a drumbeat, it tracks away from the room, along the hallway and then down the stairs, bodies and guns and blood. Then, out the door to the street where we see a crowd gathering and more police cars coming, as the camera pulls back, watching from above.

That would be the last image for most films, but not this one, for there is an epilogue.

Panning over the walls of an apartment, we see newspaper clippings as a voice reads a letter from Iris's parents thanking Travis for saving their daughter. The newspapers call Travis a hero who killed gangsters and pimps. Travis is well and recuperating, we hear from the letter, and Iris is home and back in school.

Then we are in front of a fancy uptown hotel, the cabbies chatting. Travis has a fare—it's Betsy. He sees her in his rearview mirror. He says nothing. She says "Hello, Travis. I read about you in the papers." "It was nothing really," he says, "the papers exaggerate. I got over that. Just some stiffness, is all." We hear that Palantine got the nomination and the election is just days away. "I hope he wins," says Travis. In the mirror her hair seems like a halo, moving with the breeze. Then he drops her off and won't let her pay. We see his eyes looking back in the mirror, and then we lose his cab in the traffic, which becomes a blur of lights.

What to make of this epilogue? Hold that thought: I'll tell you what I think a bit later.

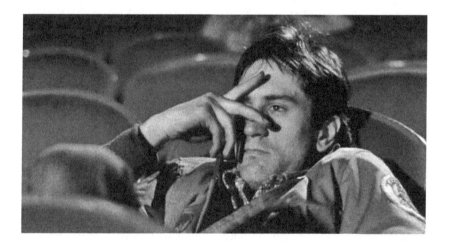

The Madness

The 1970s was a tough decade for America and for New York City. The Vietnam war ended, and soldiers returned home, not as heroes but often shunned and shamed for atrocities that occurred and a war that was lost.

Post-traumatic stress disorder (PTSD) as a reaction to war was not yet fully understood, but the sleeplessness, hyper-vigilance, recurrent images of violence, and mood swings of the disorder were all too common. There was, too, a sense of rage at the government that had chosen to fight this war for what many thought were the wrong reasons. This fed into the events of Watergate, where conspiracy and corruption at the highest levels, both locally and nationally, were revealed again and again.

New York City was on its heels financially, at risk of having to declare bankruptcy. Crime was rampant. Homicide rates had doubled in ten years. Thefts, burglaries, and rapes increased. There was gang violence, violence on the subways, and terrorist attacks by groups like the Black Liberation Army, a group of former members of the Black Panthers who gunned down two policemen. Middle-class folks were fleeing to the suburbs, and the tax base was eroding. So, the city froze hiring, slashed spending on social services, closed hospitals and fire stations, and reduced the number of police. Then there were the garbage strikes.

In 1976, President Gerald Ford refused a financial bailout to the city, leading to the famous *Daily News* headline, "Ford to City: Drop Dead."

This was the world of *Taxi Driver*. Travis was not wrong in seeing the moral and physical decay of the city. It was all around him. But he took it personally. He became convinced that only he could do something to fix it, that there was only one path possible for him: to cleanse it of its filth. This was his madness.

Is Travis just mad-angry, or are we really seeing a mental illness? I think it's clear we are seeing both: the anger becomes an expression of his madness.

In the job interview at the start of the film we learn Travis is having trouble sleeping. We don't know the nature of his insomnia, which would help us to narrow down our understanding of his problems. For instance, if he falls asleep easily but then wakes up in the middle of the night and can't get back to sleep, that might point to depression. If he has trouble falling asleep at the outset, we might be dealing with an anxiety disorder. If, on the other hand, he has nightmares that wake him up, and especially if the nightmares are of his experiences in Vietnam, we might think of PTSD, something many vets of this war experienced.

All we know is that he doesn't sleep. We also learn that he probably didn't finish high school. He is guarded about it and doesn't want to admit his lack of education. When asked about drugs, he says "I'm clean . . . like my conscience." This is obviously meant to be a joke, but it's useful to notice how badly he judges whether this is the time and place to make a joke. Also, the joke declares his conscience is clear: Why is that the idea that comes to mind for him first? His reading of the situation is off.

In the interview he says that he was honorably discharged from the service. Travis is not a good liar, as we see when he clumsily pretends he is interested in joining the Secret Service, so his answer here is probably honest. We can assume that his behavior did not cause concern when he was in the service, but I'm not sure that tells us much of value. The military culture then was problematic: racism about the Vietnamese was routine (often referred to as "gooks") and the threat of violence was everywhere, so a level of paranoia was considered normal, even necessary. Vietnam was a guerrilla war; you never knew where the enemy was or when they might attack. One of the symptoms of PTSD is an anxious hyper-vigilance, as though the sufferer is still in the jungle and might be jumped at any time. We don't see that with Travis, but we do have a sense that, for him, "out there" is the "enemy."

We see his preoccupation with the sleaziness of the city. As much as it dismays him and makes him angry, he seeks out the worst of it, spending his days watching porno movies, cruising the streets in the worst parts of town, paying closer attention to the Black pimps and gangsters in this sordid world than to anyone else. The slow-motion camera often tells us what Travis is obsessed with, not only this evidence of "scum," but also how he sees Betsy at first as an "angel," uncorrupted by what is happening around her.

Travis seems to need to mechanically learn the rules of personal interaction. For instance, when he tries to chat with the girl selling candy at the porno theater, asking her name when she clearly wants to be left alone; we see it again in much of his conversation over coffee and pie with Betsy, and when he first talks with Sport and doesn't understand that Sport suspects Travis is a cop.

Travis is often at sea with a cultural reference or the meaning of a word ("What's 'moonlighting'?" "I don't follow music." "I don't follow films."). He doesn't know who Kris Kristofferson is although he was well known at the time as a country music singer and composer (he wrote "Help Me Make It Through the Night" and "Me and Bobby McGee," which was a hit for Janice Joplin). Travis takes offense when Betsy says he reminds her of the Kristofferson song "The Pilgrim," about someone who seems a prophet and a pusher. "I'm not a pusher," he protests, but she is just referring to him as complicated. He doesn't seem to get irony or metaphor.

Travis tries hard to learn to be a "person," someone with routine interests and experiences, but he constantly comes up short. He has little insight into how he comes across. But we see him trying. When he approaches Betsy, telling her he sees her as lonely and needing a friend, he is projecting his own needs. But these are also universal needs, so his "insight" (it's not really an insight, it's a guess and a statement of his own condition) hits home, and Betsy is intrigued, not only with his comment, but also with his directness. She is used to people like Tom, who is only able to declare that he loves her when he knows she isn't listening. Travis is direct because he doesn't know how to be subtle. In that moment it works for him, and he gets a date for coffee. Soon, though, his lack of awareness backfires, and Betsy runs from the "dirty movie" he takes her to. Her rejection becomes a turning point. He denounces her and abandons his project of trying to be like other people. Now, instead of wallowing in the tawdry, nursing his anger and disgust with the way things are, he will "do" something. He prepares for assassination.

Travis shows a profound paranoia as well as increasingly focused delusions. Someone who is paranoid sees the world as against him. He or she is convinced that other people are out to get them, wishing them harm. A paranoid person is suspicious and wary; when he walks into a room and sees people talking, he will assume they are talking about him and that they are saying something bad: critical, demeaning, hateful. That they are even plotting to do him harm.

People with paranoia are usually loners because they find it impossible to trust the goodwill of others. The cabbies that Travis joins in the cafeteria after work are colleagues; they don't come across as friends. He sits at their table, but he is separate; he doesn't join in their chat about Errol Flynn's bathtub or about the rights of gays in California. His attention is elsewhere—in a glass of fizzing Alka Seltzer and the Black pimps at the next table.

So, he begins to train. This is finally something he knows how to do. He was a Marine. But even here there is a distortion, and we see the beginning of his further decompensation into madness. He declares he will stop taking pills and eat well. But we see his dinner: bread, milk, whiskey, a lot of sugar. We often see him walking the streets, drinking alcohol. He continues taking pills. What pills, we don't know. I'm guessing he would take uppers (amphetamines) for energy, for courage; drugs he would have bought on the very streets he finds so ugly.

We see him from above, lying in bed, staring at the ceiling, eyes wide open. He still can't sleep. He doubles over from headaches, says that the smell of decaying flowers is distressing and that he thinks he has stomach cancer.

These are signs that suggest that, with everything else, Travis is becoming psychotically depressed. Not the sort of depression where you take to bed and cry, but a depression that increases your sense of emptiness and hopelessness, with a conviction that the sickness and corruption you see outside in the world is now inside you. What complicates this interpretation is that, rather than withdraw into inaction, which is more typical of someone who is depressed, Travis has found a purpose in his life: that he must train to kill someone important, to change the world. Also, that in doing so, he must die. Travis is suicidal, expecting to be killed for his efforts.

Why would he want to assassinate Palantine? It's true that there is the connection with Betsy, whom he now sees as the embodiment of evil, someone who is "just like the others." And Palantine is very much present everywhere: on TV and billboards and in the newspapers, with rallies in the city that are hard to avoid. Palantine comes across as a standard Liberal, a "man of the people" who promises to fix much of what bothers Travis. But he also represents power and the government, whose authority and righteousness are increasingly questioned in the repercussions of the war in Vietnam. He cannot be trusted. And he is so powerful. If Travis can kill him, he will be erasing Palantine's power and generating his own. He will get noticed and will show Betsy how wrong she was to reject him. So, to Travis, he is the enemy, as much as the "scum" on the streets, as much as the "gooks" were in Vietnam.

The killing of the robber in the market gives Travis a chance to see the effects of his preparations: the guns he has bought and customized, the test of strength and ability to withstand pain, the practice sessions in front of a mirror challenging an imagined foe, and then outdrawing him. That he acts on impulse, shooting the robber as he turns around, tells him that his training is good. He is now a killing machine. It breaks whatever reluctance he might have had about vigilante violence.

His mohawk look at the rally, while effectively announcing to the world "there is a killer here," also makes it so that the Secret Service immediately sees him as a threat and chases him away. All his preparations are defeated by the fact that he is not very smart. He has no plan except to dress the part and walk purposely toward his target. It might have worked (such bare-bones plans have worked in the past in real assassination attempts, such as the one on George Wallace), but for Travis, it didn't.

Though thwarted at the rally, he is still determined to kill (and be killed?). He runs home and restlessly prowls his room, popping more pills. What is he to do with the adrenaline rush, with all that training, with such a need to do something big? So he drives across town to rescue the young prostitute, Iris.

This is his other delusional relationship. He first sees Iris when she is trying to run away. She is dragged from his cab by Sport while

Travis sits passively watching. Here was a chance to do something good, to counter the ugliness, and he did nothing. He sees Iris later, and after watching her from his cab, he approaches her and tries to convince her to leave Sport, stop being a hooker, and go back home. It seems a good-hearted venture, but she tells him she doesn't want to be rescued, that she likes the way things are. His conviction that Betsy is an uncorrupted angel, and that Iris is corrupted but can be saved, mirror each other. They are both untied from reality; that is, they are delusions.

Travis's original rescue plan is to offer to pay Iris's way to a commune in Vermont, or even to take her there. The note he writes her before he leaves for the Palantine rally includes money and tells her he will likely be dead when she reads it. Killing Palantine is also a suicide mission; Travis intends to die.

That seems to be his intention with this new Iris rescue plan too. He will kill whomever is in his way, then he will kill himself. He almost accomplishes that, except for the empty chambers in two guns.

This is the moment to discuss the epilogue. It is presented as a summary of what happened after the bloodbath. Travis is lauded in the newspapers as a hero, killing gangsters and pimps. He has recovered from his wounds and there are no legal consequences to his actions. He receives a grateful message from Iris's parents telling him that she is home and adjusting. Betsy becomes a passenger in his cab and tells him she knows he is a hero.

Does any of this seem likely? I don't think so. My best way to understand this is that the entire epilogue is the fantasy of a dying man—the man whose head we saw fall back onto the couch after miming shooting himself in the head. To me, this checks all the boxes—Travis is finally recognized, attention is paid, he has no need to be "God's Lonely Man" anymore. He has put the world right and been congratulated for it. Best of all, Betsy acknowledges just how special he is. Now he can go off into the night (in other words, die) content.

In interviews about this film both Scorsese and Schrader insist that they intended the epilogue to be real, not a fantasy or delusion. They intended it to be a comment on how the media can make a celebrity of a killer. Scorsese points to the way Travis looks at the world one last time through his rearview mirror to suggest that nothing has changed and that he will likely try to kill again. Scorsese may have thought that when he was making the film, but a glance in the mirror is not much to hang your hat on. The creators of a film can only tell you what they intended, not what you, the viewer, make of it. It is a film, a work of art, and you can interpret it as you choose. I find it more satisfying—and more convincing, more interesting—to see it as Travis's last musings before he dies.

Where does this leave us, diagnostically? Travis presents as someone with schizoid traits. This is suggested by his isolation and lack of intimacy with other people, his decreased range of emotion, and his inability to read verbal and behavioral cues. We see his separateness, that he is very much alone with no real friends, and that his attempts at connection are awkward and often odd, even when, briefly, as with Betsy, they seem to work.

He also clearly has paranoid delusions. As mentioned above, with paranoia there is a tendency to personalize, to take casual references as insults or condemnations, or to find hidden meanings that are threatening. When this is a personality disorder, it presents as lifelong, often showing in childhood or adolescence. We don't know if Travis showed these tendencies then. With Travis I think what he presents in addition to his schizoid personality symptoms would be best described as a delusional disorder, paranoid type. The prominent symptom is his pervasive preoccupation with the sleaziness of the city and his developing delusion that he is chosen to do something about it.

There is no doubt that parts of New York at that time were ugly with crime, drugs, and garbage. But, drive a few blocks and there were lovely, clean neighborhoods, with parks, culture, and the sort of smart, rich, creative neurotics that peopled Woody Allen's films from that time. Travis's New York is only part of the story. New York in the 1970s is both worlds, and Travis never looks beyond the depravity he sees every night. At first, he is a watcher, wallowing in the worst of the city. We never see him searching for the light, for something redemptive. He doesn't sleep and he spends his nights, when he is not watching "dirty movies," searching for scum to wash away in the sewer. Watching porn or the ugliness around him is not stimulating or a release; it feeds his anger. He is not just "God's Lonely Man." He is God's angry man.

The anger is there. We see it in bursts: when he turns on Betsy, in his increasingly uncontrolled rant to Palantine, when he assumes the martial arts position when challenged. But it's channeled too. He shows an unnatural calm as he prepares his weapons, tests his ability to withstand pain, or practices in the mirror, "You talkin' to me?"

Choosing to drive a taxi allows him to remain isolated but be in the world. There are people around him all night, but they are separated by their status as customers, and by sitting behind him and behind glass. Someone whose paranoia was not so narrowly defined would be wary of allowing anyone to sit behind them, for fear that they might attack. Travis can tolerate this because he is always watching in the rearview mirror, and because his primary concern is what he sees outside his taxicab.

There is a version of paranoid delusion called grandiosity, when the person thinks people are after him because he is special, with unrecognized talents; that he is important enough to deserve attention: "Those invisible black helicopters are hovering above to protect me from harm." This is paranoid and is also a delusion: there aren't any invisible helicopters. What makes it still paranoia is that it is an assumption of attention from other people that is not based on reality. No one is really watching Travis; in fact, no one seems to really see him at all. But Travis watches intently and is increasingly convinced (his delusion) that what he sees needs to be fixed and that he is the man to fix it (his grandiosity).

Travis's paranoia started out as generalized: his reaction to the sleaziness of the city. He focuses on Blacks, whether it's the pimps, the street toughs, the teens throwing eggs at his cab, or on interracial couples dancing together: though they are never labeled as such in the film, his preoccupations are racist and pervasive.

Over time his delusions become more focused: that Betsy and then Iris need to be rescued—Betsy from the likes of Tom, the Albert Brooks character, and from her loneliness, and Iris from Sport and life as a prostitute. With Palantine he develops a sense of mission and his paranoia becomes organized ("organiz-ized") and increasingly specific.

Do his paranoid delusions suggest schizophrenia? What is missing for this diagnosis to apply to him is *pathognomonic*: hallucinations. I try to avoid ten-dollar words, but *pathognomonic* is a good one to know. It means a symptom that defines an illness. If you don't have that symptom, even if you have others that are suggestive, you don't have that illness. Travis's off-center and extreme ideas of the world might suggest schizophrenia, but his madness is one of delusion and he shows no evidence that he ever hallucinates (seeing or hearing things that aren't there).

Does Travis's behavior fit with the antisocial personality diagnosis of the psychopath? You might think so, since he shows little empathy; he doesn't seem to register that he might be hurting the people he wants to rescue, and he has no sense of the humanity of the "scum" he finds disgusting and wants to "flush down the drain." But I see this as more a measure of his limitations socially, the schizoid avoidance of close personal connections, even as he seems to want to figure out a way to make them happen. He doesn't empathize with people because he seems to have so little experience of others. What in his background might explain that we simply don't know. His paranoia enforces his distance from other people (they are the enemy) and makes it that much harder for him to find in himself sympathy for others. The other aspects of the psychopath are out of his reach: he has no ability to con, he lies badly (making the Secret Service more, not less, suspicious), and it seems that he hasn't been in trouble with the law before.

A final note: Sometimes real life imitates fiction. John Hinckley, Jr., became obsessed with Jodie Foster after seeing her as Iris in *Taxi Driver*. He began stalking her, and when Foster moved to New Haven at the age of eighteen to attend Yale University, he moved there, too, and would slip poems and messages under her door. She did her best to avoid contact with him. He supposedly began to fantasize about ways to attract her attention: hijacking an aircraft carrier, killing President Jimmy Carter. Then he came up with the idea of killing newly elected President Ronald Reagan. Just before his attempt, he wrote Foster again: "the reason I'm going ahead with this is because I cannot wait any longer to impress you." On March 30, 1981, Hinckley shot at Reagan six times as he was leaving an event in Washington, D.C.; he also critically wounded several police officers and Reagan's press secretary, James Brady (who was permanently paralyzed). Reagan was seriously wounded and required an operation, but he recuperated. Hinckley was tried and found not guilty "by reason of insanity." He was incarcerated in a psychiatric hospital and released in 2016. After his trial he wrote that the shooting was "the greatest love offering in the history of the world." I am sure that Jodie Foster, who managed the terrible consequences of his infatuation with remarkable equanimity, would disagree.

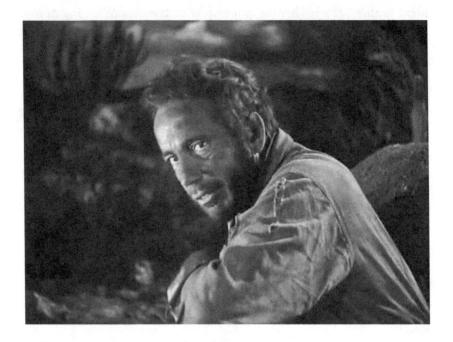

The Treasure of the Sierra Madre (1948)

Humphrey Bogart, Walter Huston, Tim Holt
Director: John Huston

This is one of the great movies. It won Best Director and Best Screenplay Oscars for John Huston, a Best Supporting Actor Oscar for Walter Huston (John's father), and it won the Golden Globe for Best Picture. You want to see this movie: it is a grand adventure, full of suspense, action, and great characters. It's the story of three misfits who join forces in search of gold in the mountains of Mexico: Howard (Huston), an experienced old-timer who's been prospecting with little luck for years; Curtin (Tim Holt), a young man out for riches and adventure; and Fred C. Dobbs (Humphrey Bogart), a born loser with an attitude. We see the hard work of finding and mining the gold, trusting your partners with the riches, and getting out of these Badlands alive.

Oh, and there are sombrero-wearing bandits too. (Confronting them when they claim to be "Federales," Dobbs asks for their credentials. Their oft-quoted reply, in a thick Spanish accent, "Badges? We don't need no badges . . . I don't have to show you any stinkin' badges!")

I want to focus on one scene, one of the best examples of paranoid thinking I've found in film.

Humphrey Bogart plays Fred C. Dobbs, moving to character parts from his leading-man days in films such as *The Maltese Falcon* (also directed by John Huston), *Casablanca*, and *The Big Sleep*. When Howard, the old-timer, has to go to help out in a Mexican village, he leaves his share of the gold with the others. They are to meet up in town. At the campfire that night, it's just Dobbs and Curtin. Dobbs starts laughing. His laugh has a nasty edge. Curtin asks, "What's the joke, Dobbsy? Aren't you going to let me in on it?" and Dobbs says sarcastically, "Sure I will, sure. I was thinking what a bonehead play that jackass made when he put all his goods in our keeping. He let us do his sweating for him, did he? We'll show him. Can't you see, it's all ours, we don't go back to Durango at all." Curtin says, "I don't follow you," and Dobbs says, " I'll make it clear to a dumb-head like you. We take all his goods and go straight up North and leave the old jackass flat!" Curtin says, "You don't mean what you are saying," and Dobbs says another line often quoted from this movie: "Fred C. Dobbs don't say nothin' he don't mean."

Curtin says that he won't touch a single grain of the old man's goods. Dobbs replies—and here is where the paranoia begins to surface—"I know exactly what you mean. You want to take it all for yourself and cut me out!"

Dobbs continues, "For a long time I've had my suspicions about you and now I know I'm right. You aren't putting anything over on me—I see right through you. For a long time you had it in your mind to bump me off at the first good opportunity and bury me out in the bush like a dog. You could take not only the old man's goods but mine in the bargain. And when you get to Durango safely you'll have a big laugh, won't you, thinking how dumb the old man and I were. " Curtin rises in protest and Dobbs pulls a gun on him, "Make another move toward me and I'll pull the trigger. Was I right or was I?" That is not a question, it's an assertion. He sees Curtin standing up as proving what he said. They scuffle and now Curtin has the gun. He says, "Listen to me. You're all wrong. Not at any time did I intend to rob you or do you any harm. I'd fight for you and yours the same as I'd fight for the old man's. . . . Considering the way things are, shouldn't we separate tomorrow or even tonight?" Dobbs says, "That would suit you fine, wouldn't it?" And Curtin asks, "Why me more than you?" Dobbs has an answer for that. "So you could fall on me from behind, sneak up and shoot me in the back." So Curtin says, "Then, I'll go first." Dobbs: "And wait for me on the trail and ambush me?" Curtin: "Why, if I meant to kill you, wouldn't I do it now?" Dobbs: "I'll tell you why. Because you're yella! You haven't got nerve enough to pull the trigger while I'm looking at you right in the eye." Dobbs starts laughing malevolently, "I'll tell you what, I'll make you a little bet; I'll bet you go to sleep before I do." The camera pulls away as Dobbs begins laughing again.

I've recorded this dialogue so fully because it beautifully traces the progression of paranoid thought. Nothing Curtin says can undo Dobbs's conviction that he is out to steal his goods. This is "projection," imposing on another what you are thinking yourself. It's Dobbs who has been planning to steal the other men's gold, but he has convinced himself they are out to get him, because that is what he would do. You can't argue away paranoia when it takes hold. It will have its own logic, and if you try too hard to convince the person that they are wrong, that they are misunderstanding the situation, then you become the enemy, part of the paranoid conspiracy.

They do go their separate ways, and things do not go well for Dobbs. I'll leave the rest of the tale for you to discover.

This sort of paranoia is different from what we saw with Travis. This is the classic "someone is out to get me" that defines the word. Travis's is more complex; his paranoia makes him focus on the most degraded parts of the city and increasingly feel a singular mandate to clean it up. It's a paranoid delusion, but a grandiose one, one that makes him feel important, not just put-upon. His paranoid thinking (it's about me, and I must respond) drives him to violence, mirroring the violence he sees around him.

Notice that Dobbs shows no evidence of hallucinations; this is not schizophrenia. His paranoia either reflects a personality disorder (if this way of thinking has been lifelong, which might fit for Dobbs, who is basically distrustful and seems to have little success in life) or it's an episode set off by greed when they strike it rich far away from the constraints of civilization.

As a therapist, the best you can say to someone like Dobbs, with a classic paranoid stance, is "I don't see it that way" and gradually suggest that there might be another point of view. Of course, if the person is Dobbs and he is pointing a gun at you, that gradual, careful approach won't wash. But if he is only laughing maniacally, then it's a place to start.

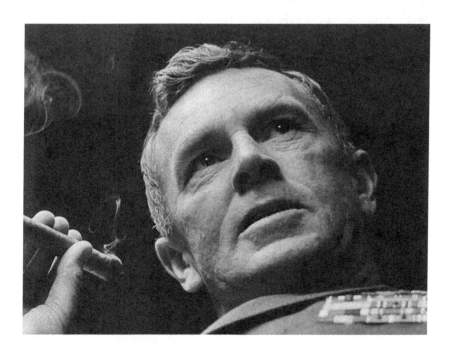

Dr. Strangelove or: How I Learned to Stop Worrying and Love the Bomb (1964)

Peter Sellers, Sterling Hayden
Director: Stanley Kubrick

This satire on the Cold War, politicians, and the military stars Peter Sellers playing three roles: U.S. President Merkin Muffley, RAF Group Captain Lionel Mandrake, and the former Nazi scientist, Dr. Strangelove. Sterling Hayden plays a mad, rogue Brigadier General Jack D. Ripper (subtle, this movie is not), who, believing that fluoridation of water is a Communist conspiracy to poison the U.S. population, sends a B-52 plane equipped with a nuclear warhead to bomb the Soviet Union. It can only be recalled using the three-letter code, and only he knows it. When the President finds out, he warns the Soviet Ambassador, who tells him that if the mission succeeds it will set off a "Doomsday Machine," which will destroy everything living thing on earth. And, yes, the movie is very funny.

Captain Mandrake confronts the General. General Ripper, casually smoking a cigar and locking the door so the Captain can't leave, explains (in another stellar example of paranoid thinking): "Mandrake, the planes will not be recalled. . . . Please make me a drink of grain alcohol and rainwater and help yourself to whatever you'd like." The camera angle shifts to a close-up from below; the General, puffing on his cigar, looks imposing and committed. He continues, "I can no longer sit back and allow Communist infiltration, Communist indoctrination, and the International Communist Conspiracy to sap and impurify all of our Precious Bodily Fluids."

A few moments later they are sitting on the couch. Soon, it will be too late to recall the planes. Ripper asks, "Mandrake, have you ever seen a Commie drink a glass of water?" Mandrake, afraid but trying to keep the General talking, says, "Well, I can't say I have." "Vodka is what they drink isn't it, never water?" Mandrake says, "I don't quite see what you are getting at, Jack," and Ripper explains, "Water is the source of all life. . . . We all need fresh pure water to replenish our

Precious Bodily Fluids. Are you beginning to understand?" Mandrake starts laughing shakily as he realizes just how crazy Ripper is.

Meanwhile, the President has ordered an attack on Ripper's base, so while they are talking there is the sound of gunfire in the background. "Have you ever wondered why I only drink rain or distilled water or only pure grain alcohol? Have you ever heard of fluoridation of water? . . . Do you realize it is the most monstrously conceived and dangerous Communist plot we have ever had to face?" Ripper pulls a machine gun out of his golf bag and sets up to begin to shoot back at the attacking force. A billboard reads, "Peace is our Profession." Ripper starts shooting, with Mandrake on the floor, cowering.

During a pause, Ripper tells him, "In addition to fluoridating water there are studies underway to fluoridate salt, flour . . . ice cream, children's ice cream. Do you know when fluoridation first began? 1946—how does that coincide with your post-war Commie conspiracy?" He continues, "It's incredibly obvious, isn't it? A foreign substance is introduced in your Precious Bodily Fluids with no choice from the individual. . . . That's the way your hard-core Commie works." Mandrake asks, "Jack, when did you first develop this theory?" Ripper says, "Well, I first became aware of it, Mandrake, during the physical act of love. Yes, a profound sense of fatigue, a feeling of emptiness followed. Luckily, I was able to interpret these feelings correctly. Loss of essence. I can assure you it has not recurred. Women sense my power, and they seek the life essence. I do not avoid women, but I do deny them my essence." There is a long pause as this sinks in. Mandrake tries to persuade him, "I drink water all the time and I guarantee you there is nothing wrong with my bodily fluids." But Ripper isn't listening. His men are surrendering and he fears interrogation. He kills himself in the bathroom.

It's discovered, too late, that the three-letter code is PBF. The bomb is dropped and the world explodes to the tune of the popular British World War II song "We'll Meet Again."

In a movie that often hits you over the head with its political points—the billboard; the General's name; the wonderful moment when the Soviet Ambassador and the Military Chief of Staff start punching each other and the President cries, "Gentlemen! You can't fight in here! This is the War Room!"; and, last but not least, the moment when Dr. Strangelove, the Nazi scientist, in a passion as he describes how the world will look after total destruction, pulls himself out of his wheelchair and cries, "Mein Führer, I can walk!"—it's not a surprise that the code is based on "Precious Bodily Fluids," General Ripper's paranoid delusion.

I've given the dialogue in some detail because it best conveys the nature of Ripper's paranoid idea. In the 1950s there was a good deal of suspicion of fluoridation of water in the United States. Fluoridation of community water sources had been proven to prevent cavities, much to the dismay of dentists, who feared it would rob them of their livelihood. There were people who thought it was a Communist plot and refused to allow it in their communities. Those people got cavities. Now it is accepted (because it works and is safe) and is, as Ripper predicted, even in our toothpaste. Ripper's concerns were not completely off-base.

However, how he came to them and where it leads him, is unique to him. His explanation is that he felt a sense of fatigue and emptiness after making love, and "knew" it was because he had lost his "essence." He goes from loss of "essence" to protecting his precious bodily fluids to being sure that fluoridation is what threatens his PBFs and that the "Commies" are responsible. Notice the reference to "1946—how does that coincide . . . ?" It coincides with the end of a war so that countries could now pay attention to something else, like improving the health of their citizens. Instead, Ripper sees "conspiracy." He is finding connections where none exist and extrapolates from there as though he has proved something. Each step sounds oddly sensible, but none of it is real. This is paranoid thinking. And in this movie, it leads to the end of the world.

RECOMMENDED READING

Fleming, Michael, and Roger Manville. *Images of Madness*. London: Associated University Press; 1985.

> Specifically, chapter 5: "War and Madness," and chapter 7: "Paranoia and Madness." This is one of the first books to examine madness in film. It is out of date, but its insights are worthwhile.

Munro, Alistair. *Delusional Disorder: Paranoia and Related Illnesses*. Cambridge: Cambridge University Press; 2006.

Shapiro, David. *Neurotic Styles* (Austen Riggs Center Monograph, No. 5). New York: Basic Books; 1973.

> Astute descriptions of various fixed ways of being, or personality styles, specifically chapter 3: "The Paranoid Style."

▪5▪

"Don't he never sleep?"

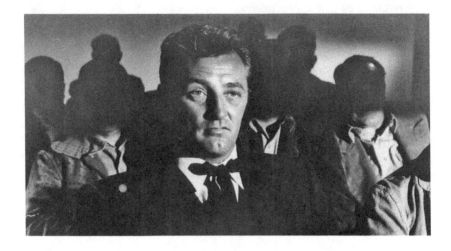

Personality Disorders

THE PSYCHOPATH

The Night of the Hunter (1955)

Robert Mitchum, Shelley Winters, Lillian Gish
Director: Charles Laughton

We are entering the world of the personality disorder.

We originally were looking at characters experiencing psychotic decompensation: for Karin, a recurrence of something that first happened before we meet her; for Carol, a first break.

Then, in *Taxi Driver*, we met Travis Bickle. He does not have the hallucinations of schizophrenia, but he is debilitated by his delusions and obsessions, delusions that he has stomach cancer, that he has to rescue two very different women who do not want to be rescued, and that he has a special mandate to somehow sweep the mean streets of the city clean by assassinating Palantine, the presidential candidate. This is a madness, a form of psychosis. They are paranoid obsessions that suggest a thought disorder and, possibly, a personality disorder.

What's the difference? Most acute psychiatric illnesses have a time of first onset. There is a time before, when you would say the person's function was relatively normal, then the madness begins—either abruptly or, more commonly, slowly and insidiously. Personality disorders, on the other hand, are lifelong patterns, formed in adulthood but with childhood precursors. They are ways of coping and dealing with the world that seem hardwired, not episodic or with a clear beginning.

We all have our eccentricities, our so-called neurotic styles. I own up to an obsessive style. My papers are in order "just so" on my desk and I have a hard time not putting things away. This style has served me well; I am pretty efficient. I get work done. It allows me to be more or less successful in life. I may well be a nuisance to my wife, who complains when I put something away that she was still using, but these are minor hiccups.

However, if my obsessive tendencies got in the way of my functioning; if I put more energy into making sure my papers were properly squared on my desk, and that my pencils were all lined up in size order, than in actually writing this chapter, it might well be called a "disorder," edging into madness.

A personality disorder, then, is a pervasive pattern of interacting with the world: a fixed style that causes trouble, most often emotional upset in those around you. For many people, such a disorder is "ego syntonic"; the person feels okay about themselves and how they behave, until someone complains strongly or repeatedly or until it causes them to fail or feel out of control, complicates relationships, or puts them in jail.

As I explained in Chapter 1, I will be referring to people with the particular personality disorder in this and the following chapter as "psychopaths." Unlike disorders like schizophrenia, depression, bipolar, and the anxiety spectrum, all of which occur to someone who has had a period of normality before episodes of the illness become debilitating, thus justifying calling them "persons with," say, schizophrenia or depression, personality disorders are essentially immutable and, as lifelong ways of being, are central to who a person is. The madness is their "normal" and labelling them with their disorder is simply describing who they are.

You won't find me referring often to Sigmund Freud, but I do find this worth sharing. Freud defined normality as the ability to live, love, and work with a certain contentment. He said that the goal of therapy was "to convert neurotic despair into ordinary unhappiness." This tells you a lot about Freud. It is likely that he had a depressive personality, that for him the glass was always half-empty, not half-full. This is a style, a worldview, and though not an ideal way to go through life, it doesn't necessarily get you into trouble. You can live with your "neurotic despair" and feel that that is your version of "normal."

But if your depressed view of the world made it so you were unable to experience any pleasure or satisfaction from your work or your relationships, then we might be looking at a depressive personality disorder. If the depressed outlook acutely worsened, so you couldn't get out of bed or get dressed or eat properly; if you could no longer concentrate or find small pleasures in daily routines; if you had no energy and were sleeping away much of the day; if you felt empty inside or frequently close to tears—and all of this was a change from how you had been—then we would be dealing not with a personality disorder but with the illness of depression. This is something we will explore in later chapters. The difference is not only in how much more extreme the symptoms are, but also that they have a beginning, and a time before that was different.

Earlier versions of the *DSM* put these different kinds of illnesses onto different axes. An Axis I diagnosis was defined as an illness like schizophrenia, paranoia, or depression, that had a distinct start and was usually episodic. An Axis II diagnosis was the personality disorder—something that defined a lifestyle, a way of being in the world. These distinctions were actually useful, though they were gross simplifications. It's not always so easy to distinguish the one from the other.

But we will try.

There are many different types of personality disorders, and to organize them (and to implicitly acknowledge how difficult pinpointing a personality diagnosis can be), the most recent *DSM* categorizes them in "clusters." There is Cluster A (odd-eccentric), including paranoid, schizoid, and schizotypal personalities; Cluster B (dramatic-emotional), including borderline, narcissistic, and the antisocial; and Cluster C (anxious-fearful), which includes obsessive-compulsive, avoidant, and dependent personalities. The fact that a person will often have symptoms from more than one cluster (called "co-morbidity" in the textbooks) underlines how porous these diagnostic categories can be.

We have few medications and few effective psychotherapy techniques to mitigate personality disorders, which, in their essence, are lifelong ways of being. These people really are defined by their madness.

We will focus here on the psychopath, a subtype of the antisocial personality disorder.

Someone with an antisocial personality disorder (more simply called a sociopath) has a history going back to childhood or early adolescence of cruelty to animals, delinquency, impulsiveness, school truancy, petty theft, and/or setting fires. These are called conduct disorders of childhood. In adulthood these individuals continue to ignore the rules of society, disregarding the rights of others, often breaking the law, and rarely showing any sense of guilt or responsibility for bad behavior.

People with the psychopathic version of this disorder display a lack empathy, con and manipulate others, take risks, behave impulsively, and rarely learn from their mistakes. They can be sexually promiscuous, though more for the sense of conquest and control than for the sex. They show little ability to feel love or warmth toward another person. They have a tendency toward violence and often wind up in prison.

Unlike people with other categories of madness, psychopaths almost never feel bad about how they function or behave. If they are distressed, it is usually a vexation with others who get in the way of them doing what they want.

The movies love villains because they are frequently more interesting than the hero. The ultimate movie villain is the psychopath. He can be charming but dangerous. And scary. Sometimes, not so charming, and rarely as murderously dangerous as the movies would portray them. In real life, most often, their danger is more subtle, more socially insidious—a danger that can disrupt a family, or a business, or a society if the psychopath gets into a position of power.

It is said that not all psychopaths are serial killers, but that all serial killers are psychopaths. This is controversial, but worth considering.

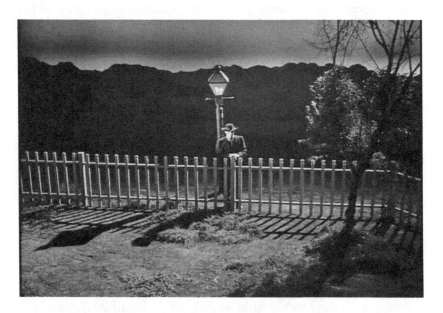

The Night of the Hunter is a strange and eccentric film. It is a favorite of mine, but one that students either love or hate.

Harry Powell (portrayed by Robert Mitchum), who we will see is a classic psychopath, pretends to be a preacher and has the words "Love" and "Hate" tattooed on his knuckles. He uses them to transfix the easily persuaded locals in the town.

But we are getting ahead of ourselves. *The Night of the Hunter* (1955) was the only film directed by the great English actor Charles Laughton, who played Henry VIII in *The Private Life of Henry VIII* (1933) and

Captain Bligh in *Mutiny on the Bounty* (1935); starred in *The Hunchback of Notre Dame* (1939); played the ghost in *The Canterville Ghost* (1944) and Captain Kidd in *Abbott and Costello Meet Captain Kidd* (1952); and was featured in Agatha Christie's *Witness for the Prosecution* (1957), directed by Billy Wilder.

The *Night of the Hunter*'s cinematographer, Stanley Cortez, had previously worked on Orson Welles's *The Magnificent Ambersons* (1942) and would later work on *The Three Faces of Eve* (1957) and *Shock Corridor* (1962). His work on this film is extraordinary: with the shadows of film noir, his lighting of the expressionistic, intentionally artificial-looking sets, and finding new ways to film underwater.

The screenplay is credited to James Agee. He was the talented, Pulitzer Prize–winning author of the autobiographical novel *A Death in the Family*, about how the loss of a father affects his young children. It is beautifully observed. The opening scene, which reads like a poem, inspired Samuel Barber's *Knoxville: Summer of 1915*, a piece for soprano and orchestra. Agee also wrote the text accompanying Walker Evans's photos of Depression-era workers in *Let Us Now Praise Famous Men*, which is considered a modern classic. He worked as a film critic for *Time* magazine and *The Nation*. His columns are collected in *Agee on Film* and are essential reading for anyone interested in film history. The screenplay he turned in for *Night of the Hunter* was nearly 300 pages long—it would have made a six-hour movie. He was told to cut it by half, then Laughton trimmed even more. However, most of the scenes in the finished film are as Agee wrote them.

The Night of the Hunter was too dark, too modern, too strange for its time: it was widely misunderstood and failed miserably when it was released. Laughton never got to direct another movie. Now, it is considered a masterpiece.

There are many reasons the movie was hard to appreciate when it first came out and is difficult to appreciate even now. It defies categorization. It's a suspense thriller that is also a child's fairytale, told from a child's point of view. It's not a film I would show to any young child; it's too scary. It's also self-consciously stylized, with reference to silent movies, cartoons, and film noir. There is an extended sequence as the children are escaping from Harry Powell that feels very much like a dream, a nightmare when time is stretched, both beautiful and sinister, and ending with an encounter with Mrs. Cooper, played wonderfully by Lillian Gish, who, taking the children in, might as well be Mother Goose personified. Who puts Mother Goose in a suspense thriller? The changes of tone and of reference throughout keep you off-balance. I find it irresistible.

The Movie

The film starts oddly. The music immediately tells us something threatening is in the offing. The music is rather dated; its emphatic signaling too on the nose. With a background of stars, we hear children sing "dream, little one, dream"; then we see the woman we will learn is Mrs. Cooper telling the children a Bible story and then disembodied faces of the children, entranced. She reads, "Beware of false prophets which come to you in sheep's clothing," and we see a bucolic small-town America from above, children playing. Then we are closer in, and a child is standing in front of a barn, looking at a dead woman lying on the floor. As Mrs. Cooper continues to read Scripture, we see Harry Powell driving alone in the countryside.

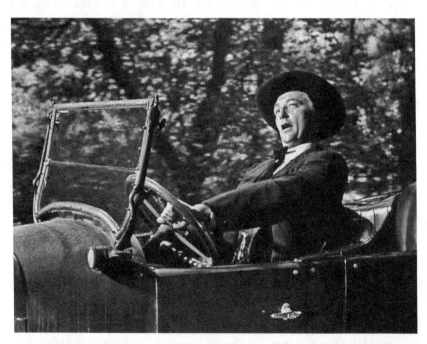

He is dressed like a preacher and is talking to himself—or is it "The Lord" he seems to be addressing? "What's it to be, Lord, another widow? How many has it been—six? Twelve? I disremember. You say the word, Lord, I'm on my way. You always send me money to go forth and preach your word. A widow with a little wad of bills hid away. . . . Not that you mind the killings, your Book is full of killings, but there are things you do hate, Lord—perfume-smellin' things, lacy things." And now we see Harry watching a striptease (pretty tame by modern standards). For the first time we see his left hand; tattooed on his fingers are the letters "HATE." He reaches into his pocket and releases a switchblade which cuts through his pocket, a not-too-subtle phallic reference. The police catch him for stealing a car.

Next, we meet young John and his sister, Pearl. Their father, Ben, arrives in a panic: he has $10,000 in one hand, a gun in the other; he has robbed a bank and killed someone. Where can he hide the money before the cops get to him? When the police come to arrest him, they force him to the ground and handcuff him, with John crying, "Don't."

Their father's cellmate in prison is Harry. He tries to get Ben to tell him where he hid the money. Ben won't tell him. When Ben asks Harry what religion he professes, Harry says, "The religion the Almighty and me worked up betwixt us."

Ben is executed for the murder.

Children in town taunt John and Pearl, singing, "Hing, Hang, Hung." Pearl doesn't realize she is being made fun of, and walks away singing the song. We meet Icey Spoon (Evelyn Varden), who runs the ice cream parlor. She is one of the more irritating characters in movie history, a small town busybody and know-it-all with a sing-song voice. She is trying to encourage Willa Harper, Ben's widow (Shelley Winters), to think about marrying again. We cut to a train traveling in the dark, accompanied by bombastically threatening music; someone bad is coming.

John is telling his sister a bedtime story very much like what happened to their dad. When he mentions a "bad man," we see the dark, oversized shadow of Harry, who is standing outside the house under a lamp. Harry is singing to himself, a hymn, "Leaning on the Everlasting Arms."

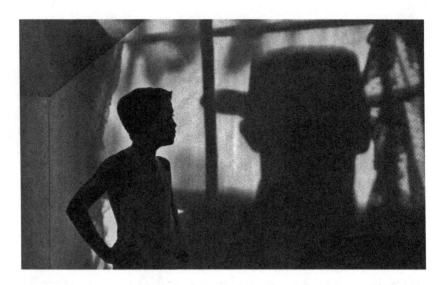

The next day, when John goes to the Spoons to pick up Pearl, he sees Harry for the first time. Pearl is sitting on the counter with her doll in her lap. Harry claims he worked at the prison and that's how he knew Ben Harper. John is staring at Harry's fingers, noticing the tattoos of "Love" and "Hate." Harry asks, "Would you like me to tell you the little story of Right Hand–Left Hand, the story of Good and Evil?" He is charming with the women. He mesmerizes them with his dramatic telling. And, of course, he is a preacher (or so they think), so he already has their goodwill. John stares at him, unimpressed. Pearl leaps into his arms: she needs a daddy.

Icey invites Harry to the town picnic, and we fade to him leading the populace in a hymn. Icey urges Willa to consider Harry as a husband. She then expounds on men and women: "I've been married to my Walt that long, and I'd swear in all that time I just lie there and think about my canning."

Willa worries that Harry might be after her money. Icey tells her to ask him directly. Harry insists that Ben told him where the money was hidden: it's at the bottom of the river. John smiles quietly; he knows where it is and the secret holds. But Willa declares, "My whole body's just a-quivering with cleanness." That's likely not what is quivering her body, but we will let that lie. It's the occasional heavily obvious line like that which dates this movie. I find it easy to forgive.

John is walking toward his house that night. It looks tiny, not bigger than one room. But when he goes inside, it's big. This is an example of the expressionistic style. The artificiality reminds you that this is a story, a fairy tale. Harry is there. He tells John he will be his new daddy. John almost blurts out the secret but catches himself, saying, "You're not my daddy!" Later Pearl asks if they can tell about the money, now that they have a new daddy. John gets her to swear she won't.

That night, Willa is getting ready for her honeymoon night. She finds Harry's knife in his jacket pocket, smiles, and fondly says, "Men," then goes out to him. Harry is in bed, claims he was praying. He tells her he has no interest in sex with her; "Marriage to me is a blending of two spirits." He tells her to look at herself in the mirror: "That body was meant for begetting children, not for the lust of men!" She is devastated but declares she wants to be "clean."

John's elderly friend by the river, Uncle Birdy, senses trouble at their house and tells John he can always come to "your Uncle Birdy" if he needs help. He's a drinker, improving his coffee with a touch of whiskey.

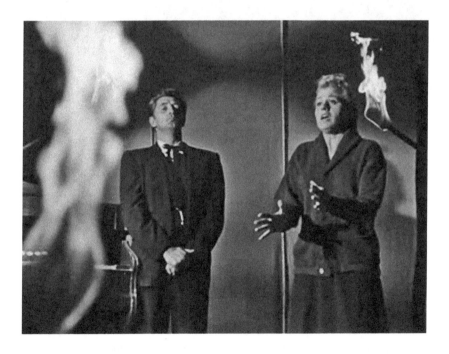

We cut to torches, a sort of evangelist revival meeting led by Harry, with Willa hysterically confessing that she drove her first husband to murder with her frilly demands. Her intensity betrays that she is one sexually unsatisfied woman.

Next, we see Pearl's doll, lying on the ground surrounded by hundred-dollar bills. She is cutting out paper dolls with the money. It was hidden in her doll the whole time. As John hurriedly tries to put the money back in the doll, Harry walks outside. As Harry stands there, a couple of bills blow past. He doesn't notice. He tells John that he knows that John told his mom that Harry asked about the money. John smirks. Harry says, "It's your word against mine. It's me your mother believes." That hits John hard.

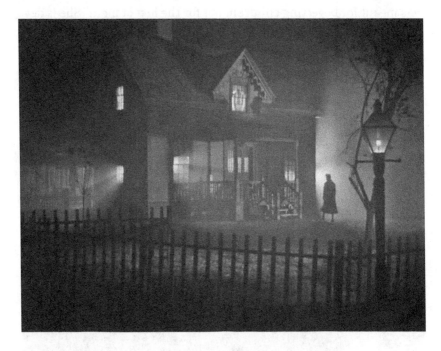

Coming home, Willa overhears Harry asking Pearl, "Where's the money hid? Tell me, you little wretch, or I'll tear your arm off!" For the first time, we see just how angry he can get. Later that night, Willa is praying in bed. We see the room from a distance, and it's obviously a set, with a black surround. The pitched roof gives it the appearance of a chapel. Harry knows she overheard. He raises his arm to the heavens, reaches for his knife, walks slowly to Willa in the bed, lifts his arm to strike—and we cut away. John wakes up to hear the sound of their old car starting and driving away.

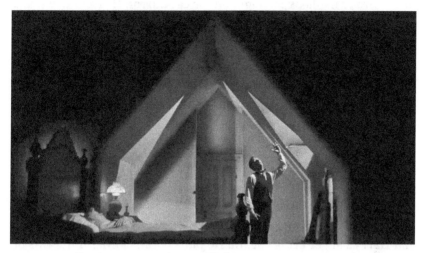

Harry tells the Spoons that Willa has run away. He pretends to be distraught. "It's my shame, it's my crown of thorns . . . from the very first night . . . our honeymooon. She turned me out of the bed." When Walt Spoon says she'll be back, Harry says, "She'll not be back. I reckon I'm safe in promising you that." They have no idea. Then he says he caught her drinking dandelion wine, so he knew she needed saving. He knows just how to play these simple people. "Can't nobody say I didn't do my best to save her."

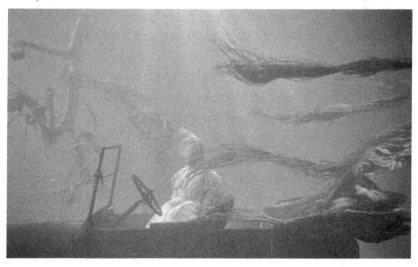

Fade to seagrass waving under the water, and Willa, sitting dead in the car, her hair waving in the water too. A hauntingly beautiful image. Uncle Birdy's fishhook is caught on the car mirror. He looks down and sees her. He says nothing, but that night he gets drunk. End of Act One.

Harry is singing "Leaning" as he leans against a tree outside the house. He calls out, "Children . . . chilllldren." It is chilling. You will remember it in your dreams. He walks toward the house, with a camera iris closing in on John and Pearl hiding in the basement (an effect from silent movie days).

Harry prowls the house looking for the children. He has them to himself now. He looks down into the basement, "Come up here, I feel myself getting awfully mad." They comply.

Harry eats dinner but refuses the children any food until they tell their secrets. When Pearl starts to tell him, John tells her to stop, and Harry's anger erupts again. He pulls out his knife: "I use this on meddlers . . . don't touch my knife. That makes me mad, very, very mad!" Harry pounds the table, "John doesn't matter! Can't I get that through your head, you poor, silly, disgusting, little wretch." He catches himself: "You made me lose my temper."

John, to protect Pearl, says he will tell. The money is in the cellar, he tells him. Go look for yourself. John is a resourceful boy, always thinking. He hopes to trap Harry in the basement. Harry lights a candle, and says "Come along, go ahead of me . . . down those stairs." He says it with great foreboding (Mitchum's line readings are a marvel; he can sound very threatening). This is not part of John's plan.

We are in the basement as they go down the steps. But this time the basement is obviously a set, like the bedroom was, all in shadows with a black surround. John points to the floor and Harry starts to dig, but it's concrete. He grabs John around the neck, looks up and says, "The Lord's a-talkin' to me now. He's a-sayin', 'A liar is an abomination before mine eyes.' . . . Speak, before I cut your throat." Pearl confesses to save John—"It's in my doll"—and Harry sits back laughing—of course! John pulls on a wooden beam and the shelf of canning lands on Harry's head. He groans like an animal. John and Pearl run up the stairs; he follows with arms outstretched, looking just like Frankenstein from the original 1931 movie. John slams the door on Harry's hand and he growls like the "Big Bad Wolf" he is.

They run to Uncle Birdy, who is too drunk to help them, so they head for the skiff on the river, with Harry close behind.

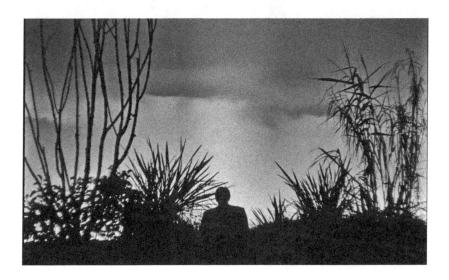

Now we are entering nightmare-dream country. They are running along the river; we see the shadow of Harry above them. He thrashes through the woods; they are slowly making their way to the boat, just offshore. Harry falls into the mud, then is in the river, as they float away, safe for now. He begins a scream of frustration to wake the dead.

The boat drifts. Pearl begins to sing to herself. We are suspended in time, like a dream. We see the boat passing a spider's web, a large toad, pussy-willows, an owl, a tortoise, rabbits. The world of nature. We watch the boat from above, the God's-eye view. Walt Spoon reads a postcard from Harry explaining that he and the children are visiting his sister. Walt mentions that "gypsies" knifed a local farmer and stole his horse. We then see Harry on a horse.

The children decide to spend the night on land and pull up to a farm. The houses look like toys, but the setting is simple and just about perfect.

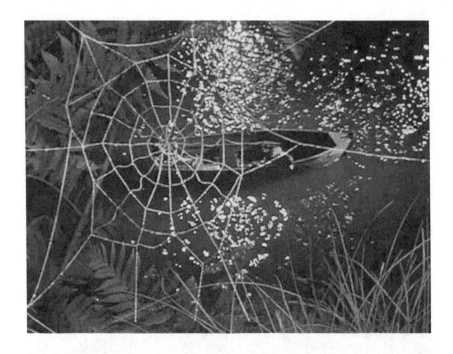

They sleep in the barn. John wakes in early morning and sees Harry on horseback silhouetted on the horizon and singing "Leaning." John says, "Don't you never sleep?" (I love that line.)

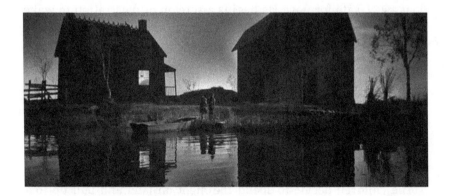

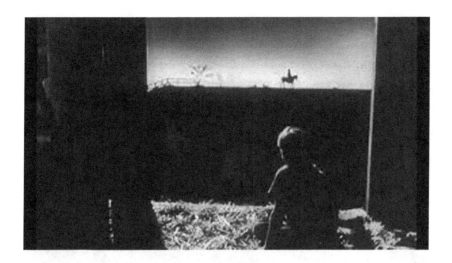

Back on the river, they finally land at Mrs. Cooper's. End of Act Two.

Mrs. Cooper is out of a nursery rhyme ("There was an Old Woman Who Lived in a Shoe," perhaps, or Mother Goose). She is a woman who cares for any child who appears at her door. Initially, she appears bossy and strict. But she is just disciplined and gently understanding. First, the children need to get washed. "Gracious, I guess I have two more mouths to feed," Mrs. Cooper says, but adds, "I'm a strong tree with branches for many birds. I'm good for something in this world, and don't I know it too." This sort of on-the-nose dialogue is quite self-conscious and overly explicit, but it fits with the way the story is being told. Though we are no longer in the dreamscape of the river, this is still a fairy tale.

Mrs. Cooper has insight, and she tells a bedtime story to the children that gets John's attention; he realizes that he is with a good person and is safe. Ruby, one of the other orphaned children, an adolescent, is in town on her own when Harry turns up and asks her about the new children at Mrs. Cooper's. When he hears her describe Pearl, he asks whether she has a doll.

Then Harry turns up at the house, and Mrs. Cooper sees right through him. When he tries to tell the story of Right Hand–Left Hand, she interrupts him: "Them kids is yours?" He says yes, and explains that their mother ran off with a "drummer" (a salesman). Mrs. Cooper doesn't believe any of it. John tells her, "He ain't my dad," and she says, "And he ain't no preacher, neither!" She comes back out of the house with a rifle and Harry runs off, threatening, "I'll be back when it's dark!"

And he is. We see him that night sitting on a tree stump in front of the house, singing "Leaning." When he sings that hymn it sounds like a threat. Then we see the children asleep in a room looking like the chapel we have seen before, but now it seems a place of safety rather than the sacrificial chamber of Willa's bedroom. Then, wonderfully, we see Mrs. Cooper in silhouette, sitting on a rocking chair with a rifle in her lap: Whistler's Mother with a gun.

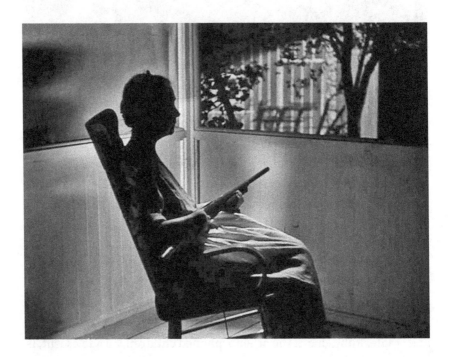

She starts singing the hymn "Leaning," too, adding, "Leaning on Jesus" to challenge Harry's ownership of the song: a battle of good versus evil. We can see Harry outside because Mrs. Cooper is sitting in the dark. Ruby comes in with a candle, which Mrs. Cooper tells her to put out. Harry is gone. Cut to an owl swooping down onto a rabbit; the rabbit squeals, caught. "It's a hard world for little things," says Mrs. Cooper.

She patrols the house with her rifle; the children stand there, frightened. She starts to tell them a story to calm them when Harry suddenly appears in the kitchen. She shoots at him. Wounded, he runs, squealing, and hides in the barn. She calls the troopers to come and get him.

While waiting, she does chores and tells John, "Children are man at his strongest. They abide."

When the police drag Harry to the ground to handcuff and arrest him, as they did John's father, John again cries, "Don't." Watching that brings back painful memories.

The aftermath seems oddly out of place and hurried. Harry is brought to trial, John refuses to testify against him, but Harry is convicted as a serial murderer. Icey Spoon gets drunk and joins a mob that wants to lynch him.

We see Mrs. Cooper ignoring the fuss, marching with all the children behind her, like ducklings all in a row.

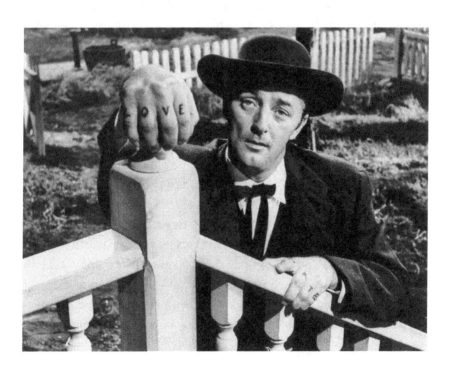

Then, it's Christmas, with picture-perfect snow. The children give her pot holders for presents; she gives them gifts that they will cherish. John feels very grown-up with his new pocket watch. They are content. Mrs. Cooper reflects, "Children abide and they endure," and the story ends.

The Madness

Let's talk some more about labels. The *DSM-5* gives several names for this disorder: antisocial personality disorder, sociopath, and psychopath.

The sociopath disregards the norms of society and the rights of others. He (it's almost always a "he") often has a history of conduct disorder when young. He often engages in behaviors that would get him arrested, such as stealing or destroying property. He is deceitful, but not always a good liar. He is impulsive and rarely considers the consequences of his actions for others or for himself. He is reckless, driving too fast or while drunk, abusing drugs, engaging in risky sexual behaviors. He can be irritable and aggressive and often gets into fights or physical altercations. He is irresponsible toward work and relationships, walking away from jobs, being careless of family, not paying debts. He has no ability to reflect, blaming others for his failures, mistreating people, and feeling no responsibility.

Not a pretty picture, and a portrait of someone likely to frequently be in trouble with the law.

This is not the psychopath, however, and not how Harry Powell presents in this movie. The psychopath, though having many of the characteristics of the antisocial personality or sociopath, is a different sort of person, and was best described by Hervey Cleckley in his landmark 1941 book *The Mask of Sanity*. This book is a classic worth seeking out (it has been in and out of print, but you can always find a copy in the library). It was revised several times, the last time in 1988. What it does, which the *DSM* fails to do, is paint a vivid portrait of the psychopath, with case histories that read like well-written short stories.

Cleckley's method is not unlike how I think of this book: an exploration of the experience of madness using the riches of storytelling and film.

The dilemma with this and some other personality disorder diagnoses, such as the paranoid or narcissistic personality disorders, is that much of the madness is hidden. That's what Cleckley was referring to when he titled his book *The Mask of Sanity*. Psychopaths, particularly, can look quite normal when you sit down with them. But underneath the facade is where the disorder lies. Psychopaths do not have hallucinations. They do not have organized or bizarre delusions, but they often have firm ideas that justify bad behavior, driving their actions. They won't imagine that angels or the devil are talking to them, but instead feel that it's okay to harass someone or steal from them to teach them a lesson. They may make the sudden decision that they don't like their job, so it's fine to just not show up; or that their family brings them down, so it is okay to just walk out on them; or that manipulations and lies are justified simply because the naive deserve whatever they get.

Such ideas take patience and skill on the part of the therapist to uncover, especially since psychopaths are wary of authority and likely to lie to see what they can get away with. People with personality disorders rarely seek therapy because they feel distress or want to change. These forms of madness have been their way of experiencing and dealing with the world for most of their lives; it is familiar and syntonic, meaning that they feel comfortable with how they are. If there is discomfort, it usually is felt by the people around them who have to deal with their problematic behaviors. At most, a psychopath will feel vexed at the difficulty that others are causing; he will see it as their problem, not his. Especially with antisocial personalities and psychopaths, if they are seeing a therapist, it is likely because it was mandated, required by a judge as part of their trial, or because they are already in prison.

Determining that someone is psychotic, like Karin or Carol or several of the patients in *Cuckoo's Nest*, is pretty straightforward. The same is true if a patient has severe depression or is in a manic high (we will see examples of these in later chapters). The person with one of these diagnoses has usually had a period of normality (maybe an extended period; maybe all their life until now) before the first episode of madness happens. First episodes are often acute and dramatic; the contrast makes the madness easier to see. But someone with a personality disorder has been that way all their adult life. This is their "normal." Getting at what underlies the behavior of someone with a personality disorder is much harder.

An additional hurdle to understanding is that, unlike sociopaths, psychopaths are usually very good liars. They do it so often and so persistently that they often believe their own lies, which makes them even more convincing. So, it is important for anyone evaluating them to seek outside information (from the authorities, from family, and associates) to discover what is really going on.

With that background, let's see how Harry Powell fits our understanding of this form of madness.

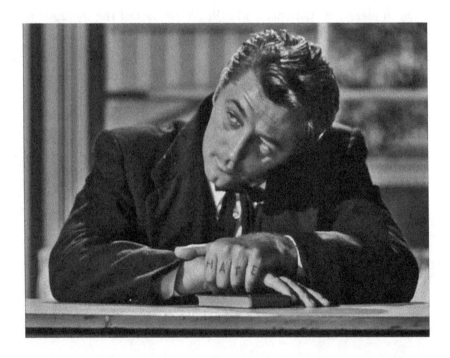

Harry Powell and Psychopathy

When we first see Harry Powell, he is driving and talking with God. If he really thinks he is talking with God and that God is answering him, he would be hallucinating, hearing voices. If he is hallucinating, then the psychopathic diagnosis doesn't fit. Similarly, if he is delusional, then it doesn't fit either.

So, what are we to make of this scene? Does this have anything to do with being a preacher?

In the movie *The Ruling Class*, a British satire on the upper classes, Peter O'Toole plays an aristocrat who thinks he is God. He is declared a paranoid schizophrenic. He is a very happy man, but he is profoundly delusional and he does hear voices. Someone asks him how he knows that he is God, and he says, "I knew I was God because when I prayed to God, I realized that I was talking to myself."

How can you distinguish that sort of delusion from simple religion? Obviously, this is a tricky question. But, actually, it's not so difficult. Much depends on the context. If the behavior is supported by the community or church, it's either a community-wide folie à deux (a shared clinical delusion) or is religiously "normal." You can only call it a madness if the behavior is clearly personalized and eccentric.

I spent some time at a psychiatric clinic in Hawaii as part of my training. There, I found how important it was to learn about the culture before rushing to diagnostic conclusions. The native Hawaiians who follow the old traditions have a ritual when someone dies. They all gather and talk about the person who has died (like a Catholic wake or the Jewish ritual of sitting shiva). What is unusual is that they believe in ghosts and it is understood that the ghost of the deceased is there in the room and can be talked to and will respond. This is accepted by the community and is a powerful mechanism for dealing with loss. It is believed by all who are part of that culture. Though it looks for all the world like they are all hallucinating, you can't call it madness unless someone there behaves in ways that the community does not sanction or understand.

Harry Powell's world does not allow for the sort of conversation he is having. His melodramatic religiosity works because he keeps his secrets about the details of the deal between "The Almighty and me."

His words in the car certainly sound more like thinking out loud than any prayer for salvation or guidance. I would understand it as a conceit of the film, a chance for us to discover how he thinks about himself. It is him, self-justifying. He is telling himself that he is doing God's work when he finds rich widows and kills them for their money. If his killings put money in his pocket, then it must be God's plan. He has a sense of entitlement and specialness that is very much part of the psychopath's view of the world. He considers it proof of God's plan that he is imprisoned with Ben Harper; he bristles when Ben asks him what sort of religion he preaches. "The religion the Almighty and me worked out betwixt us," he says.

He is rehearsing that relationship, getting ready for the next widow, and confident that she will come. When he is threatening to kill John in the basement, having discovered that he lied about where the money was hidden, he again talks as though the Lord is telling him what to do. But, again, he is not hearing voices; this is how he justifies whatever violence he is about to commit, and makes "the Lord" responsible for the consequences.

Like Travis in *Taxi Driver*, Harry wallows in what he professes to hate. We next see him at a strip show. We will later learn that he professes to have no interest in sex. In fact, he seems to find women disgusting and hides behind a religious excuse to avoid intimacy.

As he talks about the widows he has killed, there is no sense of remorse, no acknowledgment that he has caused pain to them or their families. He doesn't see people as people. Widows with money are pieces to be moved about or to be taken off the board. He does not allow himself to share the emotions of another person. This emotional coldness is a lack of empathy, and it gives him power. If you are not touched by the feelings of others, you can more easily manipulate them. Harry's ability to read people—to see their needs and their weaknesses, and to be able to turn them to his advantage—is the mark of the psychopath. His preacher disguise immediately gives him credibility in this small, mid-American town and makes his ability to con them that much easier.

What is it all for? He is willing to court a vulnerable widow, marry her (even tolerate her annoying children), and finally kill her, all to get money. It's a plan that has mostly worked for him. But he does trip himself up, and more than once. For instance, he is arrested, not for murder but for stealing a car. We know he was planning on killing Willa once he had the money, but he does it sooner than expected when she overhears him angrily asking the children about the money. His temper, an anger that flares up often and easily, gets him into trouble. Yet, when he kills Willa, he does so without passion. The whole scene in the bedroom has the look of a place of sacrifice; the room looking like a chapel, and Harry wielding his knife as though this was a ritual killing. He has never shown any tenderness or sympathy toward Willa and certainly shows no remorse after he kills her and dumps her in the river.

His crocodile tears at the Spoons, when he tells them that Willa has run away, fool them because they are ready to be fooled. Harry is a very good liar, though with these folks he doesn't have to work very hard at it. He can also be clever at covering his tracks. For instance, he sends them a postcard saying that he and the children are visiting his sister to explain his sudden disappearance. Of course, what he is really doing is chasing them along the river; it's all about the money.

He shows no sense of anxiety (psychopaths rarely feel anxiety in situations that might cause us to feel it, in part because they care so little about what others think or feel), but he is often annoyed and is easily frustrated. His patience with the children is almost nonexistent. He goes from acting friendly with John, telling him he will be his new daddy, to abruptly and nastily demanding "Where's the money hid?" in just seconds. He tries to sweet-talk Pearl, but when she acts her age or says "John told me not to tell," he loses it and yells at her, pounding the table and calling her names. The intensity of Harry's rage at these times is impressive. But so is his short fuse.

In the film that rage is exaggerated: the howl of pain and frustration when his hand is caught in the basement door and the children escape; the animal-growl when they are just out of reach on the river; and his squeal, more animal than human, when he is shot by Mrs. Cooper and runs to the barn. These are all larger than life and remind us that this is a very dark fairy tale. But, though the way Harry's emotions are expressed in *The Night of the Hunter* seems cartoon-like, they fit well with those of the psychopath.

There are, however, some aspects of the psychopath that we don't see in Harry. Most particularly, as far as we know, he doesn't drink or do drugs.

Harry basically has one shtick, one character he knows how to play: the preacher with "LOVE" and "HATE" on his fingers and the story of Good and Evil to tell. When his claim to be the children's father fails to convince Mrs. Cooper, and she dismisses his "LOVE" vs. "HATE" display, like most psychopaths he has no backup plan. So, he resorts to violence, chasing John with his switchblade drawn, until Mrs. Cooper comes out with a rifle. Then he runs away. He is purposeful when ingratiating himself with widow Willa and relentless pursuing the children, but when confronted with someone who sees through him (and happens to be holding a rifle) he turns coward and runs.

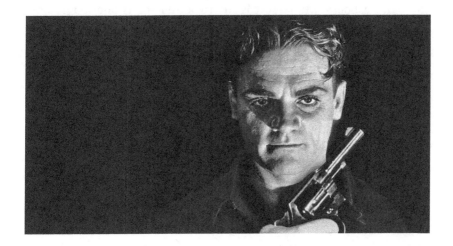

White Heat (1949)

James Cagney, Edmond O'Brien
Director: Raoul Walsh

This was James Cagney's return to the gangster roles that had made his name in the 1930s. It's the gangster film to end all gangster films, and it did, arguably, until *The Godfather* twenty-three years later. Cagney starred in tough-guy classics like *The Roaring Twenties* and *Angels with Dirty Faces*. Always playing the most ruthless of gangsters, in *The Public Enemy* he angrily smashed half a grapefruit in his girlfriend's face. His background as a dancer in vaudeville made him equally effective in musicals like Busby Berkeley's *Footlight Parade*, and later, playing George M. Cohan in *Yankee Doodle Dandy* (one of the greatest musicals ever made). He had an energy, a balletic grace, and a rat-a-tat way with dialogue that was unique. He is one of my favorite movie actors. And he is in clover here.

He plays Cody Jarrett, a psychopath, who kills easily and has no loyalty to anyone except his mother. He is the leader of a gang of train and bank robbers. Ma Jarrett is his rock and she is one tough lady. Cody suffers from migraine headaches and only she seems to be able to soothe them.

The movie opens right in the middle of a train robbery. Cody shoots the engineer with a sardonic smile and when one of his gang is injured, he just says, "Let's get out of here," and leaves him. Later we see him sitting with the gang and he begins to groan with a migraine. One of the gang says, "He's crazy, just like his old man." His Ma ushers him into another room, massaging his neck. As the headache eases, he starts to leave and she holds him back, saying "Don't let them see you like this, it might give some of them ideas." He sits on her lap, "Always thinking about your Cody, don'tcha." She hands him a drink and says, "Top of the World, son," then sends him out and tells him to show them he's all right. Cody is awfully close to his Ma; she is a gangster at heart.

There are several iconic scenes in this film. Cody has put himself in prison for a lesser crime to avoid a murder charge. While there, he asks a new arrival at the end of the mess table for news of his mother. We see and hear the inmates whispering the news down the line, until the last one tells Cody that his mother is dead. He begins to whimper, it turns into a wail, he climbs onto the table, crying uncontrollably, and punches the guards until he is wrestled to the ground. It's incredibly powerful and disturbing.

Later, out of jail, Cody is getting ready for another heist. There is a hostage locked in the trunk of a car. Munching on a chicken wing, Cody walks past and asks how he is doing. The man says, "it's stuffy, I can't breathe." Cody says, "I'll give you a little air," and shoots into the trunk until he is out of bullets. Doesn't give it a second thought.

The final scene is a classic. Cornered by the cops at a chemical plant, abandoned by his gang, he more and more crazily declares, "They think they've got Cody Jarrett, well they haven't got him," and he climbs to the top of a gas tank, laughing to himself and challenging the cops. From there Cody shoots a member of his gang who is trying to surrender. Then, a police sniper shoots him several times. Cody, crawling and then defiantly standing, fires his gun into the tank. Flames burst out, and Cody cries to the heavens, "Made it, Ma, Top of the World!" The tank explodes, and explodes again, with mushroom clouds looking every bit like an atomic bomb.

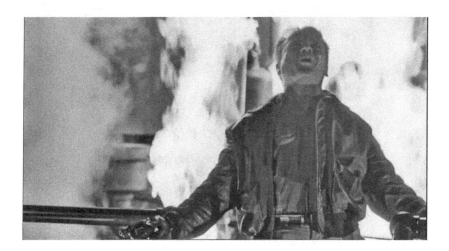

Cody has all the earmarks of the psychopath. He has a long criminal record. He robs and kills without guilt or remorse. He has a big ego and is intelligent, coming up with the plan to put himself in jail as an alibi against a murder rap. Except for his migraines (which are not part of the diagnosis), he doesn't display anxiety or problems with mood. He lies easily and treats his gang members with disdain. He has a girlfriend and treats her badly. We don't know if he uses drugs or alcohol. His only meaningful relationship is with his Ma, and that is a disturbing one. There is no evidence that he is psychotic, though he does seem on the edge at the climax, when he climbs the gas tank. Is that a suicidal act? You could make the case for it. But it looks more to me like psychopathic recklessness, the need for a grand gesture. It's one hell of an ending.

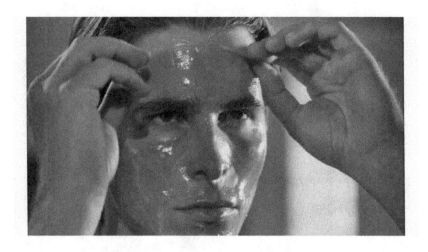

American Psycho (2000)

Christian Bale, Chloë Sevigny
Director: Mary Harron

This film was based on Bret Easton Ellis's novel of the same name that very controversially equated the greed and materialism of 1980s Wall Street with serial murder. The movie is stylish and brutally violent. Christian Bale is Patrick Bateman, a rich, young broker on Wall Street, preoccupied with getting the right restaurant reservation, having the most expensive-looking business card, and wearing the most elegant suit. The movie makes a botch of showing a real or consistent madness, but it is brilliant in several moments when Bateman, in voice-over and image, exposes his inner world.

In the opening sequence we see his spotless, white apartment at the most coveted address in New York City. He describes in detail and shows us his morning grooming ritual. We see his demanding exercise routine; then he showers (he has a sculpted body that we are invited to ogle) and applies moisturizers, cleansers, and an exfoliating facial mask. He says, "There is an idea of Patrick Bateman, some kind of abstraction, but there is no real me," as he begins to peel the mask off his face, "only an entity, something illusory. And though I can hide my cold gaze and you can shake my hand and feel my flesh gripping yours . . . I am simply not there."

That is as good a description of the internal world of the psychopath as we are going to find. Patrick is dressed well, his hair is perfectly coiffed, he is graceful, the picture of elegance. But when no one is listening (and in his world no one ever really listens) he will calmly say, smiling, "You're a fucking ugly bitch and I want to stab you to death and play around with your blood." He passes in society, but his hidden world is filled with violence.

One evening, he randomly kills a homeless person. Then, he carefully invites Paul Allen, an envied rival, to dinner and gets him drunk. Donning a raincoat to protect his expensive suit, Patrick kills Allen in his living room with an axe. There is blood everywhere.

Each day he goes to his office (doing no obvious work) and joins his shallow colleagues to make jokes about women and discuss what difficult-to-get-into restaurant or club they will go to that evening.

He has call girls come to his apartment, films them having sex with each other and with him, and then murders them brutally. His idea of conversation with these women as he prepares to kill them is to expound on the songs of Huey Lewis and the News, or Phil Collins, or Whitney Houston. We will discover that he keeps the head of one victim in his refrigerator and the bodies of another two hanging in his closet. Later we hear him say, in voice-over, "I have all the characteristics of a human being; flesh, blood, skin, hair, but not a single clear identifiable emotion except for greed and disgust. . . . My nightly bloodlust has overflowed into my days, I feel lethal on the verge of frenzy. I think my mask of sanity is about to slip."

I don't think the use of this phrase is accidental: whoever wrote this film read Hervey Cleckley.

This film is a satire and is knowingly over-the-top. Bale's performance is smart and sharp and he carries the movie. But it goes off the rails when he is at an ATM machine and gently picks up a stray cat. The machine beeps and reads "feed me the stray cat" and he prepares to shoot the cat and try to put it in the credit card slot. When a passerby interferes, he shoots her. This begins a shooting spree that ends with him blowing up a police car. Overwhelmed (the first time he doesn't appear fully in control), he calls his lawyer and confesses his murders.

And then we discover, as he does, that Paul Allen isn't dead, that none of the other murders happened, and that the lawyer doesn't recognize him. Suddenly the movie is not about a psychopath but about someone who has been living a psychotic fantasy—and this doesn't work at all. For many reasons.

He is presented to us as a psychopath. His lack of empathy is something he glories in. We see him easily manipulate people, either telling them what they want to hear or simply offering them money to go along with his wishes. He has porn videos playing continuously in his apartment and seems obsessed with sex, but has no real relationship with anyone (an exception seems to be his secretary, whom he resists killing and sends home; a rare moment of self-control). He abuses cocaine along with his colleagues, but it's not clear if he even gets high. Though he goes along with his colleagues, he doesn't seem *with* them. He is apart, observing, feeling superior. He is an atypical psychopath, since the sort of random bloodthirsty murders we see him commit are unlikely, but a psychopath, nevertheless.

But then we are led to think it's all been in his imagination, a form of psychosis. So, which is it: did he kill people or not? Confusions abound. The film does little to foreshadow that every violent thing we have seen might be a psychotic fantasy. Perhaps it's suggested by the fact that the apartment remains pristine and white even after several bloodbaths and that people seem oblivious to his murderous actions (for instance, he drags Allen's body out of the apartment building in a duffel bag, with blood leaking onto the floor, but the doorman doesn't notice). I think this is too little to hang such a reversal on.

Serial murderers do exist and though many of them are psychopaths, others indeed have schizophrenia, with psychotic delusions. But the delusions drive their behavior: they aren't the stuff of simple fantasy. Patrick quotes Ed Gein in the film; he was a real person who pretty much did what Patrick Bateman is shown doing. A farmer in Wisconsin, Gein was arrested in 1957. It was discovered that he had dug up bodies from cemeteries and put their skulls on his bedposts and made clothes and upholstery out of human skins. He also killed. There were nine vulvae in a box, a belt made from human nipples, and a lampshade made from the skin of a human face. Gein's story became the basis for Robert Bloch's novel (and Hitchcock's film) *Psycho*. It inspired the creation of several other movie serial killers, including Leatherface in *The Texas Chainsaw Massacre* and Buffalo Bill in *The Silence of the Lambs*. In *American Psycho* Patrick mistakenly quotes Gein saying, "When I see a pretty girl walking down the street, I think two things. One part of me wants to take her out, talk to her, be real nice and sweet and treat her right . . . the other part wonders what her head would look like on a stick." That quote is actually from Ed Kemper, another serial murderer and diagnosed paranoid schizophrenic, who murdered ten people, including his grandparents, his mother, and a series of female hitchhikers, whose bodies he would bring back to his home to decapitate, dismember, and sexually violate.

These serial murderers didn't suddenly discover that the murders never happened, that they were all some psychotic fantasy. *American Psycho* doesn't quite know what it wants us to understand about Patrick. Is he just having violent thoughts he never acts upon? If so, we are left not knowing how to make sense of the ending. This is a seriously flawed film but, I think, worth watching for Patrick's on-point observations about his psychopathic inner world. The rest, though fascinating, is, I'm afraid, pop-culture balderdash.

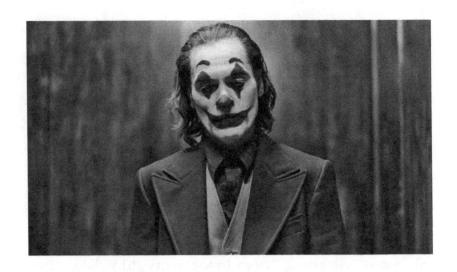

Joker (2019)

Joaquin Phoenix, Robert De Niro, Frances Conroy
Director: Todd Phillips

This blockbuster film (the first R-rated film in history to earn one billion dollars world-wide) is the origin story of the Batman villain the Joker, previously played by Jack Nicholson and Heath Ledger. Phoenix definitely makes it his own. He dominates the movie with a combination of grace and gravitas.

He is Arthur Fleck, a professional party clown. While promoting a store closing, a group of young hoodlums steal his sign. When he chases them, they beat him up, kicking him as he lies there. The city is a mess—called "Gotham" but looking very much like 1970s New York: garbage everywhere, crime up, and services down. We see his journal (one of many details that mimic *Taxi Driver*): "I hope my death makes more cents [sic] than my life." He tells a social worker that he felt better in the hospital locked up then he does now (we see a brief moment of Arthur banging his head repeatedly against a door). Then he asks about increasing his meds: "I don't want to feel so bad anymore." So, we know early on that he has been hospitalized for mental problems and that the meds he is taking now are not helping.

On a bus he starts laughing inappropriately when a woman scolds him for "bothering" her child (he was entertaining the boy, making faces). He hands her a card that explains that he has a condition that causes uncontrolled laughter.

Arthur lives with his mother (Frances Conroy), who is ill in bed and needs his care. They talk about how she worked for the rich Thomas Wayne years ago, and that she has written him many times asking for his help, with no reply.

They watch *Live! with Murray Franklin* on TV together, a regular pastime. The show is modeled on NBC's *The Tonight Show* with a host like Johnny Carson or Jimmy Fallon. We see Arthur in the audience. When he calls out "We love you" to Murray (Robert De Niro), he talks about how he takes care of his mom who always tells him to "smile and put on a happy face. I was put here, she says, to spread joy and laughter." The audience loves this, and Murray says to him, "I'd give all of this fame up . . . to have a kid like you," and hugs him. Then we cut to Arthur watching with his mother, and we realize that this was all his fantasy. Not a hallucination, but an imagining, a wish.

On the elevator he connects with the young, single mother in the next apartment by miming shooting himself in the head, an image that also brings to mind Travis in *Taxi Driver*. They share a sense that "it's crazy out there." As far as I can tell we never actually hear the woman's name in the film, but in the credits she is called Sophie.

In his journal, Arthur writes: "The worst thing about having a mental illness is that people expect you to behave as if you DON'T."

After his beating, one of the other clowns at work gives him a pistol for protection. Performing a few days later at a children's hospital, the gun falls out of his pocket. He talks to his boss from a phone booth, who berates him and tells him he is fired. Arthur slams his head against the glass, shattering it. There is a lot of anger waiting to come out.

It does when, on the subway, his uncontrolled laughter draws the attention of some young Wall Street types, who tease him, singing Stephen Sondheim's "Send in the Clowns," and then start beating him.

Arthur pulls out his pistol and shoots and kills two of them, wounding the third. He chases this last one off the subway, shoots him in the back, then one more time as he lies there on the staircase. He runs, hides in a public bathroom, and begins a graceful balletic dance. He is both exhilarated and at peace.

Afterward, he walks boldly to the apartment of his neighbor Sophie, and as soon as she opens the door embraces and kisses her. She yields. He is a new man.

In therapy Arthur says, "All I have are negative thoughts." Then he says, "For my whole life, I didn't know if I even really existed. But I do. And people are starting to notice."

His first try at a stand-up comedy gig goes pear-shaped when he can't stop laughing, but Sophie is there and she thinks he is funny. Later, when she sees the newspaper account of the subway killing by someone wearing a clown mask, her comment is, "Three less pricks in Gotham City." Not realizing it's him, she says she thinks the clown is a hero.

Two new developments bring things to a boil. First, on his TV show, Murray shows a tape of Arthur's disastrous comedy performance and ridicules him, calling him a "joker." Second, Arthur reads the latest letter his mother was about to send to Wayne and discovers that Wayne is his real father. When Arthur goes to the Wayne estate to try to speak to him, the butler tells him that his mother was delusional and had been in hospital, and that Arthur was adopted.

Meanwhile, the clown killer has become a symbol of rebellion by the downtrodden of the city. Wayne, who is running for mayor, calls them "clowns," and the slogan "we are all clowns" goes viral.

Arthur's mother has a stroke. Arthur goes to find out the truth about his mother. He tells the chart-room clerk in the hospital, "I took out some people. I thought it would bother me, but it really hasn't. I fucked up, did some bad shit." The clerk urges him to "see someone." His mother's chart from the mental hospital reads that she was delusional and that the child, Arthur, who was indeed adopted, was found bruised, with head trauma, and chained to a radiator.

Upset and sad, he goes to Sophie's apartment, letting himself in. When she comes to see who is there, we realize that she doesn't know him except as her neighbor. Images flash showing us the moments with Sophie, only now we see that she wasn't there. All the interactions we have seen between them, except for the first mimed shooting-in-the-head, were hallucinations. Shades of *A Beautiful Mind* and *American Psycho*.

Arthur goes to the hospital and kills his mother, suffocating her with a pillow. "I used to think that my life was a tragedy—but now I realize it's a fucking comedy."

Live! with Murray Franklin calls him. The video of his performance got a lot of reaction, and they want him on the show in person. He agrees, and we see him practicing how he would be, bantering with Murray and reading one of his jokes.

On the day of the show, he dyes his hair green and puts on his clown make-up. Randall, the clown who gave him the pistol, stops by, ostensibly to give his condolences for Arthur's mother's death, but really to be sure Arthur doesn't tell anyone where he got the pistol. Arthur stabs him to death with scissors. Blood is everywhere. The dwarf who worked at Arthur's clown job is also there, but Arthur assures him that he won't hurt him because he was always kind.

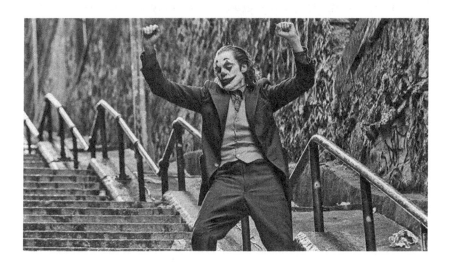

Heading toward his moment with Murray on TV, Arthur dances on the outside staircase—a moment of joy and freedom, until the cops start chasing him. They follow him onto the subway, which is filled with people wearing clown masks headed to a rally downtown. There is chaos with the cops trying to find which one is Arthur, and someone gets shot. Arthur is more and more cocky.

Murray greets him in the greenroom as he waits to go on. He asks Arthur why he is dressed as a clown, and Arthur says it's for his act and that it is not part of the protests: "I don't believe in the protests. I don't believe in anything." He asks Murray to introduce him as "Joker" since that is how he referred to him when first showing the video.

The show is broadcast live. Arthur dances on, kisses the previous guest, Dr. Sally, on the lips, sits down to chat with Murray, and almost immediately tells him he killed the Wall Street guys. Is this a joke? No, it isn't. "I have nothing left to lose," says Arthur. "Everyone is awful. It's enough to make anyone crazy." He then pulls out his pistol and shoots Murray in the head.

Arthur is arrested. In the police car, he contentedly watches an increasingly violent mob on the streets, most wearing clown masks. An ambulance crashes into the police car. The men in the ambulance are wearing clown masks too. They pull Arthur out of the car and lay him on the hood. He is okay, gradually coming to, the Leader of the Clowns. Meanwhile, we see those same men watch as Thomas Wayne, his wife, and his son, Bruce, leave a movie theater and walk into an alley. They shoot and kill Wayne and his wife. Young Bruce Wayne (who will become Batman) watches in horror.

Then we have an odd epilogue with Arthur in a mental hospital, briefly talking with a therapist, walking (are those bloody footprints?) and then running in the halls, chased by orderlies. What this tells us, I have no idea.

This story channels *Taxi Driver* and *The King of Comedy*, two films by Martin Scorsese, who was originally approached to direct *Joker*. *The King of Comedy* stars Robert De Niro as Rupert Pupkin, obsessed with a late night TV host played by Jerry Lewis. When Lewis ignores his pleas to get a chance to do stand-up comedy on his show, Rupert kidnaps him. Another small man who wants to be big.

Arthur seems, like Travis, "God's Lonely Man." He is not preoccupied with the degraded state of the city as Travis is, but it reflects his life: it's ugly, unhappy, uncared for. That mimed gunshot to the head, which is a climactic moment in *Taxi Driver*, becomes here shorthand for the desperation and isolation that Arthur and others of the underclass feel.

Arthur's words convey the sense that no one sees him, that his therapist doesn't listen, that unless he wears the clown make-up, he feels invisible. He only has his mother. And when he discovers that she has been lying to him, that he was adopted and that she was hospitalized as delusional and for neglecting and abusing him, his reaction is to kill her. She means nothing to him now.

When he allows himself to strike back, to kill his tormentors, he becomes light as air—he dances. He tells us he thought it would bother him, but it doesn't. He tells us that he doesn't believe in the protest, that he doesn't believe in anything. And we can believe that.

None of these killings is planned, except killing Murray on TV, but each one makes him feel more real, more worthwhile, more seen (you can't be more "seen" than killing someone on live television). All of this would fit the diagnosis of antisocial personality disorder, especially not feeling guilt or remorse after doing harm and not believing in anything. I would not consider him to be a psychopath because he doesn't manipulate, he doesn't con, and with the one exception, he doesn't plan. He reacts.

Interestingly, he is not that smart, which some fans have complained doesn't fit with the comic book personality of the Joker. We also don't see any random acts of cruelty. His killings aren't random. When he kills someone, he does it because that person has attacked or humiliated him. Or, in the case of his mother, profoundly deceived him.

There is much we don't know. Why was he hospitalized the first time? Was he depressed, psychotic, suicidal, manic? What meds is he taking and why does he feel better without them? Many medications for mental illness, especially those for psychosis, can slow down your thinking, make you sleepy, make you gain weight. People are glad to rid themselves of those and other side effects, at least until the benefit of the medication is also lost and the hallucinations or disturbing delusional thoughts return. Is this what Arthur means by "feeling better"? We don't know. Most problematically, if his relationship with Sophie was all hallucination, if they were never a couple, if she was not at his side with his mother in the hospital, or at the comedy club, or in his bed, then how do we understand his diagnosis?

If we discovered that he had a psychotic episode before or that he had been profoundly depressed or even suicidal, we would think of him very differently. We are surprised when it is revealed in the "now" of the movie that he is psychotic, hallucinating his relationship with Sophie. But I'm not convinced. Unlike *American Psycho*, we know that the murders he commits are real (we see newspaper headlines, for instance), but we are left to wonder what else that we have seen might be a hallucination, an expression of psychosis.

By definition, an antisocial personality or a psychopath is not psychotic; they do not hallucinate, though they certainly may show signs of delusion (as Travis does, for instance). Arthur does not seem paranoid, unlike Travis. He does not see himself having some mission or special purpose, though we may be seeing the beginning of that as the film ends (he is, after all, becoming Joker). Is his ordinary behavior unusual enough to call him schizotypal, another personality disorder worth considering? I don't think so. He is isolated, sad, unsocial, but without the clown make-up he would not draw attention to himself.

Except for the uncontrolled laughter. What to make of that? There have been commentators who give a diagnosis for that, which is a new one to me. It's called pseudobulbar affect, PBA, a rare neurological condition of uncontrolled laughing or crying. This usually occurs in people who have had a brain injury or something like multiple sclerosis. We do learn that Arthur as a child was abused and that he had head trauma. So that might fit. However, as I watched the film recently, it seemed to me that his laughter always happened when he was upset, anxious, or angered; that, instead of allowing himself to feel angry or anxious, he laughs in a way he can't stop. It seems inappropriate because those around him don't see where it originates. He can't stop the laughter any more than he can stop his anger from erupting in murder once he has a weapon he can use. I don't think we need to look for a neurological explanation; an emotional one is enough.

Phoenix so effectively shows us Arthur's pain that we feel sympathy toward him even when he is being most destructive. At least I do. But I think that, like *American Psycho*, the film lets him down, melding incompatible forms of madness. They are overdetermining that Joker is mad. They toss a grab bag of symptoms at us but leave us guessing what his real story might be.

RECOMMENDED READING

Agee, James. *James Agee: Film Writing and Selected Journalism: Agee on Film / Uncollected Film Writing / The Night of the Hunter / Journalism and Film Reviews.* New York: Library of America; 2005.

Agee's film criticism is perceptive and convincing. His original screenplay for *The Night of the Hunter* is fascinating to contrast with the finished film.

Cleckley, Hervey. *The Mask of Sanity: An Attempt to Clarify Some Issues about the So-Called Psychopathic Personality.* Brattleboro, VT: Echo Point Books; 2015.

This is the classic, first detailed examination of the psychopath. The case histories read like short stories. There are multiple editions since the first in 1941. See especially chapters 1–3.

"You know Bruno, sometimes he goes a little too far."

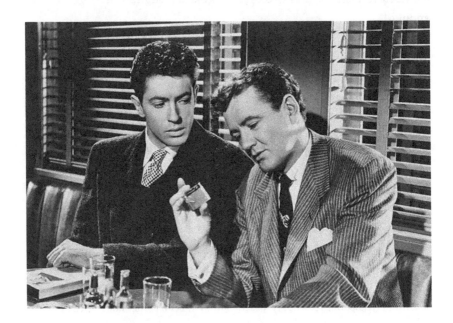

A Different Kind of Psychopath

CHARMING BUT DANGEROUS

Strangers on a Train (1951)

Robert Walker, Farley Granger
Director: Alfred Hitchcock

In the previous chapter we saw the psychopath portrayed in broad strokes. We know that Harry Powell is trouble as soon as we meet him and hear his self-justifying conversation with God about killing widows. His charm offensive, wearing religious camouflage, works for the small-town folk in the story, but we see how thin that civilized veneer is. The anger and evil intent are just below the surface.

Now we are going to meet Bruno, a character from a very different world—the modern city, among the rich and privileged. He is someone who is socially adept, intelligent, entitled, and looking for excitement, and he has one very clever idea. The portrait here is more subtle but reveals someone with all the characteristics of the psychopath.

As I mentioned before, psychopaths are not usually violent. They will break the law and leave people and institutions in ruins, but in movies like *The Night of the Hunter* and, now, *Strangers on a Train*, they are killers.

This film is based on the novel by Patricia Highsmith, who also wrote *The Talented Mr. Ripley* and several other novels featuring Ripley. Ripley does not appear here, but Bruno is much like him. In most of Highsmith's novels the protagonist is a psychopath, fascinating and convincing.

Raymond Chandler is credited with the screenplay for *Strangers on a Train*, but Hitchcock did not like what he wrote, so he trashed it. After being turned down by several other well-established writers (among them Thornton Wilder and John Steinbeck), Hitchcock settled on a young unknown named Czenzi Ormonde who, working with Hitchcock's wife, Alma, wrote what we see on the screen. I would love to see Chandler's version, but I believe it was destroyed. He tried to get himself removed from the credits for this film, but the studio insisted the credit stay because of the prestige of his name.

Raymond Chandler pretty much invented the private-eye murder mystery. Philip Marlowe was his detective, and the mean streets of Los Angeles his turf. His novels are compelling and were turned into very good movies. Most famous is *The Big Sleep*, starring Humphrey Bogart and Lauren Bacall. The screenplay for that film is credited to William Faulkner. These heavy-hitter writers did get around (the money was good). Much of the dialogue is directly from the novel and it's terrific: verbal seduction filled with sexual innuendo. But Hollywood (because of censorship, prudishness, and convention) can play havoc with a screenplay, often assigning multiple writers and then cherry-picking the details. Through no fault of Faulkner, who turned out to be one of many writers, the plot is almost impossible to follow. Don't let that faze you—just enjoy the ride. It's a very entertaining film.

What I find intriguing in the history of *Strangers on a Train* is how very different it is from the novel, and how it improves on it. The basic conceit remains (strangers swapping murders), but almost every other detail including all the dialogue (unlike in *The Big Sleep*) have been changed. Movies are a different form of art from novels and if you are too faithful to the original work you may well create a second-rate film. But using the original work as an inspiration, to be translated into the language of film, can sometimes produce a masterpiece.

Alfred Hitchcock, called the "master of suspense," started in the days of silent movies with *The Lodger*, inspired by Jack the Ripper, and effortlessly moved into "talkies." He was a major influence as a director for his entire career. After great success in his native England with the spy thrillers *The Lady Vanishes* and *The 39 Steps*, he moved to Hollywood, where his catalogue includes *Foreign Correspondent*, *Notorious*, *Shadow of a Doubt*, *Rear Window*, *North by Northwest*, *The Birds*, *Spellbound*, *Vertigo*, and *Psycho*. Madness is woven through many of Hitchcock's films, including these last three, which I will be discussing later. All his films are characterized by suspense, a darkly witty sense of humor, and brilliant and often iconic images and set-piece moments. He has influenced generations of filmmakers as well as a psychiatrist teaching Yale students about Madness at the Movies.

With Hitchcock, you are never confused about what is happening unless he wants you to be. A camera placement or a glancing edit can speak volumes. He always storyboarded his movies (a way to visualize the film before actually making it, a storyboard is a series of cartoon-like panels showing each moment in the movie, where the camera might be positioned, what it might see, what it might choose not to show), and he famously said that once the storyboards were complete, the actual filming was a letdown. Of course, the filming allowed the actors to bring something to the production, but Hitchcock, though his films were populated by some of the best and most famous stars of the era (Cary Grant, Jimmy Stewart, Michael Redgrave, Janet Leigh, Kim Novak, Grace Kelly), always claimed that the actors got in the way.

Hitchcock makes a cameo appearance in every one of his films (a way of signing them, as an artist does a painting). Briefly glimpsed, his famously rotund profile is always easy to find.

The Movie

Immediately after the credits we see the entire scheme of the film summarized. We are at a train station. A taxi pulls up and a man steps out, seen from the knees down. His shoes are polished, two-tone, fancy; another cab pulls up, another man steps out, also seen from below, his shoes are brown, ordinary, unremarkable. We see the first man cross left on the screen toward the tracks; the second man crosses right, both viewed now from the waist down. We see the rail-road tracks ahead of the train, they intersect and cross each other. Each man walks the aisle inside the train; the first man sits down, and then the second man sits across from him, and in crossing his legs, bumps the other's shoe.

We see them in full for the first time. "Excuse me," one man says. Bruno, the other man, leans forward. "I beg your pardon, but aren't you Guy Haines? . . . I certainly admire people who do things." The story begins. Bruno introduces himself, shows his tie clip with his name on it: "My mother gave it to me, and I have to wear it to please her." They don't know each other, are thrown together by chance, but their actions mirror each other. This will happen repeatedly as the story unfolds.

They are Guy, a tennis player, and Bruno, a rich young man about the same age, at loose ends. Bruno ingratiates himself with Guy, says "I don't talk much" but then talks up a storm, tells him how much he admires him, that he has read about him in the newspapers, knows he is about to marry Anne, the daughter of a senator, but that Guy needs to divorce his wife first. Guy would rather just read, but Bruno insists they dine together. Bruno orders a pair of double shots of whiskey, one for him and one for Guy. This is the first of many references to "double," a parallel to the mirroring we will see again and again, and to the concept of crisscross, visualized earlier with the crossed railroad tracks.

The movie will show repeatedly how tied together these two men, strangers until now, will be.

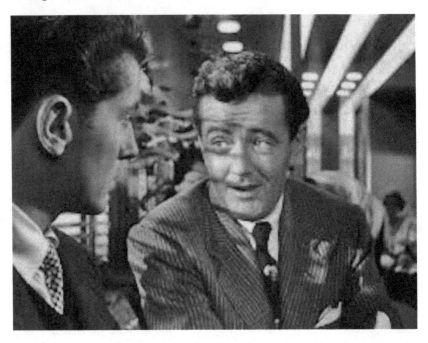

Over lunch in Bruno's compartment, Bruno tells Guy about his life. He was kicked out of three colleges for drinking and gambling. "My father calls me a bum, he hates me!" "I've got a theory," Bruno says, "that you should do everything before you die." He asks Guy if he ever drove a car blindfolded at 150 miles an hour as he has, then claims he flew in a jet plane and that he has a reservation for the first rocket to the moon. It's doubtful that any of these things are true, but he needs to think big. Bruno declares, "Guy, I'm your friend, I would do anything for you." This, after he has known him for maybe half an hour.

Bruno begins to make very good guesses about Guy's situation with his wife: that he needs to ask her for the divorce, that she was unfaithful. He can read a situation and isn't shy about saying what others might not. He begins to tell his ideas for a "perfect murder." Guy says, "I thought that was against the law" and Bruno suddenly shows some anger: "What is a life or two? Some people are better off dead. Like your wife and my father . . . I used to put myself to sleep at night with the wonderful idea I had about murder. Let's say you would like to get rid of your wife . . ." Guy says, "That's a morbid thought." But this doesn't stop the conversation: in fact, it encourages Bruno, who replies, "Just suppose. What would trip you up? The motive. Imagine two fellows meet, never saw each other before, each has somebody that he would like to get rid of. So, they swap murders! For example, your wife, my father: crisscross! We do talk the same language, don't we?" Guy wants to get away, he has to leave, "Sure, Bruno, we talk the same language." Again, he doesn't say stop, this is a bad idea; he allows Bruno to think he is agreeing with him. Bruno asks, "You like my theory?" and Guy tells him, "I like all your theories." Guy thinks he is dismissing Bruno, but Bruno hears it as agreement. Guy accidentally leaves his lighter behind with crossed tennis rackets and inscribed "A to G," and Bruno picks it up, quietly muttering, "crisscross."

This scene brilliantly defines and sets up the whole movie. We learn much about Bruno and Guy. Bruno is outgoing, pushy, rich, a wastrel; he loves to chat with strangers, and with no real sense of boundaries declares himself their new friend. He is resentful of his father and is full of off-center ideas. He admires "people who do things" and is looking for something important to "do." And he concocts murder schemes, including this one. Guy is quiet, passive, conventional, but he has a career and a fiancée, he is making something of himself. In being overly polite, in not controlling the situation, he allows Bruno to think he agrees with his ideas.

The next scene begins with a joke. As Guy gets off the train in Metcalf, a fat man carrying a big bass violin gets on. That's Hitchcock—his cameo. The joke is that the profile of the bass violin matches his fat belly, the sort of doubling we will see throughout this film; of course, the other name for a bass violin is a "double bass."

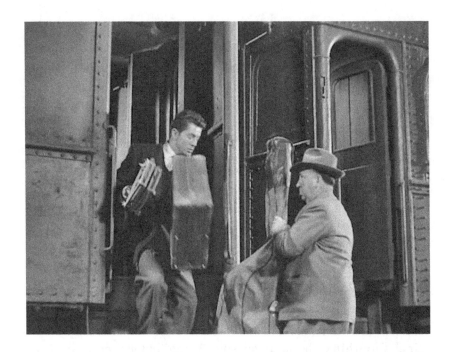

Guy meets his wife, Miriam, at her workplace in a music store. They were supposed to see her lawyer. They go into a record listening booth at the store for some privacy. He gives her money and she tells him she won't divorce him. He calls her a double-crosser. They argue; he angrily grabs her; the other customers notice. Then he calls Anne and tells her what happened, "I'd like to break her neck," he says, "I could strangle her!" and we fade to a close-up of hands, looking like they are ready to strangle someone, only to discover that it's Bruno getting a manicure from his mother.

He is wearing a flamboyant dressing gown. His mother seems distracted and confused, not quite there. She says, "I hope you have given up that silly little plan of yours to blow up the White House—you're a naughty boy, Bruno . . . you can always make me laugh." She is played by Marion Lorne, who usually plays ditzy old ladies (she was in the cast of the Broadway comedy "Harvey" (1944—49) and was the bumbling witch Aunt Clara in the 1960s television series *Bewitched*). Here, there is something sinister about her inability to see Bruno for what he is.

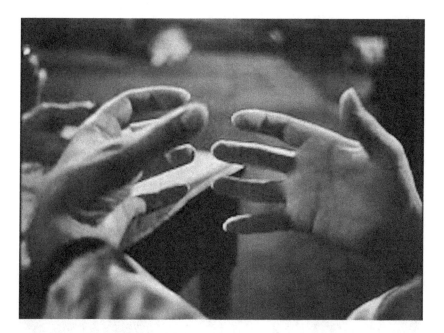

Bruno calls Guy and has to remind him who he is. Guy tells him that Miriam is refusing divorce, then he hangs up on him.

Next, we see Bruno getting off the train at Metcalf. What happens now is almost entirely without dialogue, a remarkable bit of visual storytelling. Bruno locates Miriam's address in the phone book and sits watching the house. She runs out with two young men on her arms, getting on a bus. Bruno follows. They get off at a carnival. He watches, and she turns and notices him looking at her. He is the only one there dressed in a suit. He looks grown-up and sophisticated. She is intrigued.

A little boy with a balloon comes up to him aiming his toy gun at Bruno. Bruno bursts the balloon with his cigarette. A Hitchcock joke. If you didn't know he was a bad guy before, you do now (my choice of words suggests what all this mirroring is pointing to—that Bruno is in many ways the "bad Guy," the id, the person who is willing to do the nasty, evil thing someone like Guy would only think of, or say in anger). We see Miriam watching at one of the games, a show of strength. She turns to see if the stranger is there and is clearly disappointed when she doesn't see him behind her. Then she turns, and Bruno is standing right next to her. Both Bruno and Hitchcock playing tricks. Bruno tries his luck, studies his hands as though measuring their strength and then hits the gong. He is showing off for her. He follows her onto the carousel, riding just behind.

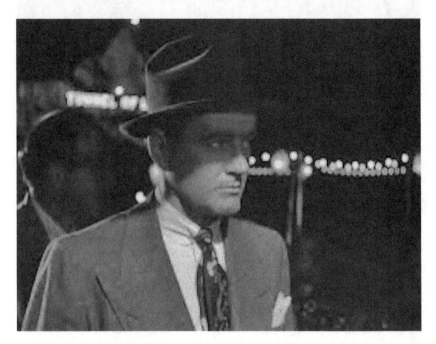

Then Miriam and her companions go for a boat ride through the Tunnel of Love. Bruno follows in a boat named "Pluto" and there is a moment when the shadows and Miriam's scream make you think the worst. But it's another Hitchcock diversion; she is only screaming in excitement.

They pull up to an island in the lake and Bruno follows. He finds Miriam alone, flicks on Guy's lighter so she can see him, and asks if she is Miriam. She says, "Why, yes," and he immediately grabs her by the throat. Her glasses fall off, and what we see from then on is through their distorting lens as, strangled, she is lowered to the ground, dead. Bruno retrieves her broken glasses and Guy's lighter. He returns to his boat as her companions find her and call for help. When he pulls up to the dock, we see that the worker there notices him. As Bruno walks quietly away, he helps a blind man cross the street, even stopping

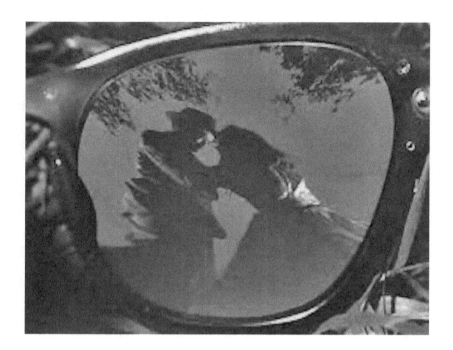

traffic. Is he doing that to not look like he is running from the scene of the crime? Probably, and also to show to himself how cool and calm he is after the murder.

Bruno looks at his watch, then we see Guy, on a train, looking at his watch (mirroring).

With this film I will skip to the more crucial scenes for understanding both Bruno and Guy. We are in front of Guy's house in Washington. As he gets out of the cab, Bruno calls out to him from across the street. Bruno is standing behind a gate. We see Guy turn, the camera is tilted for the first time, something is wrong. Guy walks across to Bruno who is in the shadows and then behind the fence, with all the appearance of him being "behind bars." "I brought you a little present," he says, and hands Guy Miriam's glasses. "It was very quick, Guy. She wasn't hurt in any way." Guy, realizing what he has done, calls Bruno a "maniac." Bruno says, "But you wanted it. We planned it on the train together, remember?" Guy says he is going to call the police and Bruno tells him, "We would both be arrested for murder." By this time Guy is also standing behind the gate: he, too, is behind bars.

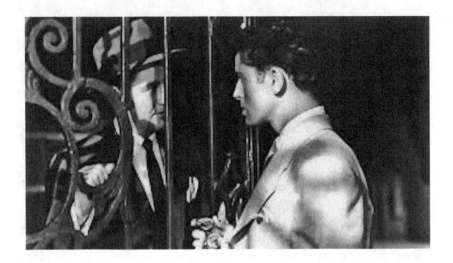

Bruno says that Guy is a free man now, but since he is the one to benefit from the murder, he would be the first suspect. Bruno never even knew her. When a police car arrives to tell Guy about his wife's murder, Guy steps further behind the gate next to Bruno: they are both hiding in the dark. Guy is acting as guilty as Bruno is (who doesn't feel guilty at all). When Guy then calls Bruno a "crazy fool," you see Bruno's flash of anger, which we saw earlier when he was talking about his father.

At Anne's house we meet her father and her sister, Babs. Babs is played by Patricia Hitchcock, Alfred's daughter, and she is quite good here. Her character is a breath of fresh air: she is someone who, usefully, says what others are too polite to say. When they are talking about the murder of Miriam, Babs says frankly that "Guy will be the main suspect—he had the motive. If he doesn't have an alibi for that night, he will have lots to worry about." And then, feeling some envy of her sister, Babs says, "I still think it would be wonderful to have a man love you so much he would kill for you."

That's the end of Act One.

As Guy is walking in Washington, he sees Bruno in the distance, a dark form against the white pillars of the Jefferson Memorial. Bruno shows up again when Guy and Anne are in a museum. He calls to Guy, and Anne notices his tie clip, "Bruno." He wants Guy to help plan his father's murder.

Later, Guy is practicing tennis at the local club. Another iconic moment: We see the crowd watching a match, following the rally, their heads swinging together, back and forth. All except one. Bruno is in the center—looking straight at Guy. The effect is powerful: Bruno will be relentless in stalking Guy until he cooperates.

When Guy finishes his match, he finds Bruno sitting with Anne and some friends. He is chatting with them in French; he is charming and seems very comfortable there. When Babs goes to introduce herself to this fascinating man, Bruno sees that she wears glasses just like Miriam's and that she looks like her. He can't help staring. We hear the carousel music and see images of the lighter's flame in her glasses. Both Babs and Anne notice his expression; intense, transfixed.

At a formal party that night, Bruno shows up uninvited. His attempts at conversation are strange. When Bruno speaks to Anne's father, the senator, he wants to discuss his idea for harnessing "the life force. I'm already developing my faculty for seeing millions of miles. . . . Can you imagine being able to smell a flower on the planet of Mars?" Speaking to a judge, he asks him how, after sentencing a man to death, he can go out and eat his dinner.

Then he begins to chat with a Mrs. Cunningham about murder. Bruno is good with elderly ladies like his mother, using charm, flattery, and attention to ingratiate himself. "Everyone would like to put someone out of the way. Now surely . . . you're not going to tell me that there hasn't been a time when you wanted to dispose of someone. Your husband, for instance." She finds him amusing. So, he continues, "How are you going to do it?" and she plays the game, "I suppose I'll have to get a gun," and her friend suggests maybe a little poison. Bruno then says he has the best tools and he shows his hands, "Simple, silent, and quick. You don't mind if I borrow your neck for a moment, do you?"

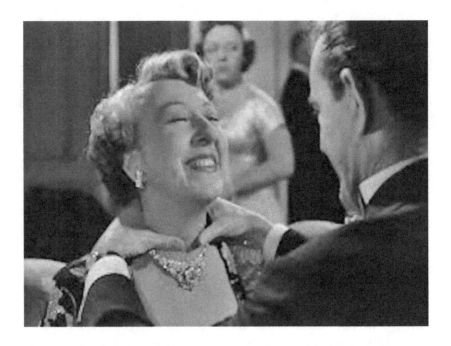

He begins to mime strangling, but Babs comes to watch, and he notices her and again we hear the carousel music, and the camera closes in on her face: he is staring at her, and she at him. Mrs. Cunningham is being strangled as his grip tightens. She cries out; Bruno faints and is carried away. Babs knows something terrible has happened. Guy confronts Bruno and punches him in the face. For once we see Guy taking charge. After that, he tells Anne the whole story—"I'd do his murder and he would do mine"—shocking Anne and not realizing his own complicity. Guy is innocent of murder, but not of the desire to murder.

When Guy goes to Bruno's house and tells him he has no intention of killing his father, Bruno vows revenge: "I'm a very clever fellow. I'll think of something."

The next day, Anne meets with Bruno's mother. She wants Bruno to tell the police that he murdered Miriam to exonerate Guy. His mother says, "I'm sure this thing must be some practical joke—you know Bruno, sometimes he goes a little too far. Sometimes he's terribly irresponsible." Anne tells her, "Your son is responsible for a woman's death." His mother asks, "Did Bruno tell you this?" When Anne answers, "Of course not," she replies, "Well, there you are! . . . I must get back to my painting." She is oblivious, unconcerned, in denial.

Bruno overhears the conversation, and he tries to convince Anne that Guy committed the murder. In doing so he talks about the lighter being left at the scene of the crime—the one piece of evidence that could convict him. He has talked about what a clever fellow he is, but he has inadvertently told Anne what he plans to do to implicate Guy.

When Anne tells Guy what Bruno said, they decide Guy needs to get to Metcalf to stop Bruno from going to the island with the lighter. (I'm not sure this makes much sense. So far, the best defense for Guy is that he was nowhere near there when the murder happened.) Guy will play his match, but uncharacteristically aggressively to be able to finish and get to Metcalf before dark, when they think Bruno is most likely to want to place the lighter there.

We begin to go back and forth between the tennis match and Bruno traveling toward Metcalf.

This sort of thing is what film does best. Cutting between simultaneous activities where something is at risk. The clock is ticking and, at some point, the separate actions will come together.

Someone asks Bruno for a light on the train—he reaches for Guy's lighter but thinks better of it and uses a match. Back to the tennis, and it's taking longer to finish than Guy had hoped.

Bruno arrives in Metcalf. Someone bumps him and he drops the lighter through a storm drain grate. Back and forth now, the tennis match intensifying, and then Bruno, trying to retrieve the lighter. He asks for help to find his "cigarette case." He is a clever fellow; he doesn't want anyone to notice the lighter. The onlookers are no help, so Bruno tries to get his hand into the grate. You see his fingers just touch the lighter and then knock it lower, out of reach. Back to the tennis; the match is at a higher pitch. Bruno's fingers are reaching deeper through the grate (are we actually rooting for him to reach it?) and he finally grasps the lighter and heads toward the carnival. Meanwhile, Guy has won his match and is headed toward Metcalf.

Bruno is waiting for it to get dark. A close-up of his face fades into that of Guy on the train. Meanwhile, the police are onto where Guy is going and are following him. Bruno is standing in line for a boat to the island when the worker recognizes him and starts talking to the police. Then Guy sees Bruno, who runs to the carousel. The police yell "Stop!" and begin shooting, hitting the man who runs the carousel, which begins to spin out of control.

The fight on the carousel between Guy and Bruno is the climax of the film. The worker points toward Bruno and says, "That's the one who killed her!," but with the two entangled in a fight, the police think he is pointing at Guy. A frantic mother cries out, "That's my little boy," and we see the boy, having the time of his life on the racing carousel (another Hitchcock joke). Meanwhile, someone is crawling under the carousel trying to get to the center control and bring it to a halt. The wooden horse hooves threaten, the horses' heads swing wildly (the editing is powerfully effective), and the carousel comes to a crashing stop, upended.

Bruno is crushed by the carousel. He's dying. Guy asks him to tell the police what really happened, to confess, to tell them that he has Guy's lighter. Bruno continues the lie, saying he hasn't got it, it's on the island. The police chief, rather incredibly, takes him at his word. Then Bruno dies; his hand uncurls and reveals the lighter.

This is another of several illogical details in this screenplay. After the climactic fight between Guy and Bruno on the carousel, would Bruno have the lighter in his hand? Not likely. That, and being able to reach the lighter through the storm drain grate, are just not credible. But I'm only registering these objections after having watched the movie many times. The first times I watched, they did not occur to me. The movie is so well made that, for me at least, it convinces from moment to moment.

Strangers on a Train presents a typical Hitchcock situation: the innocent who is caught in some intrigue that he doesn't understand. That's Guy. His name suggests that he is "Everyman." The intrigue is Bruno, who is doing Guy a favor, something that Guy might have wished for but would never do. Guy would never have thought of killing his wife when she refused him the divorce. He might have wished it, wished that she would be hit by a car or would run off to Australia, but murder, no. When Bruno tells him his idea, Guy is too nice, too well-behaved, to simply say "no." He is passive, he lets others control his agenda, and he allows Bruno to think he approves of his ideas by not saying what he means. Bruno represents the uncivilized id. If unchecked, it causes havoc. In this case, someone is murdered.

Bruno is Guy's dark side. We see this not only with the frequent mirrored activities between them, but with the scheme of light and dark. Guy wears white; he is a tennis player. Bruno is always seen in dark colors or standing in the shadows; he lives for the night. He is reaching into a sewer when Guy, all in white, is playing tennis as if his life depended on it.

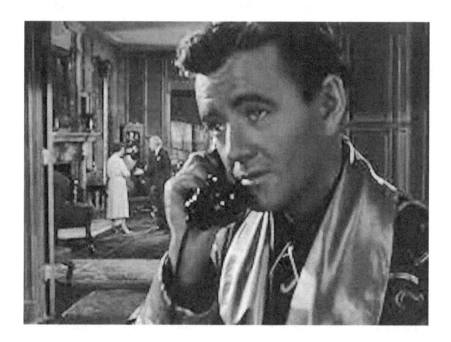

The Madness

In the previous chapter I referred to Hervey Cleckley's *Mask of Sanity* as a guide to understanding the psychopath. Cleckley's study of psychopaths led him to summarize what he saw as their most prominent and identifying characteristics. They exhibit many of the aspects of the antisocial personality, but with additional pathognomonic elements. Will these fit our understanding of Bruno? Let's take a look at the most defining features (which I will highlight in *italics*) and see.

Superficial Charm and Good Intelligence. Bruno shows this in many ways, especially the charm and the intelligence when he is in elegant company—at the tennis club and the senator's party. He is easily able to ingratiate himself with Guy when they first meet on the train. Their encounter is random but seems inevitable. Bruno knows all about Guy because he reads the newspaper's sports and social pages. He tells Guy he looks up to him: "I admire people who do things." He tells Guy he doesn't talk much, then can't stop talking, showing off. This is first-date behavior, the first of several hints that there is a sexual attraction going on. He recounts his own exploits with no sense of how damning they are. He reports examples of *Recklessness, Risk Taking, Irresponsibility* as well as *Excessive Drinking and Gambling* (all psychopathic characteristics): being thrown out of three colleges, driving a fast car blindfolded (if true, it's risky behavior in the extreme; more likely it's a lie, one of many), flying a jet plane (really?), and booking the first flight to the moon (a grandiose claim, but also declaring his love of danger and risk).

Bruno is good at getting people's attention and getting them to listen to him, especially "little old ladies." He has had plenty of practice with his mother, who finds him funny and entertaining, even at his most outrageous. He has her wrapped around his little finger. And he engages Mrs. Cunningham at the party just as easily, getting her to play the game of "how to murder your husband." That only gets out of control when Babs turns up looking too much like Miriam.

On the train, when he first meets Guy, he insists that with all his father's money, he should never have to work, much less work his way up from a lowly position. He feels entitled, and in spite of being correctly called a wastrel by his hated father who sees his inadequacy, he thinks he is quite something. Bruno appears self-assured, cockily convinced that his conversation is fascinating to anyone who listens, even as he puts himself down as someone who never "does anything." That's part of his charm; he engages by making the other person feel "big." He loves his ideas and is eager to share them to prove how clever he is. His latest: thinking of the best way to commit a murder and not get caught.

Lack of Empathy. This is the inability to imagine yourself in someone else's situation emotionally, to feel their pain. This shortcoming allows Bruno to read people more easily; his own feelings don't get in the way of seeing them, recognizing in others what they don't even know about themselves.

Even though he has never met her, Bruno has absolutely no trouble tracking Miriam down and then coldly killing her. Though what he hears about her makes her sound shallow and manipulative, that isn't a reason for her to die. Even after watching her show some joy at the carnival, which you might think would have reminded him that she is a human being with a life ahead of her, his inability to feel empathy makes him see her not as a person but as an obstacle in Guy's way, to be gotten rid of. So, he kills her in the most intensely intimate way, choking her to death with his bare hands. Then, he walks away calmly as though nothing has happened. When he hands Guy her broken glasses as proof of the deed, you hear only pride and satisfaction in his voice. He shows *No Remorse*, no suggestion of guilt. Another characteristic of the psychopath.

When he says to Guy, "I have a murder on my conscience," we really can't believe he is feeling remorse. He is trying to get Guy to keep his end of the bargain, what he is convinced Guy agreed to on the train. When Guy makes it clear he has no intention of carrying through with this and when he calls Bruno a "maniac," we see a flash of the *Anger* that underlies much of the psychopath's behavior. But Bruno is quick to push it away, declaring that he will get his revenge.

At the party, what is Bruno feeling when, as he is pretending to strangle Mrs. Cunningham, he becomes fixated on Babs? Is he feeling guilty then, reliving the murderous moment with Miriam? I think that, instead, he is remembering the intense high of that moment, the adrenaline rush of murdering someone, of embracing someone until they die. I think that is what causes him to fall in a faint.

The whole plan is falling apart. Central to Bruno's so-called brilliant idea is that he and Guy stay strangers, that they never be seen together so nothing can connect them to each other's crime. Though he loves his "crisscross" idea and is convinced Guy does too, it's Bruno who can't make it stick.

When Guy doesn't follow through, Bruno steps out of the shadows and begins to intrude on Guy's world. He calls to him in the museum, even with Anne there watching; he shows up at the tennis club and chats with Anne and her friends; then he goes to the party. Now, having been seen together in public, they are connected. Like with most psychopaths, his *Best Laid Plan Falls Apart* because of his *Impulsiveness* and not being able to follow through. He shows *Poor Judgment* in thinking that Guy would go along with the plot in the first place. He shows poor judgment, too, when he goes to the party and the club and behaves so oddly, drawing the wrong kind of attention to himself.

At the party his conversation is decidedly strange. He tells the senator about the "life force" that allows a person to see millions of miles and smell a flower on Mars. Does he really believe this? If so, he would be delusional, and this is not part of the psychopathic picture. It may be that his guard is down because he has been drinking. We know he *Drinks Too Much* (another psychopathic characteristic). I think he is just being grandiose: this is not unlike his bragging about driving the car blindfolded at 150 miles an hour. He is lying for effect. He may even believe his lie, which happens if someone repeats a lie often enough. *Habitual Lying* is a psychopathic trait too.

We know nothing of Bruno's sex life. In fact, we know nothing of his connections with anyone besides his mother and father. Does he have friends; a lover? The movie doesn't tell us. There certainly seems to be a sexual overtone to his devotion to Guy and to his instant declaration of admiration and friendship after only moments together. When they are fighting on the carousel, they are as often entwined as they are hitting each other; the pumping pistons of the wooden horses and the accelerating speed of the carousel itself until the final explosion are a not-so-subtle metaphor. Movies of the 1950s could not directly show homosexual behavior; they could only hint at it. There are lots of hints here. Bruno dresses in a flashy, flamboyant way that doesn't just say he is rich but may suggest he is gay. His manicure and his dressing gown and his relationship with his mother "say" the same thing. And his fey, "toodle-loo" finger wave to Anne speaks volumes. These are all stereotypes of the period when the film was made. Perhaps this is one reason his father holds him in such disdain (nothing in the film suggests this directly; it's just surmise). Whether Guy feels anything sexual toward Bruno is harder to say. There is certainly little passion in his relationship with Anne. But that may be due more to the rather wooden acting of Farley Granger than anything else. Robert Walker is a much more subtle actor, and he can convey in a gesture layers of meaning.

When Babs says how wonderful it must be to have someone love you so much they would kill for you, she might well, without knowing it, be describing what Bruno does for Guy.

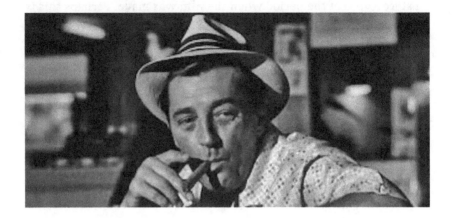

Cape Fear (1962)

Robert Mitchum, Gregory Peck, Polly Bergen
Director: J. Lee Thompson

This is one scary movie. Robert Mitchum is Max Cady, a rapist just out of prison and intent on getting revenge against Sam Bowden (Gregory Peck), the lawyer in a small Southern town he blames for his eight years in jail. At first, you know he wants to do something bad, but you don't know what. With his slow movements and sleepy eyes, Mitchum is all insinuation. He is smart, keeping just on the right side of the law, implying what he will do without saying it outright.

Early on we see him beat up a woman he has just had sex with. Bare-chested, he doesn't seem angry, just intent. It's what he does. Bernard Herrmann's music adds to the sense of dread.

Then he poisons the Bowden family dog but, of course, they can't prove it. At the marina he talks about Bowden's "juicy" young daughter, just inviting her father to punch him, then backs away. He will fight him on his own terms, when he is ready. Meanwhile he says to Bowden, "You're not going to force me into a sucker play. Just have your innings. Mine are coming." Then, to the people watching, "Guess you folks saw this, huh? You notice I naver laid a hand on him. I'm standin' here mindin' my business and this guy attacks me."

When Bowden meets with him at a bar, Cady is in his element. "Sweatin' a little, huh, Counsellor? Well, just remember, I waited eight years. Ordering drinks, he asks for twelve-year-old whisky, "My rich cousin here says the best is none too good for me." When Peck offers to pay him to leave town, with great sarcasm Cady says, "Now that's heartwarming, ain't it? A poor ex-con comes to·a new town to make a fresh start, and a leading citizen steps right up and offers him financial help. It renews your faith in human nature. . . . That would take some figuring, wouldn't it? What would you consider eight lost years worth, Counsellor?"

Then he tells a long story about the first thing he did when he got out of jail. He found his ex-wife, who had divorced him while he was in prison, kidnapped her, got her drunk, "kept her pretty busy for three days," and made her write him a "love note full of dirty words." Then he left her naked by the side of the road for her new husband to find. "I like to put values on things. The value of eight years, the value of a family. . . . Now I got what you call complate peace of mind about Mary. . . . So it's no deal."

At first when he was in jail, he tells Bowden, "All I could think about was bustin' out to kill a guy. I was gonna kill him with my bare hands, slow; so he could taste it. I killed him every night for seven years, but the eighth year I realized I was lettin' him off too easy, too fast. You know, in China or someplace, they cut off a toe, the little one, and then pretty soon they cut off the next, and so on. That's better," Calling him a degenerate, Bowden walks out. But this is only the prelude for what Cady has in store for him and his family. When Bowden hires some thugs to beat him up, Cady has the upper hand: the law is now on *his* side.

Cady is a classic psychopath. Unlike Bruno, he has only a thin veneer of the civilized about him, but enough to pass, to make himself look like the victim instead of the predator he is. His anger is barely contained, but it wells to the surface. He feels no guilt or remorse about the rape that got him in jail, but only blames the lawyer whose defense didn't keep him out of jail. He easily poisons their pet dog, enjoys beating up and degrading women, but, even more, takes pleasure in the "death of a thousand cuts" that he intends to inflict on Bowden, his wife, and his daughter. He is a man with a plan.

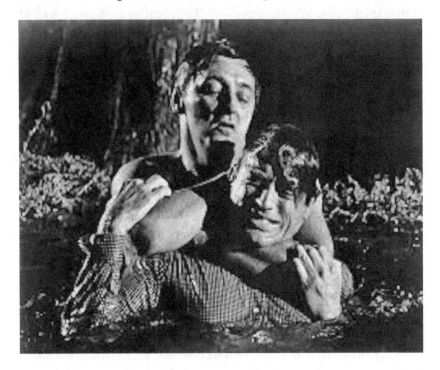

But his anger gets the better of him. When he corners Bowden's wife, he is the looming, bare-chested epitome of sexual threat. He tries to force her to consent to being raped as a way to protect her daughter and quotes the law to her. But as she resists, terrified, suddenly he can't stop beating her—this is not going to look like consent.

The final confrontation, in a nearby swamp, with Sam Bowden having to take things in his own hands, is thrilling. Mitchum's performance is one for the ages. This is a very good movie.

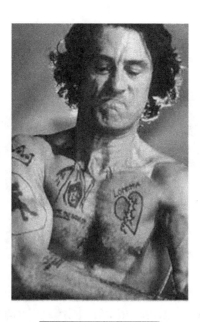

Cape Fear (1991)

Robert De Niro, Nick Nolte, Jessica Lange
Director: Martin Scorsese

A brief word about this remake. Thirty years later it was possible to say and do things onscreen that were not accepted in the early 1960s. This film demonstrates how that is not always a good thing. What makes the original *Cape Fear* so effective is how much of the suspense is created by the suggestion of violence until the final confrontation. The remake is too obvious, too much in-your- face, too much the blunt instrument. I have great respect for everyone involved. Scorsese's camerawork and editing can be very effective, but what the filmmakers added to the original script, though it does add complexity to the characters, seems too by-the-numbers: suggesting, for instance, that Sam, the lawyer played now by Nick Nolte, did a bad job defending Max, justifying Max's anger. Making the good guy less good to my mind, lessens the impact.

With Max Cady, they make blatant what the 1962 version so powerfully implied. Look at De Niro as Max Cady. They are simply trying too hard.

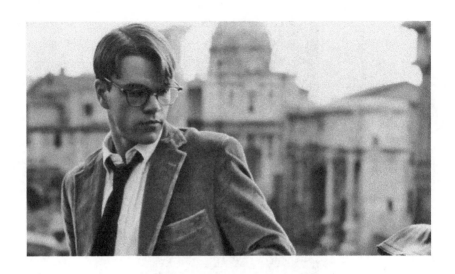

The Talented Mr. Ripley (1999)

Matt Damon, Jude Law, Gwyneth Paltrow, Cate Blanchett
Director: Anthony Minghella

This story, based on the first of Patricia Highsmith's novels about Tom Ripley, has had several incarnations in the movies.

The Anthony Minghella version is as wonderfully seductive as Tom Ripley himself, played by Matt Damon. I find it quite entertaining, with a convincing portrait of Ripley as someone who responds to every cue by changing who he seems to be to get the best advantage.

Tom, working at a high-end party and wearing a borrowed jacket, is mistaken for a Princeton graduate. One of the guests says, "You'll most likely know our son, Dickie Greenleaf." After the briefest pause, Tom asks, "How is Dickie?" Under the credits we see he is now chatting with Dickie's father, who says disdainfully, "Dickie's idea of music is jazz. . . . To my ear jazz is just noise." Next, we see Tom walking with Mr. Greenleaf, who owns a shipping company. "Could you ever conceive of going to Italy, Tom, persuade my son to come home? I'd pay you a thousand dollars." When Tom says he had always wanted to go abroad, Mr. Greenleaf says, "Now you can go for a reason."

We hear scat singing and fade to a record turning. Tom is in a basement tenement apartment, trying to identify the jazz performers, to be able to pass as a fan. Preparing for his voyage to Italy, he studies the Princeton yearbook page on Dickie. At passport control in Italy, he meets Cate Blanchett as Meredith, the daughter of another rich family. He introduces himself as "Dickie Greenleaf." She asks him, "You're not the shipping Greenleafs?" and he says, "trying not to be." Notice how often he allows the other person's assumptions to lead them without actually lying. We will see that this is his method, and it is very effective.

She notices that his luggage was in the "R" section. His answer, "My father . . . builds boats. I'd rather sail them. I travel under my mother's name." She asks, "Which is?" and he says, "Emily," which she takes as a clever joke. She is charmed and admits she travels under her mother's name too. Matt Damon's performance here would disarm anyone.

Next, we see Tom at the beach. Dickie is sunbathing with his girlfriend Marge (Gwyneth Paltrow). Tom walks by them and pretends to notice Dickie, "It's Tom. Tom Ripley. We were at Princeton together." Dickie, of course, does not recognize him. He asks, "Did we know each other?" and Tom says, "Well, I knew you, so I suppose you must have known me." Another non-answer that lets the other assume a connection.

Next Tom shows up at Dickie's apartment and is chatting with Marge when Dickie arrives. In conversation Dickie says, "Everyone should have one talent—what's yours?" And Tom does something that I think is both totally unexpected and brilliant to his purpose. He tells the truth. He says, "Forging signatures, telling lies, impersonating practically anybody." When Dickie challenges him to do an impression, Tom does a spot-on impression of Dickie's father, featuring his put-down of jazz, and then follows up with the father's offer to Tom to get Dickie to return home. Dickie is really impressed.

Later, Tom comes back to say goodbye and "accidentally" drops his collection of jazz records. Suddenly, he's not leaving—he is staying with Dickie and Marge as their new best friend.

Seeing how hard Tom works to prepare himself for his deceptions, it's hard not to root for him to succeed. At least until we discover where it all leads.

We see him studying Dickie, copying his mannerisms, trying out his voice, putting on his clothes when he is not around. And soon, when, while sailing, it becomes clear that Dickie would like to see the back of him ("You can be a leach and quite boring"), Tom accuses Dickie of rejecting him because he is afraid of the feelings he has toward him. They fight and he kills Dickie. He forges a letter to Marge breaking off her engagement to Dickie, and, moving to Rome, Tom "becomes" Dickie.

Things get complicated since Marge is still around and Dickie's friend Freddie (Philip Seymour Hoffman) is looking for him. There will be more killings, as Tom does what he needs to do, even if it means killing people he supposedly loves, to keep the impersonation going and to live Dickie's rich life.

Tom Ripley is the ultimate fictional example of the cunning, smooth-talking psychopath. He is a shape-shifter, easily mimicking others and finding ways into their world. He is charming, engaging, and ruthless, without remorse or guilt. The homosexual subtext is more obvious here than in *Strangers*. Tom's attachment to Dickie is romantic, sexual (though never acted upon), and opportunistic as he steals Dickie's things, tries on his clothes, and after eliminating him, moves into his life.

But of course, there are people who will know he is not Dickie, and they are a continued threat, either to be avoided or killed. So, in what seems a carefully considered plan, we see that once again, the psychopath cannot quite get it right. He has to kill or abandon this adopted world.

The first movie of this novel was French, *Plein Soleil*, also known as *Purple Noon*, starring Alain Delon as Ripley and directed by René Clément. It made Delon a star and followed the book closely, except for the ending—much like what happened with *Strangers on a Train* (in the novel, Guy kills Bruno's father).

Patricia Highsmith wrote several other novels featuring Tom Ripley, and some were turned into quite good films. I would particularly recommend *Ripley's Game* (2002), with John Malkovich as a middle-aged Ripley, wealthy and cultured, but still a con man willing to kill to get what he wants.

RECOMMENDED READING

Cleckley, Hervey. *The Mask of Sanity*. Brattleboro, VT: Echo Point Books; 2015.

Specifically, chapters 20, 21.

Highsmith, Patricia. *Strangers on a Train*. New York: W. W. Norton & Company; 2001.

A noir classic. The novel is interestingly different from the film.

Hitchcock, Alfred, and Truffaut, Francois. *Hitchcock*. New York: Simon and Schuster; 1967.

Director Truffaut (*The 400 Blows, Jules and Jim, Day for Night*) interviews Hitchcock about his films. A remarkable conversation between two masters.

▪7▪

"A boy's best friend is his mother."

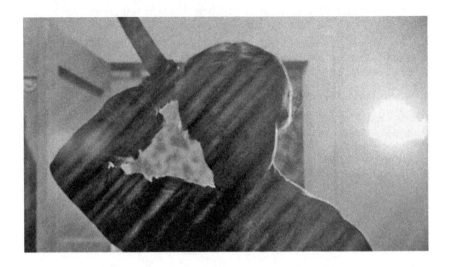

Dissociative Identity Disorder

WHO ARE YOU REALLY?

Psycho (1960)

Janet Leigh, Anthony Perkins, Martin Balsam, Vera Miles
Director: Alfred Hitchcock

Though we will explore the madness suggested in *Psycho*, I first want to describe how this one film changed the way we thought about movies and the movie-going experience. We will also look very closely at how *Psycho* works and why it works so well.

I strongly urge you: *do not read this chapter until you have seen the complete film.*

As with all the other movies here, I will walk you through the details of the action, commenting as we go along. That means that there are lots of spoilers. It would be better for you to see every film before reading about it so you can have an unmediated first reaction to it, but knowing the plot turns that occur in the other films in this book is less of an issue than it is with *Psycho*. With the other films, you might lose a sense of surprise, but in many cases knowing what is coming (as though you are watching the movie a second time) will only deepen your appreciation of the characterizations, the story, and how it is told.

That is not the case with *Psycho*.

I grant it is hard to be totally naive to *Psycho*. Some iconic moments are part of the culture. But seeing these moments in isolation doesn't prepare you for their effect in the movie. I don't want my revealing its surprises and plot twists to get in the way of you experiencing the movie fully for the first time yourself.

An essay I usually assign my Yale students to read for my class on *Psycho* is Harvey Roy Greenberg's "The Apes at the Windows," from his book *Screen Memories: Hollywood Cinema on the Psychoanalytic Couch*. His close analysis of the movie is very different from mine. He is not looking for a diagnosis or studying the structure of the movie so much as applying principles of psychoanalysis to the story. The essay is interesting and persuasive and I recommend it to you. But read it after you see the movie, not before—he includes the same spoilers I do.

I mentioned in the Introduction how much of a difference it makes if you can see movies as part of an audience. Other people's reactions can reinforce our appreciation. To hear a gasp, a muffled scream, or laughter can cue and intensify your own reaction. Such reactions make watching a movie a shared experience instead of an isolating one.

Watching by yourself on your computer, or even on a large-screen TV in your living room, is just not the same, especially with a film like *Psycho*. So, if you can manage it, see this movie in a theater. Or at least, if you can, gather some friends to watch it with you. You will be glad you did.

Almost all of my Yale students had seen at least part of the shower scene online, but interestingly most of them had never seen the whole film. I was delighted to find that many of them found it quite scary and unsettling (after all, why watch a scary movie unless you want to be scared?). The movie is more than 60 years old, and it still works. Watching the movie for the first time for my class, many students thought that Marion was going to be the "psycho." The film seemed to be all about her; she was hearing voices in the car and she certainly looked paranoid with the policeman, so, they figured, she must be the one the title was referring to.

Let me remind you what it was like going to the movies when I was a kid in the 1950s. At my local movie theater, there would always be a double feature: two full-length movies separated by a series of shorts—newsreel, cartoons, previews of coming attractions, maybe a nature documentary. Usually one feature movie was an "A" film, with a big star and a matching budget. The second feature was a "B" film with lesser stars and budgets; it was usually a genre film, like a mystery or a Western.

"B" films weren't necessarily less good; in fact, many of them are now considered of greater interest than the "A" movies of the day, and some of them are classics. They were often a training ground for actors and directors who later had major careers. Val Lewton's horror movies *Cat People* and *I Walked with a Zombie* are examples. They are considered the best of their type. The original *Little Shop of Horrors* (inspiration for the later musical) had an unknown Jack Nicholson playing the small role of the masochist at the dentist's office. Another "B" picture, Don Siegel's *Invasion of the Body Snatchers*, was a sci-fi horror film, now considered a classic, that channeled the paranoia of the McCarthy era. The first movie that Francis Ford Coppola (director of *The Godfather*) directed was one he wrote overnight called *Dementia 13*, stealing much from *Psycho*. It was a "B picture" success and kickstarted his career.

This whole double feature package cost 25 cents. Around the time of *Psycho*, the cost went up to 35 cents.

These movies were shown continuously, with no announced starting times. You would just come in when it was convenient, often in the middle of one of the feature pictures. If you were lucky, it was near enough to the beginning so that it was easy to figure out what was happening. But not always, and it didn't seem to matter. You would watch that movie to the end, watch all the shorts, stay for the second feature film, watch different shorts, and then watch the first film from the start. At some point in the middle, you would say to your family or your friends, "This is where we came in," and you all would leave, bumping knees on the way out of your row. If the first feature was particularly good you might stay until the end, seeing the last part a second time.

Back then, it was unusual to see a movie from beginning to end. There were two exceptions: roadshows and art films. For these longer, star-studded, heavily advertised movies, you bought your $1 ticket in advance for a showing at a set time.

The other exception was the art film, usually a foreign or independent movie. They might be double-featured with another art film, but the audience for those was much more likely to want to watch them from the beginning. At the few theaters that specialized in art and independent cinema, standing in line to get in at the beginning was normal.

Alfred Hitchcock's movie was not an art film; it was for the masses. He knew he had a problem. *Psycho* had two major stars: Janet Leigh and Anthony Perkins. Leigh was the bigger star with many major pictures behind her, including *Little Women, Scaramouche, Touch of Evil* (directed by Orson Welles), and *The Vikings*, with her husband, Tony Curtis. Anthony Perkins was a teen idol and an up-and-coming star, portraying Jimmy Piersall, a baseball player with father issues and bi-polar illness, in *Fear Strikes Out,* and a young Quaker in *Friendly Persuasion.*

If people did what they usually did and came into the theater in the middle of *Psycho*, they would miss Janet Leigh, and spend the rest of the movie waiting for her to appear, getting confused or angry. What to do?

Hitchcock's idea was to insist that no one would be admitted to *Psycho* except at the beginning. He persuaded the owners of local theaters to sign a pledge committing themselves to this rule. There were posters showing the queen of England and the president of the United States saying that even they would not be admitted after the movie started. This was revolutionary!

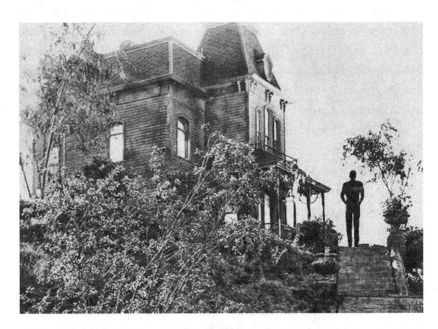

The coming attractions trailer for *Psycho* starred and was directed by Hitchcock. This was unusual; a major director did not make coming attractions shorts. Hitchcock took advantage of the fact that he was now a fixture in everyone's living room because of the success of his TV program, *Alfred Hitchcock Presents.* This anthology show was a collection of stand-alone mystery stories, usually involving a murder and often ending with an unexpected twist. Hitchcock introduced each episode, following the silhouette image of his rotund figure. He became instantly recognizable. With a droll wit he would make fun of the commercials, and after the story would often add a comment that reversed the twist, getting past the censors who always insisted that "crime must not pay." The trailer he made for *Psycho* (which you can find online) is almost jolly, as he takes us on a tour of the motel and Norman's house and keeps almost telling us what terrible thing will happen there. It's funny and properly unnerving. It sure makes you want to see the movie.

Even before the reviews, this campaign generated interest in *Psycho*. The requirement to arrive only at the beginning meant that people would have to wait to enter the theater until the previous showing was done. That meant they had to stand in line, often outside, extending down the block. This made the movie seem very popular: "Look at all those people waiting to see this!"

In the foyer of every theater showing *Psycho* there was a full-size free-standing cardboard cut-out photo of Hitchcock with his finger to his lips, saying, "Please don't tell anybody the secret of our ending. It's the only one we've got." Another masterstroke. Years later, the producers of the British film *The Crying Game* did the same thing for their movie which also had a jolting reveal. That worked too.

The reviews for *Psycho* were generally good, though there were some who complained that Hitchcock was slumming, that making a horror picture was beneath him. The reviewer for *Time* magazine called the picture "expertly gothic," and also said that "it was a spectacle of stomach-churning horror" and that "the nausea never disappears." But people seemed to like the idea of "stomach-churning horror"; reviews like that didn't hurt the box office. It was a big hit. Later, *Time* magazine listed it as one of the best pictures of the year. I think the box office may have changed their minds.

All this permanently altered the way people went to the movies. From then on, local theaters posted starting times, and people would wait in line before going inside (this was not usually "required" as it had been for *Psycho*—if you didn't care to see a film from the beginning you could ignore the line, but arriving late was now looked down upon as disruptive and a distraction to the people already watching the show). That, and the end of the studio system in Hollywood (which had often required the added "B" picture if a theater wanted to show the well-promoted "A" film), effectively ended the double feature. If people were going to wait in line for the start of a movie, then the people in the theater had to leave after the feature to allow the new patrons in. That eventually led to the demise of short features, too, such as the cartoons and newsreels that had once completed the double-feature package.

The movie industry in the 1950s was in a panic because of television. Television was free, and in more and more homes. People were losing the movie-going habit. In the decades before, families would go to the movies as often as once a week, which is why the double-feature programs would change weekly. As television became more popular, the movies needed to offer something different to compete. Since TV back then was only in black and white, films were made almost exclusively in color. Since TV screens were small, movies developed wide screens like CinemaScope and VistaVision, and the three-projector super-wide surround system Cinerama, which brought people out to see film spectacles like *Around the World in Eighty Days* (three hours long, with dozens of stars, including David Niven, Buster Keaton, Frank Sinatra, and Marlene Dietrich).

Psycho challenged that trend. It was in black and white, and projected close to the standard 4:3 screen ratio of movies from the 1940s. Hitchcock did it in black and white because of his experience making the television series. He saw how efficiently the technicians worked, turning out half hour episodes every week.

Initially, because it was a horror film and radically different from the Hitchcock "brand," he was not able to get any studio to agree to make *Psycho*. Paramount would not give him the budget he needed to make and distribute the film, so he agreed to use his own money in exchange for a significant share of the profits. The film cost about $800,000 to make. Hitchcock used the camera crew from his TV show. They were cheap compared to the crews he used for his earlier Hollywood films from the 1950s, like *North by Northwest*, *Rear Window*, and *Vertigo*. The other performers in the movie, such as John Gavin and Martin Balsam, were all studio contract players and much less expensive than the two stars. Another cost-saving measure was making the film in black and white. It's said that Hitchcock was afraid that the blood in the shower scene would be too disturbing if it was in color, but I think the main reason was that black-and-white film costs so much less. After all, he was using his own money.

And boy, was that a good decision! *Psycho* grossed some $32 million during its original run, when a million dollars was real money. It made Hitchcock very rich.

Hitchcock didn't make only inexpensive choices. He knew when it was important to get value. He hired Bernard Herrmann to compose the music. Herrmann wrote the soundtrack music for Hitchcock's *Vertigo*, *The Man Who Knew Too Much*, and *North by Northwest*, as well as for *Citizen Kane, Cape Fear, Taxi Driver*, and many other films. He also wrote music for *Alfred Hitchcock Presents* on TV. Herrmann's score for *Psycho* is one of the most famous in movie history. He decided to use only strings to increase a sense of tension and anxiety. The pounding, obsessively relentless music grabs us right away.

Hitchcock told him he did not want any music during the shower scene. Herrmann disagreed and composed it anyway. He showed Hitchcock the rushes of the shower scene with and without the music. Hitchcock was smart enough to change his mind. The shrieking, jagged theme stayed in and became iconic. Try watching the shower scene without the sound—you will see what a difference the music makes.

The other expensive choice was Saul Bass. Bass was a graphic designer who made some of the most dynamic and memorable credit sequences of the 1950s and 1960s. He designed the opening credits for *Psycho*. He was also listed as "pictorial consultant," which is unusual. Bass has claimed that he was responsible for designing the shower scene; and it seems true that he did storyboard the entire sequence. As I explained in discussing *Strangers on a Train*, storyboarding is how a film is planned before they actually start shooting. It looks like a series of cartoons, often posted on separate panels on the walls of a room, showing in sequence each camera angle and each shot. Sometimes the drawings are detailed, sometimes they are sketches. Hitchcock was not a fan of improvising on set, or asking anyone's advice. It's likely that Bass's storyboard was a collaboration with Hitchcock, created together after much discussion.

Janet Leigh and others insist that Hitchcock himself was there to direct the shower scene, which took about a week to shoot, with its sixty-some cuts (different camera placements) for one minute of screen time. Making movies is a collaboration, with many people contributing. But the director makes the final decisions; the "buck stops" with him. It's said that "success has a thousand fathers, but failure is an orphan." Because this scene became so renowned, it's not surprising that Bass would want credit. But unless he was there for the filming, he can't justifiably say making the moment by moment decisions, he directed it, (The Bass storyboards are available online. A url is in Recommended Reading at the end of this chapter. Take a look, and decide for yourself who deserves the credit.) Unfortunately, this contretemps ruined their relationship and they never worked together again.

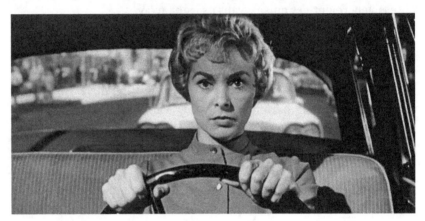

The Movie

After the driving strings and the dizzying lines of the credits, we are given a very specific place and time, Phoenix, Arizona, December 11, 2:43 PM. The camera scans the cityscape and closes in on a nondescript building, pausing and then hopping through a seemingly randomly chosen open window. We are voyeurs spying on a half-dressed couple: love in the afternoon.

Marion Crane (Janet Leigh) is unhappy with these secret meetings; Sam is okay with the status quo. She says this is the last time. Sam is burdened by money worries, paying alimony and settling his father's debts. Marion wants respectability. This is the stuff of soap opera.

When Marion arrives at the real estate office where she works, her colleague, Caroline, played by Patricia Hitchcock, chats about her newly wedded status. Then Cassidy walks in. He is a rich oil-man client, drunk and flirting and talking about buying a house for his daughter as a wedding present. So, weddings and being married are very much in the air. "My baby," says Cassidy, "and she has never had an unhappy moment in her life. You know what I do about unhappiness? I buy it off." When he flashes the $40,000 in cash he is paying for the house, Caroline stares and says, "I declare," and Cassidy replies, "I don't, that's how I'm able to keep it." So, it's illicit money that is fending off unhappiness. No wonder it gives Marion ideas. When her boss tells her he is uncomfortable having so much cash in the office, he asks her to take it to the bank. She tells him she has a headache, that she will put the money in the bank, then go home to spend the weekend in bed.

We next see her in her apartment. She has changed her white bra and slip for black. (Not too subtle—she is now on the "dark side"—but here, I think it works. It speaks volumes without saying a word, something Hitchcock is very good at.) The camera moves from her to the envelope with the money sitting on the bed; then we see a suitcase. She is getting dressed and packing for travel. The music is obsessively repetitive. She has made a decision.

In her car, heading to see Sam in Fairvale, Marion imagines what he will say. At a stoplight, her boss and Cassidy walk past. Her boss notices her. Now the driving music starts, jagged and insistent. Lights in her eyes. Next morning, she is parked by the side of the road. A policeman stops to check on her. She wakes with a start—he peers down on her with his dark sunglasses, looking threatening—but he is only there to help. She tells him she was almost falling asleep while driving, so she pulled over to rest. He says it would have been safer to stop at a motel (ironic, considering what will happen when she does). He asks her, "Is there anything wrong?" and she says, "Of course not, am I acting as though there is anything wrong?" "Frankly, yes," he says, and he is right. She looks like she is hiding something. And she is—the envelope with the money is sitting on the seat next to her.

When she leaves, he follows her. The intense relentless music continues. She stops at a used car dealer to switch cars. She will be paying cash. She checks a newspaper to see if there is anything there about her and notices that the policeman is across the street watching. She goes to the ladies' room, and we see her from above (the God's-eye view) counting out the money. The salesman feels rushed and is suspicious as she pushes to buy the car right away. As she starts to drive away in her new purchase, the salesman yells—she has forgotten her suitcase and coat, which they then put in her new car. The whole point of switching cars is to avoid notice, but her behavior has drawn attention from both the salesman and the policeman.

Now we have a sequence that is reminiscent of the dream-like journey in *The Night of the Hunter*. She imagines the salesman comparing notes with the policeman, and her boss wondering where she is and trying to locate her. Then, her imagination working overtime, she envisions her boss telling Cassidy that the money is missing. "A girl works for you for ten years, you trust her," he says. Cassidy says, "If any of it [the money] is missing, I'll replace it with her fine soft flesh." Marion smiles. She knows she deserves to be punished for what she has done. But she enjoyed stealing his money and likes the idea of Cassidy's anger and threat.

It's night and it starts to rain, hard. The windshield wipers can't keep up, it's hard to see, everything is a blur. The car slows down and so does the music. She notices some lights: it's a motel, the Bates Motel. She pulls in. This is the end of Act One.

Marion stops at the motel office and sees a house on the hill behind, with a woman standing in the window. The house is dark and foreboding. When Norman Bates (Anthony Perkins) bounds from the house, he is friendly and chatty—and chooses to put her in the room right next to the office. She doesn't realize that she is so close to Fairvale; if it wasn't for the rain, she could have driven all the way. Norman shows her the room, pointing out the facilities. His manner is eager but hesitant; embarrassed, repressed, he can't quite say the word "bathroom."

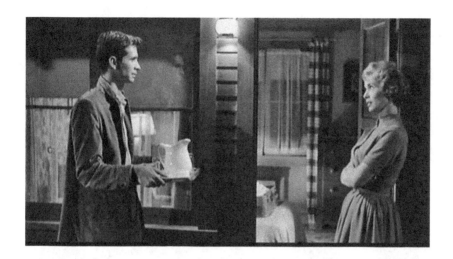

He offers her dinner at the house. When he leaves, she overhears his mother chastising him for wanting to bring a woman into the house. Meanwhile, Marion wraps the money in a newspaper and leaves it on the bedside table. A few moments later Norman returns with a sandwich dinner on a tray and suggests they eat in his office. He is too uncomfortable to sit in her room. "His mother "isn't quite herself today," he tells her.

The scene in the parlor room behind the office is crucial. It is the most dialogue-heavy in the movie. There are taxidermied birds on the wall. Birds of prey. They are his hobby. "A man should have a hobby," says Marion, but Norman demurs. She asks, "Do you go out with friends?" Norman responds, "A boy's best friend is his mother." Norman asks where she is going and she tells him she is looking for a "private island." Norman tells her, "We are all in our private traps, and none of us can ever get out . . . I was born in mine, I don't mind it anymore—I do mind, but I say I don't." His changes in mood are quick and disturbing.

Marion comments on how his mother berated Norman. Norman says he can't leave her or even defy her (and we see a stuffed owl on the wall behind him, looking ready to pounce), "She is ill . . . I can't run away . . . If you love someone you don't do that to someone even if you hate them. I don't hate her; I hate what she has become." When

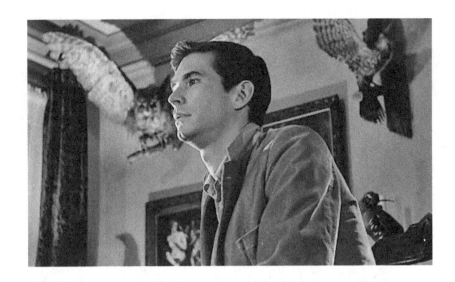

Marion suggests that it might be better if he put his mother "some-place" there is a transformation in Norman's face. Suddenly he looks intense, angry, a bit crazed: "You mean a madhouse? . . . Have you ever seen the inside of those places? . . . the cruel eyes studying you . . . my mother there?—but she's harmless." He admits he has considered it. "She needs me . . . she just goes a little mad sometimes. We all go a little mad sometimes. Haven't you?" We see Marion making a decision; stealing the money was a mistake and she wants to fix it. "I stepped into a private trap [back in Phoenix] and I want to try to pull myself out of it," she says, and leaves for her room.

We have been following Marion closely until now (she has been in every scene), but for the first time we are exclusively with Norman. He sees that she signed in with a different name. Back in the parlor, with stuffed birds everywhere, he removes a painting from the wall: there is a peephole behind, and he begins to spy on her as she gets undressed. He looks up toward the house; it's hard to read his expression—intense, guilty? He heads there. We see him enter the house, hesitate at the stairs, and then sit down in the kitchen.

Now we come to the famous shower scene. Marion takes off her bath-robe, we see her bare back, and she steps into the shower. She pulls the curtain and turns on the shower. The water cascades down and she is washing herself, cleansing herself of her mistake, her crime, her guilt, looking for a fresh start. The only sound is the shower. We see a shadow through the curtain. Suddenly, it's pulled aside, and the shrieking strings begin. It's an old woman with a knife held high ready to strike.

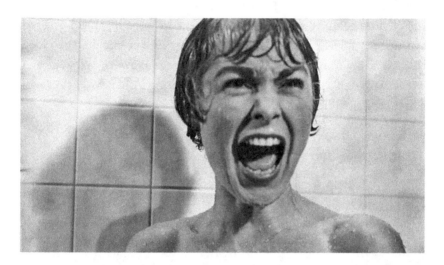

Marion screams and the knife slashes at her again and again. We hear it enter flesh, but only once see the knife against her belly. We never actually see the knife cut. But we see blood begin to mix with the water and Marion screaming. The woman leaves, and Marion's hand is grasping the wall; she turns and slowly slips to the floor, her

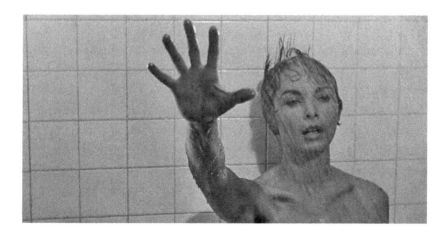

eyes fixed and staring. She reaches out and grabs the curtain, the hooks breaking one by one.

The music stops. Her body falls forward over the edge of the bathtub, and we see the blood and water swirling into the drain. This image dissolves into a matching close-up of her eye, dead and open, with the camera turning and pulling away until we see her head pressed against the floor. There are drops of water on her cheek—they look like tears, but they are just the water from the shower. We have been witness to a violation, both terrible and exciting. And never again will a bathroom feel the same.

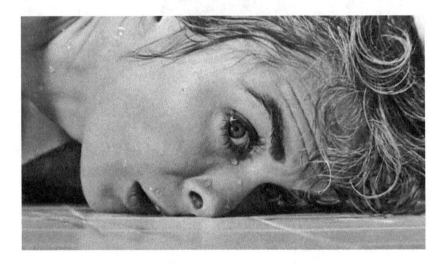

The camera moves from Marion's face to her room and the money, wrapped in the newspaper, then to the open window, and we hear Norman cry, "Mother, oh God, Mother ... blood." Norman rushes back from the house. Now begins a fascinating, essentially silent sequence (except for the obsessive repetitive strings, no longer shrieking, but marking time). When Norman sees Marion's body in the bathroom, he turns away, hand over his mouth, knocking over a bird painting from the wall. The shower is still on. He sits for a moment and then begins a careful, obsessive cleaning of the room, removing any evidence that Marion had been there. He drags her body onto the curtain, wraps it and puts her into the trunk of her car. He washes the blood from his hands and scrubs the bathtub and bathroom floor clean. He removes her clothes and her suitcase. The camera reminds us that the newspaper with the money is still there. Norman does one last survey of the room, notices the newspaper, grabs it and tosses it into the trunk too.

The money is Hitchcock's "MacGuffin"—a term he used for the thing that first drives the plot but isn't really what the story is about. Most of his films have a MacGuffin. When Norman tosses the newspaper, we understand that Marion's murder was not about money. It was a crime of passion, seemingly sparked by jealousy at Norman's sexual interest in Marion.

Norman then drives around behind the motel cabins. We see the car slowly driven to the edge of a pond. Norman gets out and pushes it forward into the muck. He watches as it begins to sink. Suddenly, it stops, half-exposed. We see his anxiety, and we share it (we have become co-conspirators, in spite of ourselves).

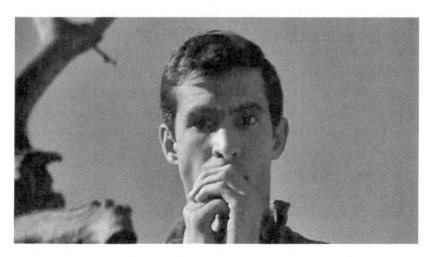

But then, as the car sinks some more, there is a half-smile of relief as it disappears under the surface. Watching with Norman, we, too, want the car to vanish. By witnessing his careful erasure of his mother's crime, our sympathies have shifted from Marion to Norman. As the car with Marion's body sinks into the muck, we almost forget she is there; the story is now Norman's story. That is the end of Act Two.

Nothing like this had ever been seen in the movies. Never before had a major star been killed midway through the film. In fact, it was rare for a major star to even die in a mainstream Hollywood movie. And this murder didn't happen in a dark, claustrophobic setting, but in the sanctuary of a bathroom, white-tiled and bright. The ultimate private place. The murder is seen up close, with the woman naked and defenseless and dying before our eyes. All of this was new, a transgression, a violation of the norms of movie-going.

We were led to believe that this was going to be a story about Marion, about her giving in to temptation and the impulsive decision to steal the money, and her attempt at restitution and redemption. After the moment of soap opera in the hotel room, the story had the shape of a typical Hitchcock suspense thriller: the innocent man (or woman) who gets caught up in something unexpected and has to use their wits to survive it. Up until this movie, the Hitchcock brand promised just such a movie, with suspense and humor in fine balance. With *Psycho*, Hitchcock broke that contract, that understanding with his audience. Suddenly you couldn't trust where the story would go. If this bad thing could happen, what else bad might happen? It was a different kind of chill and was a risky thing for Hitchcock to do. But the audience loved being kept off-balance and not being able to imagine what would happen next. And there was more to come.

The next act is less revolutionary, though it certainly has its moments.

Marion's sister, Lila (Vera Miles), approaches Sam at his hardware store. She is looking for her sister, thinking that Marion was with him. He convinces her that he doesn't know where she is. Arbogast, a detective, interrupts them. He is looking for Marion too. So, the movie now becomes a detective story. Arbogast makes the rounds and finally ends up at the Bates Motel. Norman is there, munching on candy corn. As Arbogast looks at the motel register and notices

Marion's handwriting, the camera watches Norman from below, an odd, disorienting angle. Norman looks more and more nervous as the detective asks him about Marion. Arbogast notices that Norman hesitates in front of Room #1, where Marion stayed. Then he sees Mother in the window of the house. He asks Norman if he is hiding Marion. If so, he asks, "You wouldn't be fooled, you'd know she was just using you." Norman's angry response is interesting. "I'm not a fool, and I'm not capable of being fooled—not even by a woman." Then he lets slip, "Maybe she could have fooled me, but she didn't fool my mother." So Arbogast asks to talk with Norman's mother. Norman refuses: "She's confined." The camera lingers on Norman as the detective drives away. He looks thoughtful and then smiles: I fooled him.

Arbogast calls Lila to tell her he thinks he has located where Marion stayed, and that he wants to try to talk to Norman's mother. Norman is not at the office when he goes back, so Arbogast goes to the house. We watch him climb the outside steps. The front door is unlocked. He enters the house and begins to climb the stairs. We see him from above, and then a door creeps open.

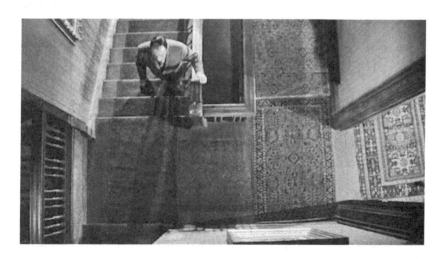

The camera rises until we have the God's-eye view of the upstairs landing, as Mother comes out, knife raised, and slashes Arbogast in the face. He falls backwards down the stairs, arms flailing, and the camera stays close until he lands at the bottom. Mother is above him stabbing repeatedly as he screams.

Lila and Sam have been waiting for Arbogast to return. Lila gets impatient, so Sam agrees to go to the Bates Motel to look for him. We see Norman, standing by the pond behind the motel—another car with a body has been submerged. Sam arrives. He too has seen Mother at the window, but no one answers the door and he doesn't see that Norman was at the pond in back. When Sam returns to Lila, they decide to talk to the sheriff.

Sam and Lila tell the sheriff the story and mention seeing Mother at the window. The sheriff tells them, "Norman Bates's mother has been dead and buried in Greenlawn Cemetery for the past ten years." If that doesn't bring chills, I don't know what will. It certainly does to me, even after so many times watching the movie. Suddenly we are dealing with a ghost story. He continues, "It's the only murder and suicide case on Fairvale ledgers. Mrs. Bates poisoned this guy she was involved with when she found out he was married, then took a helping of the same stuff herself . . . strychnine. Ugly way to die." He tells them that Norman found them dead together, in bed. Sam insists there was an old woman at the house, and Arbogast had said so, too, on the phone. The sheriff mulls, "Well, if the woman up there is Mrs. Bates, who's that woman buried out at Greenlawn Cemetery?" More chills.

Now, we are back with Norman. He goes into the house. We see him from behind, climbing the stairs with an odd swishing gate. He enters Mother's room while the camera stays outside. We hear Norman plead with her to hide in the fruit cellar; people are asking questions. She berates him and says she won't go. Her voice is rough but strong. The camera rises toward the half-opened door and then up to the ceiling, pivoting over the landing. Norman says, "I'll carry you," and she yells at him not to touch her. Then, we see him carrying her down the stairs. We can't see Mother clearly; we are too high, too far away.

Sam and Lila are determined to go back to the motel. They concoct a plan: Sam will detain Norman while Lila goes up to the house to talk to

Mother. First, they look in Room #1, knowing that Marion was there. Sam notices that there is no shower curtain and Marion finds torn paper in the toilet that Marion had used to calculate how much of the stolen money she had remaining. Sam tells Lila, "I don't like you going into that house alone," and she says, "I can handle a sick old woman." Hitchcock likes his jokes.

While Sam engages Norman, Lila goes toward the house. The camera is placed so that the house looms above. It seems to be moving toward Lila as much as she is headed toward it. She enters, goes upstairs, knocks on Mother's bedroom door, and walks in. There is no one there. The room is overloaded with Victorian knick-knacks. There is a startle when Lila sees herself in the mirror. Then she notices a depression in the bed, where Mother presumably spends most of her time. Lila goes upstairs to Norman's room, filled with childhood toys, a record player with the Eroica symphony, and a book that she has a strong reaction to (but we never see what's inside).

Meanwhile, Sam has accused Norman of stealing the money. Norman, of course, doesn't know anything about the money—he tossed it, unknowingly, into the trunk of the car. Suddenly Norman realizes that Lila must be in the house. He and Sam struggle and he hits Sam on the head with a bookend. Lila is coming down the stairs when she sees Norman coming up.

She looks for a place to hide—under the stairs is a door. Her curiosity is aroused; she opens it and sees Mother from behind, sitting in a chair. She touches her shoulder, the chair turns, and we see a shrunken skull. Lila screams, and flings her arm up knocking the overhead lightbulb, the violins shriek and Norman enters the room, wearing a dress and hairpiece, holding a knife, ready to attack. Sam rushes in and wrestles Norman, who shakes his head to conveniently make his wig fall off (so the slower members of the audience can be sure to realize it's him— one of the few really clumsy moments in the movie). The light from the swinging bulb makes it look as if the eyes of the taxidermy Mother are moving. It's both shocking and deeply unsettling.

Then we have an epilogue—to help the audience stop their own screaming and to give a logical construct to what seems so primal, so irrational, so disturbing. We are at the police station and the psychiatrist will explain all. He says, "I got the whole story, but not from Norman. I got it from his mother. Norman Bates no longer exists." Lila asks him if he killed her sister and the psychiatrist says, "Yes," but then launches into a digression with little sense of the terrible news he has just confirmed. He is too full of himself, too sure that he got it all, and quite insensitive to the implications of his story. This does not make psychiatrists look good.

He tells them that Norman killed his mother and her boyfriend, unable to tolerate that she had turned her attentions away from him. Then, he tried to "erase" his crime, the ultimate taboo: matricide. He stole her corpse, kept her body intact with chemicals, and began to "be her," keeping her as though alive and dressing in her clothes. When Norman would become attracted to a woman, the mother part of his persona would take over, and in her jealousy, she would attack and kill the object of his desires. The psychiatrist explains that Norman would not know that this had happened, but when he discovered what Mother had done, "like a dutiful son," he would cover all traces of her crime. "When the mind houses two personalities there is always a conflict; in Norman's case the battle is over and the dominant personality has won."

This whole sequence is the least energized, least convincing aspect of the movie. Was it necessary? For an audience of that time, very probably. They had never seen anything like this film, and the psychiatrist's explanation makes it seem rational and less disturbing. Its flatness also gives the audience time to catch its breath, to regroup, to settle. After all, this has been quite a wild ride. Before we see Norman/Mother for the last time, we need a pause, a moment of calm.

A guard brings Norman a blanket. He is sitting alone. The voice we hear is Mother, speaking as the camera closes in on Norman: "They know I can't even move a finger, and I won't. I'll just sit here and be quiet . . . They are probably watching me. Well, let them see what kind of a person I am." Norman looks down; there is a fly on his hand. Mother says, "I hope they are watching. They'll see . . . and they'll say, 'Why, she wouldn't even harm a fly.'" Norman looks up with a diabolic smile; the image of a skull is superimposed on his face and then we see a large chain: it's pulling Marion's car out of the muck of the pond. The End.

The viewer has been provided a visual image to match the psychiatrist's explanation. The dark forces that created this evil are being exposed to light. All will be well.

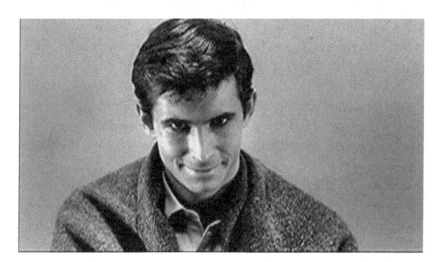

The Madness

The psychiatrist in the movie makes a compelling case for his formulation about Norman. But what exactly is he suggesting was wrong with him? What was his madness, separate from his being driven to kill women to whom he was sexually attracted? That's harder to pin down.

I've included this film in the book mostly because I find its effect on the history of our movie-going experience fascinating. Also, it points to the interesting diagnosis of multiple personality disorder, what is now called dissociative identity disorder or "DID."

I have never in my clinical practice seen a convincing case of this phenomenon. But I have colleagues who see it frequently. The *DSM* is aware of the difficulty making this diagnosis and the possibility of feigning the madness, especially for those who would use it to escape responsibility, and suggests ways of detecting someone who is pretending (those faking DID seem to enjoy having a second or third personality; they don't display the depression and shame that patients with this madness can experience; the amnesia that is a common symptom is often too conveniently placed, etc.). It made me wonder how much the clinician's interest might encourage patients to report the experience.

Patients want to please their therapists. They want to hold their doctor's attention; they want to be special. It's commonly part of the therapeutic process, especially with longer therapy relationships. Many treatment models are particularly interested, for instance, in the study of the dreams of their patients, the well-known "door to the unconscious." It's been shown that therapists can subtly show their patients what aspects of their dreams are most interesting, and over time, some patients will alter their dreams to match the therapeutic expectations of their doctor. So, the patient of an analyst who is a classic Freudian might report phallic or Oedipal dreams, while the patient of an analyst whose training follows the work of Carl Jung (with his universal archetypes) might wallow in myths. Whatever will keep your analyst awake and interested.

Could this be what happens with my colleagues who seem to specialize in multiple personalities? They perk up when something that looks like an alternate personality presents itself, so patients (particularly borderline or dependent personalities who can center their lives around their therapies with a desperate energy) are more likely to present those symptoms, almost like a gift.

Of course, the opposite could well be true. I might have simply had a blind spot to this because I was a skeptic. DID is notoriously difficult to diagnose. So, conceivably, because I wasn't looking for it, I might have missed the diagnosis even when it sat in my office. It happens.

Current literature has convinced me that DID is indeed real, but rare. Research suggests it is seen in 1 percent of the general population, close to the percentage of people with schizophrenia. Many of the review articles emphasize that the diagnosis is not easy to make: the therapist often has to dig deep because patients with this diagnosis often look like they may actually be suffering from other forms of madness (such as psychosis, rapid-cycling bipolar disorder, autism, or borderline personality disorder). This is one of the reasons the concerns about therapists encouraging the behaviors of DID were so persistent in the past.

DID rarely looks like it does in the movies, with dramatically different and separate identities, switching in real time; versions that have been compared to "possession." The multiple personality as seen in the films of the last fifty years or so is an exaggeration that seems encouraged by the public's fascination with the possibility of living other lives. First there were the fictionalized true stories starting with *Three Faces of Eve*, progressing to *Sybil* with her thirteen personalities, or "alters." The television film of her story starring Sally Field as Sybil and Joanne Woodward as her therapist was a major media event. Woodward portrayed Eve in the film that started this trend and won the Oscar as Best Actress for her performance (after the success of *Sybil* upped the ante, the real Eve later said that she actually had twenty-two alters, not the three in the title). Then, there were the completely invented stories, including the Showtime series *The United States of Tara* from 2009, starring Toni Collette, about a woman with DID who accumulated seven alters in the four seasons of the show.

These parts are catnip to actors, opportunities for them to display their ability to inhabit more than one character at a time, and sure to get awards recognition. That, and audience enthusiasm for the genre, has made this diagnosis very much a "flavor of the month" in movies and long-form television. What could be more seductive than, instead of being limited to one existence, you could try on a dozen distinct people and see how others might respond to you if you were very different—bolder, sexier, more confrontational, more sensitive, a different age, another gender?

How to understand this complicated diagnosis? I think of DID as an extreme version of the relatively common experience of "depersonalization." This is a symptom of anxiety: a sense that you are separate from yourself, that you are observing yourself from outside, as though you were watching yourself in a movie. It is related to "derealization," the sensation that people and things around you (your room, the furniture in it, the street outside, the people) are all somehow different, strange, not themselves, not real. Usually these are transient experiences, often at times of high stress; when the stress or anxiety decreases, so does this strange sensation of separation and oddness. But, for some, especially those who were traumatized early in their lives, it can develop a permanence, a particularity that resembles a different self—the "alter" of the DID diagnosis.

How might this apply to Norman? In DID as defined in the *DSM-5*, the patient displays two or more distinct personalities, and it is rare for the different personalities to be noticeably distinct to the observer. The way the disorder normally presents itself is with a hard-to-define discontinuity of your sense of who you are and with repeated episodes of amnesia. The dissociation is felt as depersonalization, the sense that you are experiencing thoughts and perceptions that you don't feel in control of, that your way of talking and thinking has suddenly changed. Some of these sensations can be noticed by others; many cannot. The amnesia shows itself by not knowing how you got somewhere, or where something in your possession came from, finding clothes in your closet that you never would have chosen, or finding writing or a drawing that is obviously yours but that you don't remember doing.

This is how most multiple personalities are said to present. The ones that make the novels and that show up in movies are called "possession-form" and are statistically very rare. Studies suggest that only a fraction of those with DID will have the sort of dramatic presentation you see in the movies, where the person seems to be "taken over" by another with a change of posture, voice, way of talking, way of dressing, and often showing a different sense of moral and personal values.

In this manifestation, usually one persona does not know what is happening, but other personalities are fully aware, so that the amnesia is specific, usually to the "original" personality, the one most friends and family are familiar with.

The idea that Norman would not know what Mother has done fits this paradigm. That he would feel a strong need to undo it, to clean up after what she has done also fits. However, we are told that Norman was disturbed long before he began to put on Mother's clothing. He was so tied to her in life that, when she took a lover, he jealously killed them both. Only then did he begin the transformation of becoming Mother/Norman. We will never know what his being "disturbed" looked like before he murdered his mother and her lover. Perhaps he was experiencing other personalities then. If so, that would strengthen the diagnosis. But we can't know—there is no one to ask.

I don't think the television shows and movie sequels based on *Psycho* are helpful here. One sequel is actually a prequel (*Psycho IV: The Beginning*, 1990), which is meant to give us Norman's backstory. The writers have a field day coming up with complications to keep us engaged: Norman's mother, Norma, was institutionalized for schizophrenia. Except she wasn't actually his mother . . . and so on. None of these sequels hold a candle to the original, and I want to limit our discussion to Hitchcock's vision.

Putting on clothes and a wig to complete the experience of being Mother doesn't fit the concept of multiple personality. The person whose persona changes may dress differently, but it's because that is the way the persona dresses, not in imitation of someone else. It's a very different dynamic.

Norman dressing as Mother and keeping her body there to feel closer to her seems to me a more psychotic solution than a dissociation. If he believes Mother is alive and talking with him, even as he mimics her voice and wears her clothes, then we are dealing with a delusion, a psychosis like schizophrenia, not a dissociative disorder. With a delusional disorder, Norman might dress up as Mother when he murders Marion, but he would remember the murder and not express such surprise and dismay at seeing her covered in blood. So, that doesn't quite fit, either.

The wearing of his mother's dress and a "cheap hairpiece" does not imply that Norman is a transvestite or has a gender identity problem.

The psychiatrist in the film rather too casually confirms that, and he is correct. What we are seeing here, I think, is a deadly, twisted psychotic version of a child's imaginary playmate. Norman is dressing this way to make more real his delusion that Mother is still alive. This is madness, but it has nothing to do with gender identity dysphoria and it does not really look like DID. However, at the end we do see a profound identity disorder: not about his gender, but about who he is. As the psychiatrist says, "He was never all Norman, but he was often only Mother."

So, once again, we have a bit of a mash-up of madness. We are left with the psychiatrist's explanation in the movie. What we have seen, startling and unforgettable, does not lend itself to a simple diagnosis. And not to impose one wisely preserves the film's impact.

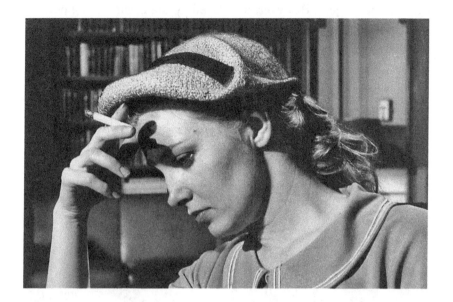

The Three Faces of Eve (1957)

Joanne Woodward, Lee J. Cobb
Director: Nunnally Johnson

Eve White, a housewife in 1950s Georgia, is brought to the psychiatrist by her husband. She has had bad headaches and episodes of amnesia. The doctor discovers that she has another personality, Eve Black, who, unlike the meek, submissive Eve White, is a bit of a hell-raiser. Her husband accuses her of buying expensive clothes and treating their daughter badly, but it turns out the culprit is Eve Black. Later, Eve tells the doctor she is hearing voices, and is reassured by him that this doesn't mean she is "going crazy." But what they discover together is that there is a third personality, Jane, who is aware of the other two personalities and is the happy medium between the two.

If this sounds formulaic, even with the unusual subject of multiple personality, it's because it is. Much of the film is like an illustrated lecture on the subject. However, it is saved by the mesmerizing performance of Joanne Woodward in only her second starring role. She is totally convincing when she shifts from one personality to the other, changing her accent, her tone of voice, her posture, her gestures. But did they have to use the music in such a heavy-handed way? Every time she changes personality the music hits you over the head to announce the change (dull for Eve White, honky-tonk sexy for Eve Black, just to be sure you "get it").

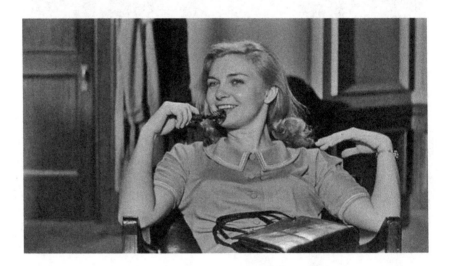

This was the first movie to feature multiple personality. It was based on a book by Hervey Cleckley, MD, who also wrote *The Mask of Sanity* about the psychopath. The producers must have thought that they had to make it absolutely clear that this really happened. They recruited Alistair Cooke to introduce the film and explain that it was based on a real person and a real illness. (Cooke was a British journalist who was well known as the presenter of a television show called *Omnibus*, a unique program of classical music, jazz, opera, and excerpts from Broadway plays and musicals. At that time in the 1950s, commercial stations were obligated to include "high culture" in the mix of situation comedies and Westerns. Cooke, with his engaging British manner, represented high-toned authenticity.)

Unlike most of the films in this book, *The Three Faces of Eve* feels dated. The pace is slow and, other than Joanne Woodward, the performances, to me at least, seem stilted. Nonetheless, it takes seriously not only the portrayal of Eve's madness but how it affects her husband and daughter. It is thoughtful about the nature of her therapy, which becomes an exploration of the childhood traumas that might have precipitated this dissociative illness. The film is worth seeing for its historical importance, and especially for Woodward's Oscar-winning performance.

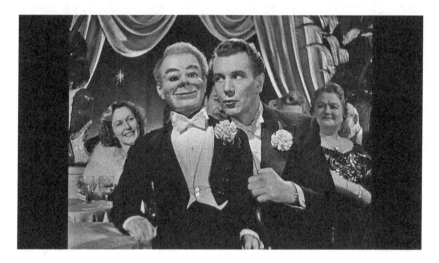

Dead of Night (1945)

"The Ventriloquist's Dummy" episode
Michael Redgrave
Director: Alberto Cavalcanti

This classic British horror film is an anthology of stories all told by a group who gather in a country house. One of the guests insists he has a sense of déjà vu, that he has been there before with these very people. Discussing whether they believe in such things and in the supernatural, they each tell a story of a strange occurrence they have witnessed. It's the final story that interests us here: "The Ventriloquist's Dummy." However, the whole film is worth enjoying. The first of its kind, it turns out that the central story of the guests in the house is a supernatural tale of its own, feeding back on itself. It definitely brings chills and is the forerunner of many other films with a similar conceit.

The last story stars Michael Redgrave (a Shakespearean actor of great reputation then, and the father of actress and political activist Vanessa Redgrave). He is Maxwell Frere, a successful ventriloquist with a dummy called Hugo Fitch. Hugo, dressed formally in tails, enjoys pushing boundaries. It's their act. But increasingly it seems that Maxwell is not fully in control of what Hugo says. Maxwell seems high-strung, very insecure, and he drinks too much. When Sylvester Kee, an American ventriloquist, introduces himself, Maxwell becomes suspicious that he wants to steal Hugo. Hugo encourages that idea. When Maxwell tries to keep him quiet by putting his hand over Hugo's mouth, Hugo bites him, leaving him bleeding. Just who is in charge here? Then Hugo goes missing and Maxwell hysterically accuses the American and shoots him. He is put in jail and refuses to cooperate with his psychologist until they give him Hugo, declaring, "He's more to blame for all this than I am." When they bring Hugo to Maxwell in his prison cell, Maxwell shudders, then embraces him, but Hugo nastily says it wouldn't suit him to wait for Maxwell while he is in jail so he'll be looking for a new partner. Maxwell, on the verge of tears, pleads with him: "You wouldn't run out on me now?" As Hugo continues to taunt him, Maxwell puts a pillow over his face and then stomps on him. The observer reacts as though he has killed a person. Afterward, Maxwell becomes silent and unresponsive, catatonic. The prison psychiatrist (who is the guest telling this story) asks Kee, who was only wounded, to approach Maxwell—maybe seeing him will bring him out of it. But Kee is wary. After all, Maxwell shot him. When he reluctantly agrees to go, Maxwell does indeed begin to speak, but in the voice of Hugo. In an amazing acting tour de force, he appears exactly as though he is now the dummy.

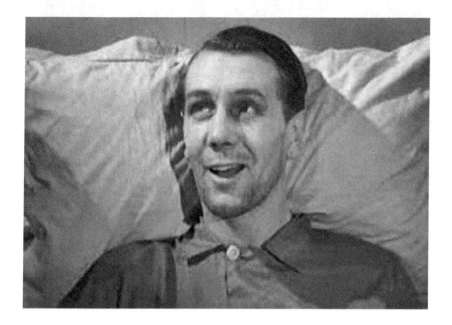

So, in this story we have a version of two personalities in one person. But in this case, the personalities are the dummy and his handler; it becomes less and less clear which is which. This idea, which is usually couched in supernatural terms, was the inspiration for many horror films to come, including *Magic,* with Anthony Hopkins the *Chucky* franchise, and even an episode of *The Twilight Zone.*

This is obviously not DID as described in the *DSM,* but it could well be understood as a variant of it, another version of dissociation, where the person feels disconnected from himself, in a world that seems strangely "wrong." Or the person could be clearly psychotic, with the delusion that he is possessed by the dummy. In many ways it's closer to Norman in *Psycho* than most other movies suggestive of DID.

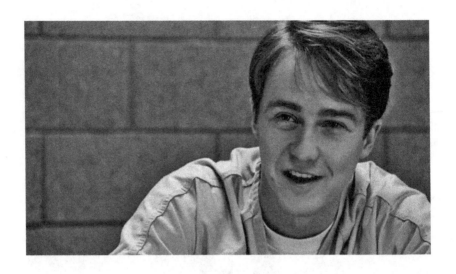

Primal Fear (1996)

Richard Gere, Edward Norton
Director: Gregory Hoblit

If you want to see a really convincing transition of personalities, then this is the film for you. It's a very good mystery thriller, with a career-making performance by Edward Norton in his first film, as Aaron, accused of murdering a priest. Aaron stutters, is hesitant, speaks in whispers, and is constantly looking at the floor. He sure looks like "he couldn't hurt a fly." He claims he was in the room when the murder happened, but that he blacked out, something that happens to him often, and he woke up covered in blood. Frances McDormand plays a psychiatrist interviewing him, and she pushes him to explain his relationship with Linda, a friend, asking him questions he says are too personal. He suddenly aggressively tells her to "leave him the fuck alone" so that she edges to the door. Then, just as suddenly, Aaron is timid and quiet again.

His lawyer, Martin Vail (Richard Gere), comes into the interview room and presses Aaron, telling him that he needs to know the truth: did he kill the priest? He will defend him whether or not he is guilty, he just has to know. In a fascinating and intense scene, Vail yells at him, "I don't fucking believe you. . . . You did it, didn't you?" Aaron turns away, hitting his head against the wall. Suddenly he turns, looking at Vail, and in a different voice says, "Who the fuck are you?" Vail asks, "Who the fuck are you?" Aaron kicks a chair and gets in the lawyer's face. We discover his name is Roy. He says, "You're his lawyer, ain't you?" as though he had not met him before. "I heard about you." Vail asks, "Where is Aaron?" and Roy says, "Aaron's crying' off in some corner somewhere—you scared him off! You've got to deal with me now, boy," then he slams the lawyer against the wall. Roy tells him never to act tough with Aaron, and Vail says, "Aaron gets into trouble, he calls you." Roy says, "Aaron don't have the guts to do nothin'. It was me, boy." Then a few moments later, Roy is gone and it's Aaron wondering what just happened.

Norton's performance is brilliant, the moments of transition well defined, the details of behavior just right. The backstory fits as well: the headaches, the blackouts, a traumatic childhood. This is what the most dramatic forms of DID, multiple personality, can look like. The story builds from there, and I won't spoil it by telling you what happens, but it's probably not what you think.

RECOMMENDED READING

Bass, Saul. Storyboard for the shower scene from Psycho. 1960.

> The complete storyboard, which certainly looks like it guided the editing. And then, selected panels comparing them with the actual film, where you can see what Hitchcock added: "Psycho 1960 - The Shower Scene: Storyboards by Saul Bass," https://www.youtube.com/watch?v=taRL9LF3XGo; "Who directed the shower scene in PSYCHO?," https://www.youtube.com/watch?v=RHas6iZ5bhE.

Bloch, Robert. *Psycho*. New York: Simon and Schuster; 1959.

> A compulsively good read. An example of how Hitchcock transformed and improved on the original.

Brand, Bethany L., Vedal Sar, and Pam Stavropoulos et al. Separating Fact from Fiction: An Empirical Examination of Six Myths About Dissociative Identity Disorder. *Harvard Review of Psychiatry*. 2016 Jul; 24(4): 257–270. Available at: https://www.ncbi.nlm.nih.gov/pmc/articles/PMC4959824/.

Greenberg, Harvey Roy. *Screen Memories: Hollywood Cinema on the Psychoanalytic Couch*. New York: Columbia University Press; 1994.

Specifically, chapter 5, "The Apes at the Windows," on *Psycho*. A remarkable collection of essays, with close psychoanalytic readings of classic films.

Loewenstein, Richard J. Dissociation debates: everything you know is wrong. *Dialogues in Clinical Neuroscience*. 2018 Sep; 20(3): 229–242. Available at: https://www.ncbi.nlm.nih.gov/pmc/articles/PMC6296396/.

Wood, Robin. *Hitchcock's Films, Revisited*. New York: Columbia University Press; 2002.

A revision of one of the first books to take Hitchcock seriously as a master of cinema.

▪8▪

"Goodnight, Daddy. Hold my hand."

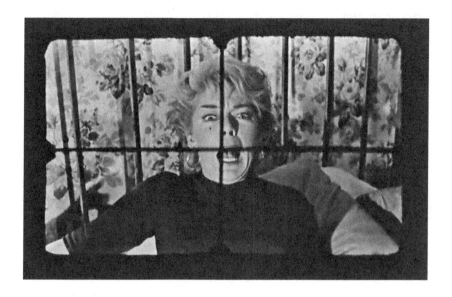

Are We All Voyeurs?

A FILMMAKER'S UNDOING

Peeping Tom (1960)

Karlheinz Böhm, Anna Massey, Moira Shearer
Director: Michael Powell; Screenplay: Leo Marks

The first image is of an eye. We've seen this before—in *Taxi Driver* and *Repulsion*, a sign that we will be getting a close look at the inner experience of a major character. But in this film, the eye will mean something more: this will be a film about "watching."

The eye here is first closed, then open, and we see a prostitute in a dark street, the figure of a man some ways away. There is the sound of whistling, a hint of what is to come. Famously, the serial killer in the early sound film "M," starring Peter Lorre, whistled as he tracked his prey. You don't need to know this association for it to affect you—it's eerie on its own.

Then, there is a close-up of a Bell and Howell movie camera tucked in a coat; the camera lens comes closer to us, blurring, and suddenly we are looking through the camera viewfinder at the prostitute, who names her price. We have shifted from "seeing" with our eyes to seeing through a viewfinder, as the camera "sees." This is new.

The camera looks her up and down and then follows her as she leads us down an alley and upstairs to her room (this is Newman's Passage, a real location associated with Jack the Ripper; these days, rather less threateningly, it houses a great place to get traditional English meat pies). We watch through the viewfinder as the prostitute, Dora, settles in the room and begins to undress. The camera moves puzzlingly away for a moment and then we see her, with a bright light shining in her face, look startled and then increasingly frightened. She screams in terror as we come closer and closer, and there is a cut to a movie projector. We see a man sitting next to the projector, watching the same scene, now in black and white on a screen. The black-and-white image becomes larger as the movie's title appears: *Peeping Tom*. As the credits continue, we watch him watching; now, we are seeing the film that fills the screen, and then the man again as he rises excited from his chair, and then sits, disappointed. Over an image of the projector is the name of the film's director: Michael Powell.

This is the remarkable beginning to a remarkable film. As we have seen in other movies by directors in full control of their effects, this one summarizes its subject and its theme in the first moments, over the credits. Think of *Strangers on a Train* with crossing views of Bruno and Guy in the train station, ending with an image of crossed train tracks, and *Taxi Driver* with Travis's eye surveying the blurred images of the city.

Peeping Tom was a radical departure from the sort of films that Michael Powell, its director, had made before. He had partnered for nearly two decades with Emeric Pressburger making prestige films, some with patriotic themes like *The Life and Death of Colonel Blimp*, following its lead character (played by Roger Livesey) through three wars, and *Stairway to Heaven (A Matter of Life and Death)* with David Niven as a pilot who dies too soon. They made very popular, grand melodramas such as *The Red Shoes*, a film that is credited with sending a generation of young girls to ballet class, and *Black Narcissus*, with Deborah Kerr as a nun in the Himalayas. These were uplifting films, ones you could take your family to. *Peeping Tom* was Powell's second film without Pressburger, and it was shockingly different from anything before.

One reason it was so different is that the screenplay was not co-written by Pressburger, as all Powell's other films had been, but by someone new, Leo Marks. Marks led a very interesting life outside of movies, one that helps us understand a lot about this movie.

Leo Marks was the son of the owner of Marks and Co., an antiquarian bookstore of some renown in England, located at 84 Charing Cross Road in the bookshop center of London. Marks grew up playing in the aisles of that store. He was an observant and very intelligent child. One day he noticed the numbers and letters written in pencil inside each book in the shop. Intrigued, he asked what they meant. He was told that it was a code, a code that indicated how much the store had paid for the book and what price they wanted to sell it for. Young Leo spent some time studying and figured out the code. It was the beginning of his life's work.

He became a cryptographer and, during the Second World War, he headed the codes office in support of agents placed behind the lines in occupied Europe. At the time, the codes were tied to famous poems, which worked but was rather too easy for the enemy to figure out. Marks came up with the idea of basing them on original poems he would write and the agents could memorize. No chance of the Germans knowing these ciphers! He also invented the use of silk handkerchiefs with ciphers on them that could be used once and then discarded, increasing their security. His work during the war was a secret until he published his memoir in 1998, *Between Silk and Cyanide: A Codemakers Story 1941-1945*, but it informed much of *Peeping Tom*, a film filled with wordplay and codes. It's no coincidence that the lead character's name is Mark Lewis, a simple inverse of Leo Marks. Or that Mark is presented as a mystery who needs to be decoded to understand why he does what he does. We will see lots of examples as we look more closely at the film.

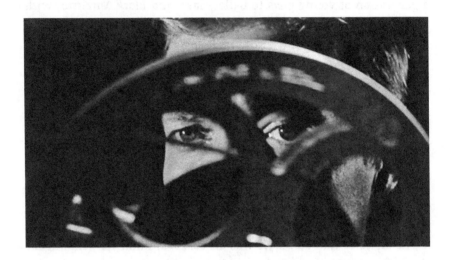

There is a lot to unpack. Aspects of the production that affect how we see the movie. Mark is played by Karlheinz Böhm (or Boehm), a German actor, the son of the orchestra conductor Karl Böhm. Michael Powell has said that when he auditioned Böhm for the part he knew he would be good because he "would know what it's like to have a controlling father." Böhm's slight German accent works well here; it's hard to pin down, but it gives him a sense of "otherness" that works.

Helen, the young woman whom he befriends, is played by Anna Massey. This was her second film. She was beginning what would be a highly regarded and long career on the stage. Her father was a famous figure too: Raymond Massey, a distinguished Canadian actor and movie star, who played Abraham Lincoln in the biographical film, *Abe Lincoln in Illinois* (1940). The little boy, Mark, whom we see in the home movies, is played by Colomba Powell, Michael Powell's son. And Professor Lewis, Mark's father, is played by Michael Powell himself. Some very powerful and demanding fathers both on-screen and off.

Moira Shearer is Viv; a small part that she makes vivid (sorry, the punning in this movie is contagious). Shearer was a major star. She played the ballerina in *The Red Shoes* and was principal ballerina in the Sadler's Wells Ballet of London. Her character, Viv, is violently killed. At the time the film was released something like this was unheard of and shocking; you just didn't kill a star. A few months later, *Psycho* came out in England, and Janet Leigh, an even bigger star, was done in too.

There was a significant difference between the two films. Leigh is introduced as the central character of *Psycho*, so that her death midway through is completely unexpected and disturbing, while we don't meet Viv until halfway through, learn little about her, and almost immediately realize she will be Mark's next victim.

The first reviews of *Peeping Tom* were devastating. Here are some examples:

The Star: "A film which, despite its brilliant technical skill, nauseated me."

The Daily Express: "Nothing—neither the hopeless leper colonies of East Pakistan, the back streets of Bombay nor the gutters of Calcutta— has left me with such a feeling of nausea and depression as I got this week while sitting through a new British film called *Peeping Tom*."

The Observer: "It's a long time since a film disgusted me as much as *Peeping Tom*."

The Daily Worker (the Communist newspaper): "From its slumbering, mildly salacious beginning to its appallingly masochistic and depraved climax, it is wholly evil."

The Sunday Express: "As a thriller, it fails to thrill. As a shocker, it succeeds only in being nauseating for the sake of nausea. This is a sick film—sick and nasty."

The Sunday Times: "He cannot wash his hands of responsibility for this essentially vicious film."

The Tribune: "The only really satisfactory way to dispose of Peeping Tom would be to shovel it up and flush it swiftly down the nearest sewer. Even then the stench would remain."

There is a level of hysteria in these reviews. "Nauseated . . . disgusted . . . wholly evil . . . sick and nasty . . . vicious . . . a stench"? Something in this film made them *very* uncomfortable. This is not ordinary disapproval.

How do we understand such extreme reactions? Granting that "the past is a foreign country; they do things differently there" (the famous opening lines of *The Go-Between* by L. P. Hartley), though the calendar said 1960 when *Peeping Tom* was released it was in fact very much a 1950s button-down time in England, a very button-down country. The cultural transformations of the mid-1960s were some years off. Even so, the vitriolic reviews take one aback with their ferocity.

Powell and the film's distributors were so demoralized by these reviews that they withdrew the film almost immediately.

I find myself wondering what might have happened if they had had more confidence in what they had produced. What if they had tried to "turn lemons into lemonade" and put up adverts (as they say in England) plastered with excerpts from the worst reviews, with the challenge to "see the movie and decide for yourself!" It's the sort of thing Alfred Hitchcock might have done. He was very good at thinking outside the box and coming up with creative and amusing ways to sell something difficult. It might not have gone down well in that time—I'm not sure how open people were to making up their own minds in the 1950s—but maybe it might have given *Peeping Tom* the audience it deserved.

These reviews pretty much ended the career of its director. Michael Powell was not able to make another major film for close to a decade, and the few films he made went nowhere. He was done.

This was a strikingly different outcome from what happened with Hitchcock's *Psycho* when it was released just a few months later. Both directors released films very different from what the public expected. Powell was famous for larger-than-life stories with a broad canvas, rich use of TechniColor, and exotic locales. Hitchcock made thrillers leavened with a sense of dark humor. His *Psycho* was a low-budget film, in black and white, and though it had genuine stars in Janet Leigh and Anthony Perkins, it seemed at first to be a small story, set in small-town America. Though it was in color, *Peeping Tom* was also a low-budget picture, but its effect was very different. Instead of an exhilarated delight in the twists of its plot, it generated a feeling of disgust in the reviewers. How the original audience felt we shall never know because they hardly had a chance to see the movie. It was pulled from distribution a week after it opened in England, and had a very short run in the States.

I think Hitchcock learned from the dismal experience of Powell. He was smart about public relations in a way Powell was not. Powell paid little attention to how his films were promoted. The name of "The Archers," his company with Pressburger, was enough to draw an audience. Though Pressburger had nothing to do with *Peeping Tom*, "The Archers" were credited as producers (the Archers logo—an arrow shot into a bullseye—is the opening credit). That gave a false impression of what sort of movie it might be, which might have been the beginning of the reviewers' violently negative reactions.

Hitchcock did not allow the press to see *Psycho* before its release. So, by the time the reviews came out, many people had already seen the film and were excitedly talking about it.

Psycho of course is a different movie, and many would consider it a more successful one (not just because it burnished Hitchcock's career and made him a fortune). In that film, we do not know who the murderer is, or why he murders, until the very end. We are kept very much in suspense. And of course, there is the shocking murder of its marquee star halfway through the movie. All this made *Psycho* a sensation.

Though I greatly admire *Peeping Tom*, it is simply not as entertaining or as clever as *Psycho*. Or, more accurately, it's too clever for its own good. All the verbal and visual puns don't sit well with the subject of a voyeur who murders women. Also, we know right away who the murderer is; there is no mystery and little suspense. There is wonderful gothic atmosphere, and we are curious about how he kills and why, but is that enough to make the murders palatable enough to recommend the film to your friends? Powell does the unthinkable—he kills off a major star in Moira Shearer. But the effect is less dramatic;

we aren't allowed to become as invested in her as we are in Janet Leigh before she takes her last shower. For all its formal brilliance, *Peeping Tom* lacks the jolts, the unexpected twists, and the occasional humor of *Psycho*. It also lacks the remarkable performance of Anthony Perkins and the sympathetic one of Janet Leigh.

So, I don't think that marketing or courting other critics to counteract the first reviews would have made that much of a difference in the box office. But it might have rescued Michael Powell's career enough so that he could have continued making movies. That he couldn't is sad.

Ultimately, Hitchcock was a better showman than Powell, both in his directorial choices and in how he sold his movies.

It is thanks to the director Martin Scorsese that we can see *Peeping Tom* today. Scorsese tells how he was haunted from his early days studying film with stories about this movie that was so hard to find after it was withdrawn. After he saw it in 1970, he thought that it was brilliant and original.

Scorsese arranged for a restored version of the film to be released in the late 1970s, and it was immediately hailed as a lost masterpiece. Today it is on several lists of the best horror films ever made; the magazine *Total Film* named it the twenty-fourth greatest British film of all time. Fortunately, Powell was alive to enjoy the new recognition, however belated. He died in 1990.

The Movie

After the opening credits, *Peeping Tom* continues the next morning, again through the camera viewfinder. We have not yet seen the face of the cameraman-murderer. At first his face remains hidden by the camera; then we see he is a quiet-voiced young man, who, when asked "What newspaper do you work for?," says with a small smile, "*The Observer*." That is a well-regarded newspaper in London; the first of many verbal and visual jokes in an otherwise serious film. He is indeed an observer . . . of the aftermath of the murder he committed the night before.

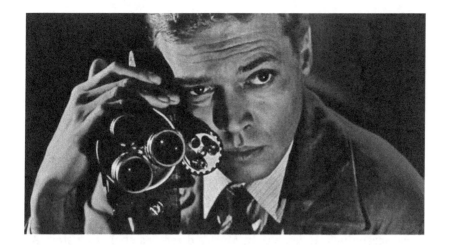

We next see him at a newspaper shop, where we watch him watching (this will be a repeated theme) as a mild-mannered elderly gentleman asks about "views," pictures of naked women, soft-core pornography. We discover that Mark is the photographer taking the pictures upstairs. The introduction of a schoolgirl who comes to buy candy returns us to the ordinary: her innocence is in sharp contrast with the sleaziness. Then we are upstairs, and we see Mark fascinated by a new girl with a facial scar. Millie, who has been doing this for a long time, asks him to photograph her so the "bruises don't show"—she has been beaten by her boyfriend. She asks him to "make us famous" and he tells her to "look at the sea"; there is no "sea" (or "see") and that confuses her, but it creates the exact expression he is looking to photograph.

Now we have one of Powell's clever transitions: as the nude model Millie pours tea, we cut to whiskey being poured at Helen's birthday party. Helen is the young woman who lives in Mark's building. They have never actually met. The whiskey is being poured by Helen's blind mother. Mark peers in the window: one of the rare moments when he really is a "peeping tom." Helen is curious about him; after all, he lives in the room upstairs. She asks how long he has lived there, and he tells her he grew up in this house; in fact, he owns it. She asks him to join her party and, when he demurs, she later comes upstairs to bring him a piece of birthday cake. Helen notices his back room, asks if he was watching films, and asks to see them as "a birthday present from you to me." She follows him into an enormous darkroom suffused with red; she bumps into things in the dark, fascinated by the cameras, the developing chemicals, the projector and screen. Mark explains, "This room belonged to my father; he was a scientist."

She asks Mark what film he was watching. We know it was the killing of the prostitute Dora which is essentially a "snuff" film, and he almost shows her that, then changes his mind. Instead, he shows her his father's movies of him as a child. Piano music accompanies these screenings. Helen sits in Mark's director's chair to watch. As Mark starts to show the film he says, "This is the first . . . twenty-first birthday present I'll ever have given."

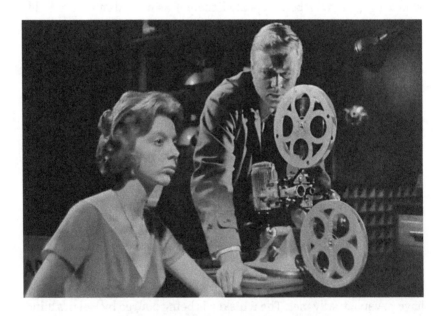

We see Mark as a boy, spying on lovers in the park (of course his father is spying on him in making this film). Then we see a lizard on the sleeping boy's bed; the boy awakens, frightened. We hear the father's voice, a whisper: "That will do Mark, dry your eyes and stop being silly." Mark wants to film Helen as she watches, but she refuses him. A smart move because we have seen what happens when Mark films a woman.

The movie shifts to the boy standing next to his mother's dead body. Mark refers to this as "the next sequence," as though moments of his life are only sequences in a movie. He then shows "her replacement," Mark's new stepmother. Mark's father, whom we see for the first time in the movie, gives him a gift—a camera—and Powell shows us that camera sitting on a shelf, the beginning of Mark's collection. Helen turns off the projector; she has seen enough. She demands, "What kind of scientist was your father?" Mark tells her he made a study of the neurologic responses to fear. He shows her his father's many books: "I'm sure good will come of it, for someone." The father seems to be fetishizing a sadistic gaze; looking at someone in pain or fear and calling it a scientific study. We will discover that Mark is doing his father one better. End of Act One.

We now see a close-up of Helen's birthday cake, we hear "cut" in the voice of a director, and we indeed cut to a soundstage where a commercial film is being made. Another of Powell's sly verbal/visual jokes. Here, in a parody of filmmaking, an actress is a victim of the dictatorial director, demanding that she faint "better," and that she do it over and over until she gets it right. The director is called Arthur Baden. Anyone English would think of Robert Baden-Powell, the founder of the Boy Scouts. Michael Powell is fully aware that he, too, is implicated in the consequences of being a watcher, as well as a maker of films.

Mark is a focus-puller at the studio. His job is to be sure the camera is always in proper focus; essentially, he is an assistant to the cameraman. But tonight he has another agenda. He will be meeting with Viv (Moira Shearer), a stand-in to the star. For the first time the film is not from his point of view. We follow Viv as she eagerly gets ready for her moment. We know she is walking into a trap. The image reminds us of Dora, the streetwalker at Newman's Passage. Viv walks hesitantly onto the darkened stage; she whistles, knowing she is being watched. Where is Mark? Then, blinded by the spotlight—a metaphor of power—we see Mark on a platform, descending from above. "I've put the red light on—they won't interrupt us."

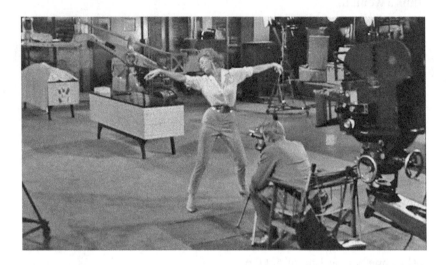

Viv dances to warm up. Shearer does a wonderful job, I think, in bringing Viv to life for the brief moments we have to know her. Her warm-up dancing to the jazz music shows a love of movement and of being in the moment. Her curiosity about Mark's filming—asking to look through the camera lens and imagining she is her own director— underscores the liveliness that is about to be snuffed out.

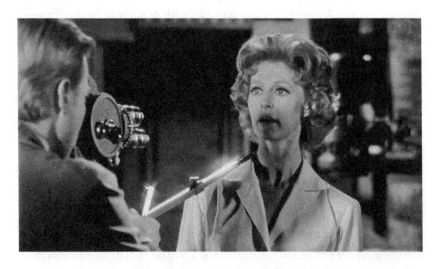

For the first time we see Mark's weapon: a very phallic tripod leg that, unsheathed, becomes a bayonet aimed at Viv's throat. And soon, once again we see the victim's terror, looking at something even more frightening than the weapon that is about to kill.

Then there is another visual joke. And here we may see a part of why the reaction to this movie was so strong. We have witnessed two murders, yet the story never gives us a moment to pause and feel proper dismay at the loss of life. In contrast, after the attack on Marion in *Psycho*, we watch her dying; we see her reach out to grab the shower curtain, which she drags over her as she collapses on the edge of the tub; we see the bloody water swirling into the drain; we fade on her dead eye; moments later, there is a long, dialogue-free sequence showing Norman cleaning away evidence of the murder. This gives us time to absorb what has just happened and serves to change the focus from Marion to Norman.

Instead, in *Peeping Tom,* we get another visual pun. Are the makers of this movie so very callous as not to realize the effect of their story on the audience? Or is the self-consciousness of these jokes a way of "not feeling," of saying, "It's just a story, don't take it too seriously?" Whichever, it begins to grate, even as you might admire its wit.

What's the joke this time? Very much the same as with the birthday cake. We see Helen's blind mother pouring out a finger of whiskey, and we cut to Mark pouring the film chemicals that will develop the movie of Viv's murder.

Now the story slows down and we see more of Mark's relationship with Helen. She is writing a children's book about a magic camera. She asks, will Mark take the photos for the book? He is delighted, with a child-like excitement. Later, he gives her a birthday present: a brooch which she tries to decide how to wear. As she puts the brooch on her left side, then on the right, Mark mirrors her movements. He is a camera, taking her picture.

At the studio, the police are interrogating everyone about Viv's murder. Mark seems very calm, chatting with his friend about the latest film playing in town. Jokingly, noticing his calm, the friend says, "Mark, are you crazy?" His reply: "Yes, do you think they will notice?"

As I pointed out before, there has been no mystery in this film about who the killer is. We know before the credits are done. The only mystery that remains is, why is he doing this? The only suspense is, will he be caught? The investigating police come across as authority figures; much like Mark's father, their job is to try to decode the crime, but they don't see what is in front of them. Mark remains calm until the policeman questioning him asks to hold his camera. As he examines it, you can see Mark desperate to grab it back from him. It's like a part of his anatomy, and this is a violation.

Compare his general calm when engaging with the police to his obvious anxiety when talking with Helen's mother later that day. She asks him about his intentions with Helen. "I feel—I can't describe it, I can only film it," he says. We hear the sound of Mark's heartbeat—Mrs. Stevens makes him nervous because, unlike the police, she can "see" him. Minutes before, when he had peeked again into their window, she knew he was there: "The back of my neck told me." There is an odd film moment here too. We glimpse a curtain being drawn to reveal his meeting with Helen in her living room. Again, a reminder of the artifice of the movies? That this is more a stage than real life? Or does it say, in another way, that Mrs. Stevens sees him with her inner eye?

That evening Helen and Mark go on a date to discuss her book. We have never seen Mark without his camera, but we have seen how very uncomfortable he is to be separated from it. So, when Helen asks him to leave it behind on their date, he is reluctant. But he does, leaving it in his mother's old bedroom. He tells her he will never photograph her: "Whatever I photograph I always lose."

As they are walking, he sees lovers kissing and he reaches for his camera, but it isn't there. As they enjoy the meal we cut back and forth to the film timer in Mark's laboratory, ticking ticking, timing the development of the movie of Viv's murder. Even enjoying a moment of normality, Mark can't stop obsessing about his project, his movies of fear and death.

After they arrive home, Helen asks him not to watch his films that night. He can't promise that. After she gives him a good night kiss, he kisses the camera lens. Creating a memory.

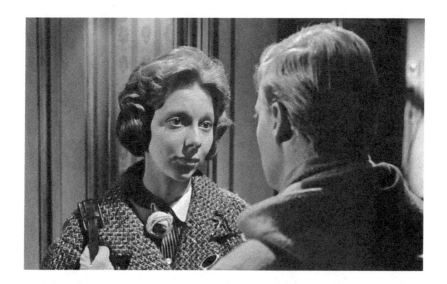

Then, back in his movie laboratory, which more and more resembles the clichéd "mad scientist's lair," he is projecting the film of Viv's death, when he realizes that Helen's mother is there. "I visit this room every night. The blind always live in the rooms they live under," she says. She sees Mark's room with her stick, also pointed like his deadly tripod, but she can't see his snuff film. As Mark stands in front of the screen, Viv's frightened face is projected on his back, and it looks like a skull. This is something that Helen's mother cannot see.

Mark begins to open his tripod weapon against Mrs. Stevens and she feels fear, backing up against the movie screen, but because she can't see, she is not frightened in the same way as the others. Mark collapses, impotent at her blind power. Her instinct, "which can't be photographed," tells her he is troubled. She insists that he get help. If he doesn't, he will not be allowed to see Helen again; in fact, they will move away. "I will never photograph her," he promises. As she leaves, she photographs his face, her hands "taking a picture." There are so many ways to see. End of Act Two.

The next day, the police are still investigating Viv's murder. A psychiatrist is watching from a low platform and Mark goes to talk to him. He tells him of his father's research. The doctor has heard of his father and admires him. Mark asks about being a "peeping tom," and the psychiatrist recognizes that Professor Lewis might indeed have been interested in such a thing—"scoptophilia—the morbid urge to gaze." This is hardly a full description of what drives Mark, but never mind for now. When asked about treatment, the doctor assures him it can be treated "four times a week, it can be cured in three or four years." This is not what Mark needs to hear. But it is another example of someone who does not "see." This psychiatrist jokes that, like Mark, he too is a focus-puller. But he doesn't focus on what is in front of him, that this is someone in despair and desperately asking for help.

We see that the police suspect Mark and are following him. So, we have a sequence of Mark being watched as we watch him being watched. At the news shop he meets up with Millie. From the window Mark films the policeman watching him. We begin to understand that his filming is not just to document fear, but to document his murders and their discovery. Then we see Millie, played by Pamela Green, a real-life pin-up model who earlier had made "naturist movies." She is posed on a bed, and we know she will be the next victim, that she will be killed even with the police just outside. We see a glimpse of her naked breasts; a first for a commercial movie in England.

The final sequence is powerful and gothic in its details and intensity. Helen's curiosity gets the better of her and she turns on the film in Mark's projector, which shows the murder of Viv. The disturbing piano theme begins, and we see a close-up of Helen's face, watching. Anna Massey gives us a master class in acting. We watch her face registering what she is seeing: first puzzlement, then shock, then fear. She backs away, not wanting to see but not able to stop looking, and is startled (as we in the audience are) by Mark. "I can't see you frightened," he says. "It's just a film, isn't it?" she asks. "What did you do to those girls, Mark?"

Mark explains his secrets. As he turns on multiple recording devices, we hear that his father has recorded every moment in Mark's life, and of the lives now in the house. "Do you know what the most frightening thing in the world is?" he asks. "Fear." He pulls out a big, distorting mirror—this is the light that each victim saw just before she was killed. Her own reflection, her own terror.

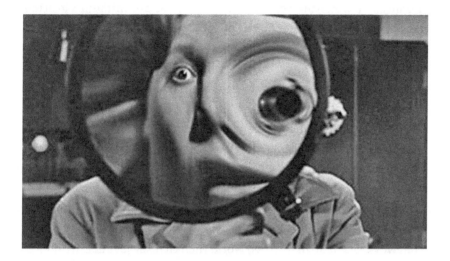

The police are outside the house, and Mark is filming them from his window. He has prepared for this moment—his suicide—an array of still cameras timed to his run to the killing tripod. Pausing just a moment, he says, "Helen, I'm afraid, and I'm glad I'm afraid" and then Mark stabs himself with the tripod-knife.

As the police arrive, too late, they find Mark dead on the floor with Helen, fainted, beside him. We hear a cacophony of recorded voices, and then his father's voice: "Don't be a silly boy, there is nothing to be afraid of." And then the child Mark: "Good night, Daddy. Hold my hand."

Fade to red.

The Madness

We need to look at madness here at two levels. The madness of Mark Lewis, of course, but first at the madness of Powell and Marks in making this movie in the first place. I don't mean that Powell and Marks were mentally ill in making *Peeping Tom*, but it is a question of judgment; how did they not realize how difficult this film would be for a perceptive audience to watch?

It is a "mad" project for one simple reason. Every chosen detail of the story implicates the viewer, accuses him or her of indulging in the pleasures of watching someone in pain, or at a minimum violating their privacy, of being not just a "peeping tom," but of taking a quietly sadistic pleasure in the watching. As Helen was not able to look away even as she backed away from the reality that she was watching a real murder on film, we, as humans, are fascinated by the catastrophes of others. Traffic slows down when there is a car accident, not because the accident is blocking the flow, but because each driver slows for a moment to see: Did someone die? Was someone hurt? Is the car wreck particularly bad? And to feel a momentary relief that it didn't happen to them. As we have seen in our discussion of *Repulsion*, a measure of Carol's not being normal in her reactions is her complete lack of interest in the small car accident she walks past on her way home from work. She is so in her own world then that she just doesn't notice. But we see that as an aberration, a measure that something is wrong with her.

At the start of *Peeping Tom*, as soon as the image becomes one with the camera viewfinder, we are watching *with* Mark; not looking at him, but seeing as he sees. This identification with a serial murderer continues throughout the movie. We are all voyeurs, it seems to say, sitting in the dark, watching the private moments of others from the safety of our seats. We take pleasure in knowing, as they are hurt physically or emotionally, that it isn't happening to us —and we keep on watching. This is one of the particular pleasures of watching a horror film. But it applies to all movies. Yes, we know this is entertainment, that it is "made up," that it is not real. And usually that is enough to allow us to enjoy the moment, without reflection. We feel safe, knowing it isn't real.

But this film doesn't give us a break. It forces us to think about what we are seeing and that we are enjoying it. We are enjoying seeing a streetwalker terrorized and murdered, a child frightened by a lizard placed on his bed, another woman murdered, and another, each dying in a moment of terror. In *Psycho*, we see someone naked in the shower being murdered—certainly a violation of privacy and more, but at no point does Hitchcock suggest we are implicated in the murder. In contrast, here we are accused of being accessories to the crime we see by the way this story is told, and by simply watching.

Of course, Powell and Marks don't let themselves off the hook. In fact, they implicate themselves even more than us. There are so many gestures toward the fact that Mark is a director like Powell is a director: Mark's chair with his name on it is a "director's chair"; the commercial director's name suggests Powell's name and we see him repeatedly abuse the actress whose fainting isn't "real" enough. We also see how Mark, when he is in a social situation, is so quiet he is invisible, but once he has his camera and is directing a scene—with Millie above the news shop, with Viv in the darkened studio—he is all business. Suddenly we see the power of the director.

Powell himself plays the sadistic father who sees his son as an experimental subject, spies on him continuously, and frightens him repeatedly. That Powell not only chose to play the part but put his son in the film to play Mark seems to magnify the offense.

I think these implications go a long way toward explaining the extremely negative reviews the film got on its first release. The reviewers didn't quite know why they found the film so disquieting, but they sure knew they hated the experience of watching it.

But what about Mark? How to understand him? In her groundbreaking book on horror films, *Men, Women, and Chainsaws,* Carol Clover posits that Mark enjoys masochistically re-viewing the pain and horror that was inflicted on him as a child—he identifies with the victim (he too was a victim, with the light in his eyes). He is compelled to repeat what is unpleasant and painful—Mark watches every night in hope of finally getting it "right." He masters his own terror by becoming the victimizer; then as he watches his movies, he can re-live his own experience, once removed. Laura Mulvey, a feminist film theorist, in her perceptive commentary in the Criterion Collection DVD of the movie, makes many of the same points, as well as underlining the "male gaze" as central to how the story is told.

Mark has been watched and filmed since childhood. His father's gift of a camera confirms that he must be his father's successor, carry on his work. He takes on this task so completely that we see that in many ways he thinks of himself as a camera. He carries it with him all the time. Helen tells him that the camera seems an "extra limb." He sees the world through the camera; it's a fetish object that he holds to him like a loved one. When he watches Helen try on the gift brooch, he mimics her movements as though he is filming them with his body; after she kisses him goodnight he kisses the camera lens. It's as though the camera must experience something to make it real.

As he watches the policeman handle his camera, we see his discomfort, how he has to hold himself back from grabbing it. It's his comfort object, his connection with his father, his way to make sense of the world. Having been raised with his father always watching, and with his mother dead and no one to counter his father's objectifying him, Mark feels compelled to continue his father's work, but in competition. To take control, he must amplify it, find new ways to generate the fear he has been taught to study. To take it to the next level, to own it, he comes upon the idea of forcing his "subjects" to watch their own death. The ultimate fear. And it's not enough that they must be frightened of dying—he amplifies it more by having them look at themselves screaming in a distorting mirror.

Of this study of fear Mark says, "I think some good must come of it," but it comes across as a wish, not a conviction. There is something delusional about his repeated disappointment with each filmed murder; something about the "light" not being good enough. He is trying to make it perfect, but what does that mean? It's an impossible dream, but it leads him to kill again.

One question that I don't think anyone considers while seeing the film for the first time, but that I have found myself wondering now that I've seen it a few dozen times, is: What starts Mark on this killing spree? Why now? It's clear that he has been living in the house, overhearing the lives of the people there, for years; that he has held a job as focus-puller and has another job making "views," semi-nude photos. Both those meet his needs to photograph, to become a "watcher." We see his fascination with the girl with the damaged face. Why isn't that enough to satisfy his need to film someone hurt, as he has been hurt?

What moves him to begin with his first murder of Dora, the street-walker? We have to think this is the first, don't we? The movie starts with it, and nothing suggests there have been any murders before. Is it something about the normal world of Helen that disturbs his equilibrium and starts the clock? Because it's clear that Mark isn't just on a project to record fear. He is on a suicidal project, knowing full well where all this leads. His final gift to his father will be to record his own fear before dying.

The easy label for someone like Mark, who seems to kill without compunction, would be to call him a psychopath. But Mark seems in too much emotional pain for that label to fit. He shows no guilt over the murders, that is true. He is a monster—but an oddly sympathetic one. He shows none of the manipulative habits of the psychopath, none of the ability to con or convince. He doesn't randomly cause harm, and he rationalizes his behavior, calling it science, not to fool anyone but because he really seems to believe it. He can't bring himself to question his father's behavior; he can only imitate him.

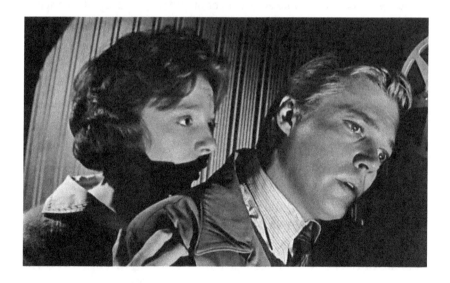

In addition to being a fascinating exploration of madness (though one that doesn't quite parse as real), a reason I think that the rediscovery of *Peeping Tom* was so successful is that it gave academics and those who study popular culture for what it tells us about human psychology something really meaty to chew on. Powell and Marks are very smart, and they created a fascinating puzzle to solve. Marks, the decoder, created a maze of clues to find and figure out. It is a treasure hunt for film buffs, Freudian analysts, and feminist writers.

The film reflects its time. There is much gesturing toward a Freudian understanding of what makes people tick. In 1960, Freudian psychology was at its height: Everyone in the movie business (at least in Hollywood) was being analyzed, and it was more accepted in middle America that it was okay to be in therapy. Back then, therapy meant Freudian analysis. So, we are presented with Mark Lewis, who struggles with the legacy of his authoritarian father and who, in trying to outdo him, crosses the line. A very Freudian concept. Would his father, whose idea of frightening a child is to put a lizard on his bed, have gone to the extreme of murder in order to study fear? Not likely. But as a victim of his father's assaults (though benign by comparison), Mark must counter them, up the ante, by the greater assault of murder. Does this make sense psychologically, or is it just a conceit, playing with the ideas of Freud? It certainly gives the writers of essays (this one included) something to talk about. The sprinkling of Mark's eccentric behaviors are codes to be broken by the analyst—or the cultural theoretician.

I think this film served dual purposes for its creators. For Powell, it was a way to think about the job of making movies and to consider what it means to watch a film. If directors are sometimes tyrants—abusers of their colleagues, tolerated because they have the power to make or break a career—and because if they are good, their works make money for the studio and actually approach "art," then what to make of the audience, sitting there in the dark, watching what the directors and their crews have made? Or even more directly, what to make of the reviewers—professional watchers, voyeurs—who are paid to watch in the dark, to "spy" on the lives of others, and tell the rest of us what to think?

I've talked about how when we watch movies (notice I've now included you and me in the conversation), we are privileged to see things that are usually private: We get to see extreme behavior, violence, intense emotions and situations. Like Chauncey Gardiner in the film *Being There*, we all "like to watch." Even when watching comedies, we are being voyeurs; we are often laughing hardest when characters are making stupid mistakes or bad decisions or getting physically hurt; it's a comedy because it all ends happily. And we laugh because the bad but funny things are not happening to us. Mel Brooks, a wise and funny man, in his *2000 Year Old Man* character, has this to say about the difference between tragedy and comedy (imagine this being in Brooks's voice of a very, very old Jewish man): "Tragedy is if I cut my finger. Comedy is if you walk into an open sewer and die." This is wisdom. It's also funny.

So, Powell and Marks played a game together. They made a Frankenstein monster of Mark Lewis—made up of parts of a puzzle, of clues to be decoded—and they did it cleverly, giving the people in the audience something to mull over, to figure out. The reviewers in 1960 weren't ready to step back and consider these clues as those of 1998 would; they could only respond to the not-so-subtle damning of themselves as watchers, and also to the complete lack of sensitivity to the experience of the victims, except as subjects of Mark's obsessive search.

What endears this movie to me are the performances. I think Mark is a construct; his madness is manufactured. What makes him sympathetic is Karlheinz Böhm's quiet manner, his shyness, his puppy-dog eagerness to please Anna Massey as Helen. And Massey's performance gives us a sense of the normal; she comes across as a lively, curious, interesting young woman who finds Mark intriguing and tries to draw him out. The actors flesh out and make convincing what otherwise might be a skeleton of smart but rather lifeless conceits. This, to me, elevates *Peeping Tom* from a brilliant curiosity into something of real value.

To reduce Mark's madness here to a specific diagnosis is a mug's game. But let's give it a try. Let's start with the diagnoses that don't fit. We see in Mark someone who does not appear to be psychotic; he does not see or hear things we can't. He does seem to hear his father's voice at times, but this is the movie's way of showing us his memories, not actual voices experienced as outside and commanding. One could argue that, but let's agree that they are not a clearly psychotic symptom.

You could certainly make the case for him being delusional. His every action is determined by his sense of having a mission to complete his father's work. A grossly distorted and dangerous idea of what that should look like, but still he holds to it. This is a version of paranoia. Not the paranoia of "they are out to get me" but the paranoia of "I am special and they want my secret." Mark's delusion is that his life must be defined by finishing his father's work. He won't write books as his father did, he will make a movie. Even better. All his decisions revolve around that.

To be intensely preoccupied with something illogical, as Mark is, is not only delusional. It is also an obsession. And if, even though it makes no sense, he can't stop himself, we are looking at compulsive behavior. The person with a delusion will say, "This is the sense it makes, you just don't understand my view of the world," and all your logic can't change his mind. To that extent, Mark is delusional. But he also shows strong evidence of obsession and compulsion. Though he does not demonstrate the more classic compulsive behaviors such as handwashing, or checking and re-checking things, or the mental activities of counting, praying, or word repetition, he does show a very specific compulsion. In his obsession with his father's work, with the idea of studying fear, with the conviction that this is important, he is compelled to film it, to find victims, to generate fear, to document in film the process of this "study," and finally to kill.

How to understand why he considers killing to continue this study of "fear" acceptable? Nothing in the film helps us understand, and it is not at all likely in this mental illness, or in most others I can think of, that such an obsession would lead to murders. His being a victim of his father's version of this study just isn't enough to explain it. His father may have taught him to be a peeping tom, he may have created or encouraged his compulsion to "watch," to find fascination (and possibly a sexual satisfaction) at spying on the private moments of others, but how does that lead Mark to kill?

The only way I can understand it is that the murders aren't really about studying fear at all; they are the means to the ultimate suicide to which his troubled childhood has led him. When we first meet Mark, we do not see someone who feels very good about himself. To say he has a poor self-image would be an understatement. As Helen's mother says, "I don't trust someone who tiptoes in his own house." His death becomes a version of suicide-by-police, since his murders will eventually attract their attention. We see him documenting the arrival of the police—as well as the ambulance, the reporters, and the curious—at the very beginning of the movie after his first murder of Dora in Newman's Passage, and at the news shop he kills Millie knowing the policeman is just outside. Their closing in forces him to the death he has prepared for—his own. What he never seems to have considered is that he would meet someone like Helen, who would bring out a sympathetic connection to another that he had never before experienced, which makes his dying, while still inevitable, much harder.

These considerations make it unlikely to think of Mark as any sort of psychopath. He is not impulsive, he is not irresponsible (he holds two jobs and does them well), he shows no tendency to con or manipulate. Though he is fascinated with bruises and damaged women, he doesn't abuse them (except to kill them; what I mean is we don't see him taking pleasure in hitting or hurting anyone but he is mesmerized by the evidence of disfiguration or hurt, as shown in his fascination with the new girl). Mark can be controlling when behind the camera, but otherwise he is extremely passive.

For him, killing is a compulsion, not a character trait. He says to Helen, "Don't let me see you frightened." He wants to film her, but he knows it might trigger something he can't stop. His not being comfortable with how he is in the world does not fit with psychopathy. Yet his lack of remorse makes you wonder. He only talks about a wasted shot with the murder of Viv. He has extinguished her life, yet all he thinks about is "the light went bad." His acts of murder seem sadistic, but he doesn't take pleasure in the killings or the pain he is inflicting—it seems not to register at all. Again, this is not the behavior of a psychopath.

I would think of this callousness as part of his obsessive preoccupations, not as proof of lack of empathy. "I can't feel it. I can only film it." This is his pathology—an invented one for the movie, not one likely to be encountered in a therapist's office. Similarly, his strong identification with his camera also seems to me a movie conceit, another one of Leo Marks's codes to be broken. Interesting and provocative, but not real.

Often the translated title of a film tells us more than the original. *Peeping Tom* as a title doesn't really tell us what to expect. The title of the film in French is not any better: *Le Voyeur*, is quite close to the English meaning. In the French edition of his very good memoir, *A Life in Movies*, Michael Powell says he would have preferred *La Cinéaste* (The Filmmaker). A revealing difference.

The title in Italian, *L'Occhio che Uccide* (The Eye that Kills) is, I think, closer to the mark.

A bad pun, sorry, I couldn't help myself—the definition, by the way, of a compulsion.

▊ OTHER VISIONS ▊

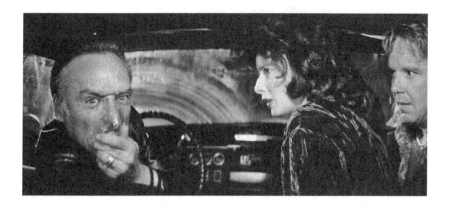

Blue Velvet (1986)

Isabella Rossellini, Kyle MacLachlan, Dennis Hopper, Laura Dern
Writer and Director: David Lynch

This film has one of the most over-the-top portrayals of a sexual psychopath in the movies. Very different from Mark in *Peeping Tom*. Dennis Hopper plays Frank Booth, and he is pure evil. The film begins with a famous sequence: a small town seen in slow motion to the tune of the song "Blue Velvet." We see picket fences, a firetruck, flowers, children at a crossing. A man watering his lawn suddenly collapses; a dog drinks from the hose in his hand. The camera closes in on the grass, then we see and hear insects under the ground. So, an idyllic scene, disturbed by the man's collapse; there is darkness just below.

Jeffrey Beaumont (Kyle MacLachlan) is called home to take care of his father, who has had a heart attack. Walking home one day, Jeffrey stumbles on a severed ear lying on the ground. He and a girlfriend from school (Laura Dern) take it to the police. The police don't seem to take it seriously, but the young people are intrigued and want to figure out what happened. Pretty soon they discover that Dorothy Vallens (Isabella Rossellini, the daughter of Ingrid Bergman), a lounge singer in town, is involved. Jeffrey finds his way into her apartment and hides in the closet. This leads to one of the most famous and disturbing scenes in the film—frankly, in any film.

Frank Booth arrives and, as Jeffrey watches—he is definitely a "peeping tom"—he sees Booth dominate, curse, hit, and sexually abuse Dorothy. We will discover that Booth has kidnapped her husband and child and she is now his sexual slave.

Frank controls Dorothy completely: "Shut up! Call me Daddy you shithead! Spread your legs so I can see. Don't you fuckin' look at me!" He puts a medical mask on his face, inhaling a gas which is never identified, and starts crying, "Mommy, baby wants to fuck" with his head between her legs. He then rapes her. Something about this degradation seems to appeal to her. After Frank leaves, when she discovers that Jeffrey has been hiding and watching, she pulls out a knife and forces him to have sex with her. Now she is in control, and it thrills her.

Frank Booth is a man who takes pleasure in violence; controlling, demeaning, and inflicting pain. This is the dark underside of this small town; he is a drug dealer with an arrangement with the police. They let him kill other drug dealers, steal the drugs that the police confiscate, and then sell them.

When Booth discovers Jeffrey with Dorothy, he and his goons force them to go for a ride. Booth drives fast, then suddenly pulls over. He asks Jeffrey, "What are you looking at?" (there is no good answer to that, it's just a challenge), inhales his gas, and sexually mauls Dorothy. Jeffrey tells him to stop bothering her and slugs him on the nose. Frank gets him out of the car, kisses him, smearing blood in his face, and proceeds to beat him up while singing along with a recording of Roy Orbison's "In Dreams."

The juxtaposition of the sweet melody with casual, brutal violence tells us a lot about Frank and is a movie conceit about psychopaths we will see in the next Other Vision too. His emotional thermostat ranges from quiet threat to eye-bulging rage. These are not the genteel, seemingly charming psychopaths of the previous chapters, nor, like Mark, are they quietly compelled to kill. These men (always men, it seems) don't mind showing their anger; they like to play with their victims, like a cat toying with a soon-to-be-devoured mouse. They are threatening and dominating; it's who they are and they want us to know.

When Dorothy tries to end her relationship with Frank, he kills her husband (whose ear Jeffrey had found earlier), beats her up, and leaves her naked on Jeffrey's lawn. Jeffrey, drawn to Dorothy and to this sordid world, loses what innocence he had. So much for small-town values.

Isabella Rossellini's performance as Dorothy is raw and brave. The emotional toll must have been enormous. Every time Dennis Hopper is on the screen, he is electric, scary, and funny too; he is such a profane caricature, striding into a room, loudly screaming, "Let's fuck! I'll fuck anything that moves!"

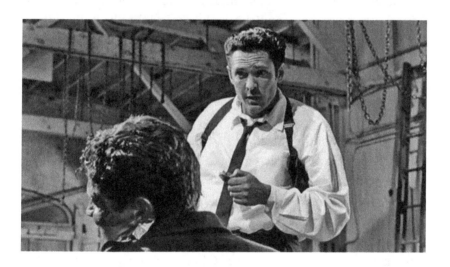

Reservoir Dogs (1992)

Harvey Keitel, Michael Madsen, Steve Buscemi
Writer and Director: Quentin Tarantino

The perfect jewelry heist goes wrong. The police confront the robbers, there is a shoot-out, and two of them are killed, in addition to a couple of policemen and bystanders. The survivors retreat to their meeting place, a warehouse.

They did not know each other before all this, and the boss kept it that way by giving them code names based on colors. They suspect that one of them is an undercover cop and they plan to torture a captured policeman to find out who it is. Michael Madsen is Mr. Blonde, and he is happy to be the one to do the torture. Early on he tells the policeman, tied to a chair, "I don't really give a good fuck what you know . . . but I'm gonna torture you anyway. . . . Not to get information. It's amusing to me to torture a cop. . . . All you can do is pray for a quick death, which you ain't gonna get." He pauses. "You ever listen to K'Billy's 'Super Sounds of the Seventies'? It's my personal favorite."

He turns on the radio and, when Stealers Wheel's "Stuck in the Middle with You" comes on, he finds it to be the perfect soundtrack for casually strutting, brandishing a knife, and then brutally cutting off the cop's ear, pretending to talk into the bloody, severed ear while the cop is screaming in pain. This scene has ruined the song for me. Mr. Blonde is right—it's catchy and fun. But now it is forever associated (for me and anyone who has seen the movie) with this scene of casual torture.

Mr. Blonde is in the same mold as Frank Booth, though he doesn't show the rage that Booth does. He is a psychopath and proud of it. He treats torture and killing as lightly as an outing in the park. He jokes, teases, chats with his victim, and then cuts him, all to the beat of the Stealers Wheel song.

This was Quentin Tarantino's first film, an independent film that was made possible when Harvey Keitel (Iris's pimp, Sport, in *Taxi Driver*) read the script and offered to back it if he could play Mr. White, the old-hand criminal. Suddenly the barely-there budget of thirty thousand dollars was upped to $1.5 million.

The dialogue and the structure of the film is vintage Tarantino, with backstories and flashbacks foreshadowing the unique smarts of his next film, the one that really put him on the map, *Pulp Fiction*. *Reservoir Dogs* is violent and bloody, but that fits the situation. We never see the heist, only the aftermath, which makes it clear the movie isn't about the heist, it's about the relationships among this group of psychopaths. Mr. Blonde is the most ruthless; Mr. Pink, played by Steve Buscemi, is paranoid; Mr. White is the cool professional; Mr. Orange, his protégé, has been wounded in the melee.

Washing up after the botched robbery, Mr. Pink says, "Tagged a couple of cops. You kill anybody?" Mr. White says, "A few cops." Mr. Pink asks, "No real people?" Mr. White replies, "Just cops." A conversation any real psychopath would understand.

RECOMMENDED READING

Clover, Carol J. *Men, Women, and Chain Saws: Gender in the Modern Horror Film.* Revised edition. Princeton, NJ: Princeton University Press; 2015.

See especially chapter 4, "The Eyes of Horror."

Hanff, Helene. *84, Charing Cross Road.* Grossman Publishers, New York; 1970. Penguin Books (Reissue), New York; 1990.

This is a wonderful book about the bookstore Leo Marks grew up in. It's a short book, an exchange of letters. Hanff was a writer in 1950s New York who loved books but had little money. She wrote a chatty letter to the Marks and Co. bookstore asking about a book she wanted to purchase, and received a friendly reply from Frank Doel, the store manager. This started a friendship by letter that lasted for twenty years. They talked about books, of course, but also about what it was like in these years after the war, about their families, about life. Hanff sent the staff food packages (things were tight in England after the war). The letters are funny and thought-provoking, filled with stories of life in postwar New York and London.

Helene and Frank never met. She had little money and didn't like to travel. By the time she made it to England, Frank had died and the shop was closed. The book was made into a lovely movie starring Anne Bancroft and Anthony Hopkins. It's good, but read the book. You will thank me.

Mulvey, Laura. *Audio Essay on Peeping Tom* [DVD]. New York: Criterion Collection; 1999.

Her running commentary on the film—from a feminist perspective, with insights into the problematic psychology of the film and of Mark.

Mulvey, Laura. *Visual and Other Pleasures.* 2nd ed. New York: Palgrave Macmillan; 2009.

See "Visual Pleasure and Narrative Cinema," 1975. This is the essay where Mulvey first explores the concept of the "male gaze" in film. Many of her ideas generated controversy and are still much discussed by film theorists.

Powell, Michael. *A Life in Movies*. New York: Alfred A. Knopf; 1987.

A personal history by the English director Michael Powell, but also a history of the film industry, with a chapter on the making *of Peeping Tom*.

Rodley Chris. *A Very British Psycho*. 1997. Available on YouTube. https:// youtu.be/ 5wkU hj7_ tYg.

A Criterion Collection documentary on Leo Marks and *Peeping Tom*.

▪9▪

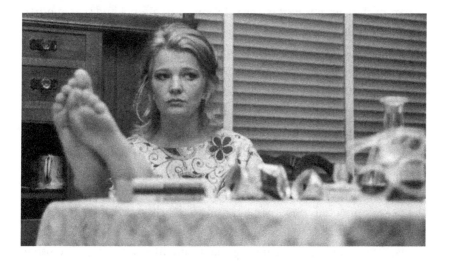

"Tell me what you want me to be ... I can be that, I can be anything."

Mood Disorders
and the Family

A Woman Under the Influence (1974)

Gena Rowlands, Peter Falk
Writer and Director: John Cassavetes

I have a confession. I dreaded sitting down to write this chapter. No, that's not quite true. What I dreaded was having to watch the movie again to prepare for the chapter. I have taught this film for more than thirty years, so I have watched it that many times and more. Each time I find it grueling; I find it difficult to sit through. It's ironic because the film centers around what I did for a living for most of my adult life—working as a psychiatrist who found it most rewarding to work with whole families, not just with one part of the family, the so-called "patient." My work orientation has been to see each person who comes to me for help as part of a family, a system that can not only help me better understand the identified patient's problems and situation, but can, more often than not, be part of the therapy, part of the solution. Very often, I find that another family member is hurting as badly as, or even more than, the patient, underscoring how important it is to see and work with them all.

What's different in watching *A Woman Under the Influence* is the level of immersion in the characters' every moment. Not just sitting with them in a one-hour therapy session, but the sense that you are living with them, experiencing every significant moment in their lives, and many of the small moments too, that define them. The other thing that makes this hard for me to watch every time is that I really like both of the film's main characters, Nick and Mabel, and I find it difficult to see them, so connected in many ways and so clearly caring for each other, yet so incapable of actually taking care of each other and avoiding this crisis. These characters feel very real to me in a way almost no other film has made me feel.

None of the horror-thrillers that we have looked at so far (portraying psychosis, paranoia, sexual violence, and the psychopath) are as hard to watch for me as this movie. It stirs up emotions of a sort of helpless pity. I would love to have Nick and Mabel in my office, together with the children, and with the mothers-in-law. As I watch the movie, becoming so involved with their pain, I imagine how a good therapist might have made a difference for them. It's harrowing.

It's also painful because it is closer to my own world, our own world. Most of us, if we are lucky, do not experience violence firsthand or suffer from severely disabling psychotic mental illnesses. And, if we are lucky, as most of us are, we don't have a psychopath or sexual predator in our midst.

But we all have family. This is what we know.

Having said all that, I think it is a wonderful movie which you will be glad to have seen, even if the seeing is difficult. The acting is amazing, and the experience of watching the story unfold is extraordinary.

A Woman Under the Influence is a dive into a particular family: they are Italian-American, working-class, noisy, poorly educated, living in New Jersey, but recognizable, and not so different under the surface from any of us. The movie is relentless in its insistence that we get to know these people intimately.

It is meant to make you uncomfortable. If you try to intellectualize it, it defeats you. An issue in the film for this family is the lack of any privacy in that house. The parents' bedroom is also the dining room. The only private room is the bathroom, with a sign to prove it. We are watching all the family members' private moments, and their public ones, too. We are voyeurs, not to the obvious secret things, but to the moments that show that they lack the emotional intelligence to know how to help each other or how to be there for each other, to understand one another.

Unlike most mainstream films, *A Woman Under the Influence* was independently made. Its techniques are very different. The scenes are long, much longer than an audience is used to. They stretch on, showing the small moments that other films ignore and the repetitions that a mainstream movie would summarize. Here, you must live it, and become just as frustrated and impatient—or as invested and absorbed—as the characters on the screen. The close-ups of their faces are too close—and held too long. There is a sense of claustrophobia; the close-ups pull the viewer in but then feel like they are "too much." The long scenes may first pull the viewer in too, but then, "enough, already," they push you away. This is very different from what most film audiences are used to.

You may be surprised to hear that most of my students like the movie, and many recommend it to their friends, but not as a fun, Friday-night watch. This is a movie you have to take seriously. It's demanding. It's two and a half hours long, as long as most Biblical epics. My students talk about it being "real," "effective," that it gets at your "guts." One student called it "honorable and honest" and said he had planned to watch only a part of it but couldn't stop: "It's like trying to look away from an auto accident."

Another student told me that he didn't like the film "because it didn't have a specific climax or focus." A good observation. But, I asked him, "Does life? Isn't life, for most of us, just one thing after another?" I think he understood my point. This movie does select what it shows; it has a focus, but there aren't the elisions to the next big moment you see in other films. Once you are in a scene, you are in it for what may feel like forever—you can't escape it any more than the family can.

John Cassavetes, the writer and director, is considered a pioneer of the independent film in America. He started as an actor and had some early success, but his real love was for writing and directing. His films include *Faces*, a portrait of a night in the life of a married couple; *Husbands*, about three middle-aged men and their friendship; and *Minnie and Moskowitz*, a comedy. He was nominated for an Academy Award as best director for *A Woman Under the Influence* but lost to Francis Ford Coppola. His wife, Gena Rowlands, who plays Mabel, the "woman" of the title, was nominated for an Academy Award for Best Actress and won a Golden Globe for Best Actress. The film was also nominated for a Golden Globe for Best Drama, Best Director, and Best Screenplay.

Because it's an independent film, Cassavetes had to find funding to cover making and marketing it. He paid for this film and most of his others with occasional work as an actor in Hollywood. He played Mia Farrow's husband in Polanski's *Rosemary's Baby*. That role helped pay for this movie. He also mortgaged his house.

Peter Falk, a long time friend who was in several of Cassavetes's films, plays Nick Longhetti, Mabel's husband. He had enormous success portraying *Columbo* on television throughout the 1970s and afterward. Since he owned a percentage of the program, Falk had become quite wealthy, and he chipped in a significant part of the cost of this movie. Among his commercial films is *The In-Laws*, with Alan Arkin, one of the funniest comedies ever made. Years later, he played the grandfather reading the bedtime story in *The Princess Bride*.

This was very much a low-budget production. It was filmed in a house rented in New Jersey. Mabel's mother is played by Rowland's real mother. Nick's mother is played by Cassavetes's real mother, and she is a force to be reckoned with.

The long, seemingly discursive scenes might make you think that much of the film was improvised. In fact, it was fully scripted. The actors playing the lead roles contributed a lot to the screenplay as they learned about their characters, but what we see on the screen is very much what was written on the page. Which, to me, makes it even more extraordinary.

The Movie

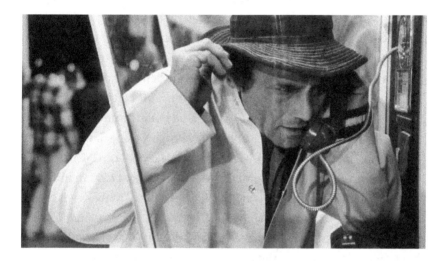

The film opens on workers up to their waists in water, and a piano theme with a strong walking bass. We see Nick among them. Then, after work at a bar. Nick is on the phone, saying, "I'm with my family tonight. . . . Forget about it. I've got an unbreakable date, with my wife." An emergency, they have to work all night. He hollers into the phone, his temper rising, "Forget about it! No way!" His colleagues applaud him but the look on his face says it all: they have to go back to work.

We see kids running out of a house, followed by their grandmother, then by Mabel, their mom. Grandma tells them, "Your mother is terribly nervous," a heavy-handed setup for meeting Mabel. Every once in a while, the movie explains more than it has to. Because we see Mabel's nervousness immediately, we don't need to be told. She is back and forth, asking do they have everything, do they have their shoes on; she is running this way and that, she has trouble saying goodbye, imagining catastrophe: "If anything happens, if they are impossible, I want you to call me. I don't want you saying, 'Mabel is having a wonderful time, I don't want to disturb her' while one of my kids is lying there bleeding." As grandma backs out of the driveway with the kids in tow, Mabel coaches her, unnecessarily, "Turn your wheel, okay, okay, okay, go."

She immediately says to herself, "I shouldn't have let them go," and runs into the house.

It's dark inside. She turns and gestures to each corner, marking her domain, at first silently, then she turns on an opera recording. She stands at the window, paces, smokes, gestures as though putting a spell on the dining table, then we see her, feet on the table, drinking and looking empty and sad. She is waiting for Nick to come home for their "date."

Nick is finishing his overtime work. He wants to talk privately to his friend: "I promised her on my life I'd be home tonight. I promised her that this night was going to be a love night, a special night." His friend says, "But you didn't even call her." Nick says, "I can't call her, she already sent the kids to her mother." When his friend says to him that Mabel is a delicate, sensitive woman, Nick tells him, "Mabel's not crazy, she's unusual. Don't say she's crazy." (He didn't.) "This woman cleans the clothes, makes the bed, washes the bathroom, what the hell is crazy about that? I don't understand what she is doing, I admit that. But I think I know. She's mad at me." Then he says he knows she is not normal, that "she might burn down the house. I don't know what she can do."

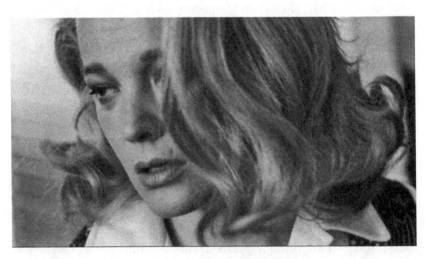

The point of view switches back to Mabel looking lonely and sad. Finally, the phone rings. It's Nick. He tells her he loves her, calls her "sweetheart," and promises that they will spend all the next day together. She is more upset than she has said, and she is already a bit drunk. The jazzy piano returns and we see her walking down the city street talking to herself and entering a bar, smiling.

She sits down next to Garson, a stranger, tapping him on the shoulder, then drumming a beat on the bar, which he copies. She says to him, "You know Nick stood me up tonight?" She downs an entire glass of whisky and begins to sing quietly to Garson, and then she calls him "Nick" while she cries on his shoulder. They go back to her house. She can barely walk, and Garson is forcing kisses on her.

The next morning, she is in bed and Garson is dressing. She wakes with a startle, calling "Nick?" She goes into the bathroom; the door is marked "Private." Garson talks to her through the locked door: "As long as the shower is on, I know you are all right—at least I hope you are." Her behavior has him worried, especially realizing that she is married. She bursts out of the bathroom: "I'm not in the mood for games, Nick. Nick Longhetti . . . Mabel Longhetti," pointing to herself and then miming an uppercut punch at Garson. She suddenly panics, realizing the kids aren't in the house: where are they?

Nick is in a car approaching the house. This looks like a setup for a confrontation, but Garson is long gone when Nick arrives. He doesn't come alone. Nick has brought his friends from work, a dozen or more, looking for breakfast.

Mabel is sitting on their bed. Nick asks, "What's the matter?" She says "Nothing . . . who's there?" "Everybody." She asks, "Did you eat. . . . I'll get something." She rallies, combs her hair, and is introduced to his friends.

Mabel is smiling, the welcoming hostess. She shakes each hand, asking, "Would you like some spaghetti?" A few of the men she knows; the rest are strangers. She walks toward the kitchen, lingering and smiling at them all. A moment later she is yelling at one of the men, a friend, sitting on the kitchen counter drinking water, telling him to get out. "Spaghetti again?" he complains.

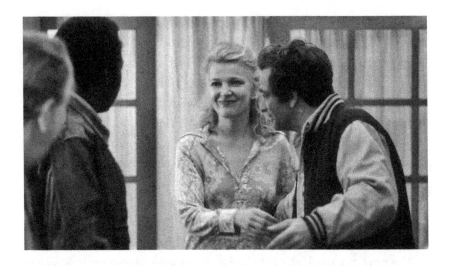

Soon they are all helping; it feels like a party. They sit down, Mabel and Nick at opposite ends of the dining table. She is smiling, but there is a forced quality, and she seems to be looking around: am I doing okay? She begins to ask each man what his name is. She doesn't recognize many of them: "I remember your wife, I don't remember you." She says to each of them, "I'm Mabel." Many of her gestures seem tentative at first, then exaggerated. She raises a toast, "Everybody eat a lot and live a long time!" Talking to herself, she keeps on trying to get Nick's attention.

When one of the men starts to sing opera, she gets up and stares into his mouth with a look of amazement. She is invading his space. She says to another man, "I love this face . . . this is what I call a really handsome face," and holds his head, then she hits his shoulder and tells him how strong he looks. The fellow is embarrassed. She asks him to dance. Nick says, "You've had your fun, it's enough," but she persists. Suddenly Nick yells, "Get your ass down!" Silence. Everyone is self-conscious.

When Nick's mother calls to tell him she has a pain, he announces this to the group. Mabel sniffs and makes a dismissive motion, then the gesture changes to something like an umpire calling "You're out." Nick is yelling at his mother on the phone, insisting she call the doctor—this is a noisy family. Mabel looks defeated, deflated, and very sad as the men get ready to leave.

Mabel and Nick are finally alone. Mabel repeats the "you're out" gesture. They look at each other. Mabel contorts her face, hands askew, miming her anger at being so dismissed by him, but she can't say it. "I was trying to be nice. I like your friends. I'm a warm person, I'm not one of those stiffs with their nose up in the air," and she mimes that, too, stiff upper lip "thenk-you" [sic].

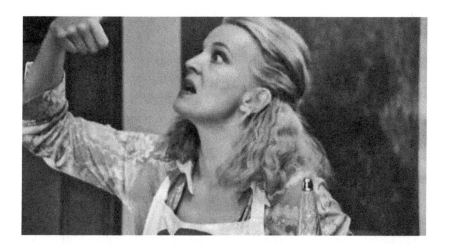

He yells back at her, "I know that." It is clear she is struggling to express herself, to tell him that she wants to make the company feel comfortable, to make Nick proud. Then she does an imitation of Nick, roughly yelling "Sit down Mabel, get your ass down," flinging her arms up. Nick tells her he knows she wasn't doing any harm, but it was the way the guy looked at her, she was embarrassing him. "He thinks you mean something; he doesn't know you don't mean it." She suddenly looks very sad again. She asks Nick, poignantly, "I didn't do anything wrong?" He smiles and throws her a kiss. She says to him, "Tell me what you want me to be . . . I can be that, I can be anything."

The opera soundtrack returns and they get ready, finally, for bed. Nick is very tender with her.

I'm describing all this in such a granular way because it defines Nick and Mabel's relationship and begins our understanding of her madness. We will learn more, but the essence is all here.

Later, grandma returns with the kids. They weren't expected. Nick and Mabel are still in bed. Nick at first says he wants to get more sleep, but then the children are on the bed and he starts teaching them to whistle. Mabel tries to rush them off to school (so she and Nick can be by themselves again). Nick continues the whistling lesson. Mabel sits on the bed, gesturing and talking to herself. Nick drags grandma into bed too. Finally, Mabel stands up and announces the children will have a party as soon as they are back from school, and off they go. Mabel jumps back into bed with Nick. He hugs her; she looks sad. He asks her twice if she will be "all right." She says to him, "Why do you keep asking? Do you think I'm wacko or something?" Then, leaving the bed, she says she can hardly wait for the kids to come home: "All of a sudden, I miss 'em." The push-pull of their relationship is apparent. She wants closeness and connection; he has a hard time being alone with her and expressing his tender feelings, repeatedly putting people between them.

We next see Mabel on the sidewalk, impatiently waiting for the school bus. She asks passersby the time, but in a way that makes them walk faster to get away from her. Her polite request quickly devolves into yelling at them for ignoring her. She starts making her dismissive, odd hand gestures, usually with a verbal snort. You, too, would avoid this woman if you saw her.

Mabel is pacing on the street, and when she sees the school bus, she flags it down and directs it as though it might not want to stop. She jumps up and down as the kids climb off the bus.

They run home together and sit on the stairs. Mabel tells them, "I hope you kids never grow up, never. You know I never did anything in my whole life that was anything except I made you guys—I made you and you and you." Suddenly she has a headache, and the children start to massage her back; clearly this happens a lot. "Can I ask you kids a question about me?" she asks. "When you see me . . . do you ever think of me as dopey or mean or . . . ?" Middle child Angelo answers, "No, you're smart, you're pretty, and you're nervous too." She thanks him, then embarrasses him asking him to show her how strong he is by flexing his muscles. He does it, reluctantly. Mabel is delighted: "You see how good this is, that we are talking like this." It is as though she is performing the role of a good mother.

She rushes them inside and they pretend to hide as someone comes to the door. It's a father, Mr. Jensen, bringing his son to the party. He says he is just dropping him off, but she is in his face, asking him if he is uncomfortable, and she makes him more uncomfortable by her closeness and touching. He agrees to stay.

Her mood and attitudes turn on a dime. She had offered him tea. He asks for it, and she says, harshly, "Oh, screw the tea, it's time to dance." The music is *Swan Lake*, the dying swan. Mabel says to the kids, "Come and die for Mr. Jensen." She begins to dance, encouraging them. She acts the cheerleader, the social director, but she is trying too hard— a common mode for Mabel—and Jensen is even more uncomfortable. Nick calls on the phone and she says to him, "It's working! Listen, I'm a great mother, I not only love the kids, I love Mr. Jensen, I'll never be mean again. He was such a stiff when he came over but I got him loosened up." The children are all hugging her. The phone disconnects (did Nick hang up?) and again, suddenly, Mabel appears to be suffering from a profound sadness. Just as quickly, she switches into social director and urges the children to put on costumes.

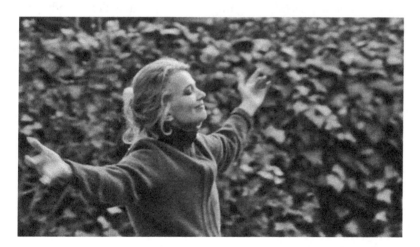

She is outside dancing quietly to *Swan Lake*. She asks Mr. Jensen, "What's your name again? Harold? You poor thing, you can't name somebody Harold. . . . Hey, would you dance with me?" She is repeatedly pushing social boundaries, making people uncomfortable. He tells her he is worried about the kids, about leaving them with her. He tells her she is acting "strange, I wonder if you have been aware of that." That hits her hard. The kids are in various stages of undress, putting on costumes. Mr. Jensen is pushing his children to get dressed so they can leave. Mabel apologizes, and Nick comes home with his mother and sees their daughter Maria running around the house naked.

Nick hurries upstairs and confronts Mr. Jensen, yells at him. Mabel tries to explain and Nick slaps her across the face, knocking her to the floor: "See what you made me do, having a party." As he tries to rush Mr. Jensen out of the house they begin to tussle. Nick is in a rage: "Get out of here, I'll kill you and your kids!"

Next thing we hear, Nick is asking for the doctor, yelling into the phone, "Nobody's sick here, Mabel's crazy." Mabel is sitting there, bewildered. Nick is pacing, drinking, yelling. "You are going to be committed. Going to the hospital until you get better." Mabel quietly says (referring to his hitting her), "You got embarrassed and you made a jerk of yourself, that's all. I do that every day. I'm not sore at you. I always understood you and you always understood me. That's how it was. Remember I said, 'It's going to work because I'm already pregnant.'" Nick quietly says to her, "Don't let your mind run off . . . don't do that," and he looks close to tears. She holds her fingers up saying they are as close as that, always have been: they are one (her face is a range of moods, from frightened to angry). Nick replies, "I don't know who you are."

The doctor arrives.

Mabel is standing, alone. Something's up. The doctor asks if she has been drinking; then, if she has taken a pill. Mabel hesitates, then says, "Is morphine a pill? Sure, I've taken pills. Vitamin pills, sleeping pills, uppers, downers, inners, outers." (This kind of verbal cascade sounds manic.) "What did you tell them, mama [addressing Nick's mother], that I drink?" Nick's mother shouts, "Yes, she drinks!" Then Mabel says, "I am upset, I do get upset, but I calm down. I do have anxiety, still." She whispers to the doctor, "Don't listen to that woman on the staircase [Nick's mother], she's got it in for me." The doctor asks her what's troubling her. She says it looks like there is a conspiracy. "He's got something in that bag," she says, pointing at the doctor, "Am I right, Nick, am I right, Nick?" Mabel is getting angrier, more agitated, and the doctor tries to calm her. Nick's mother glares at her and yells, "Doctor, aren't you going to give her a shot?" and in a nasty, know-it-all voice, declares, "Mabel, we are trying to help you." But Mabel knows better and starts making noises at her, appearing even crazier. Nick lies to her: "The man is here on a social call, nobody's sick." Mabel asks him if he loves her. As Nick starts to answer yes, his mother shouts, "This woman has to go, think of the children . . . you can't stay in this house! My son tells me stories of the talk, the little things . . . he says you give him nothing, you're empty inside . . . my son is a good boy, doctor, this woman is crazy!"

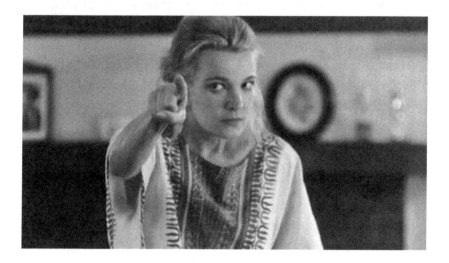

This scene is really painful to watch. And there is more. Mabel is shaking, standing on the couch. She quietly, hesitantly, says, "I have five points. I've figured it out. For me, one is love, two is friendship, three is comfort, four is I'm a good mother, Nicky." He says, "Mabel, I love you." She continues, "Five is, I belong to you." She seems in a trance, far away. Nick slaps his hands, and she looks startled, confused, and then faint. He embraces her and says, "I love you, you've made me happy, take deep breaths." When the doctor approaches with a calming medicine in a syringe, Nick turns on him: "Sit right down, I'll throw you right on your ass!" but Mabel is in her own world, talking to herself, gesturing; she holds her fingers in a cross as though keeping the vampires away. She becomes hysterical, more and more upset, suddenly worried about what will happen to the children if she has to go to the hospital. She can't stop talking, obsessing: "I want to take the children with me, they're mine and I want to protect them." Nick hugs her again, "I love you, I would lie down on a railroad track for you. If I made a mistake, I'm sorry, but so what . . . come back to me." She mimes a threatening fist—first pointed at Nick, then at the doctor. She runs upstairs to the children. Nick stands there, overwhelmed.

The children hug Mabel while Nick's mother tries to pull them away. The doctor tells Mabel he is committing her to the hospital.

End of Act One. The film is only half over. Frankly, I'm emotionally exhausted writing about it.

Time has passed. We are at Nick's work at a quarry. Several of his fellow workers tell him they have heard there was trouble at his house. He angrily tells them not to ask about his affairs. They are just trying to be helpful. He tells one of them, "She's got a screw loose. She needs some time in the hospital. Is that what you want to hear, you asshole?" He is fuming. When another worker doesn't say anything to him about Mabel, he assumes he's thinking about it and starts yelling at him too. Later, that same worker is rappelling down a cliff. Nick angrily bumps into the rope and causes him to fall. Nick is dumbfounded but oddly, no one blames him.

The next day he tells a friend at work that he needs to spend time with his kids: "It comes to mind I don't know my kids. They are a little shook right now; I want to take them to the beach." His friend offers to go with him. Nick picks the kids up from school; they ride in the back of the truck. Nick is in yelling mode, bossy: "Wear your clothes. Nobody gets pneumonia when I'm the father." It's chilly, not a beach day. Nick drags the kids from here to there. The girl Maria is running, she wants to play in the sand. Nick picks her up: the kids must play what he wants them to play. On the way home his friend drives and Nick sits with the kids in back. He opens a beer and Tony, the eldest, asks if he can taste. "Sure," and before you know it, they are all drinking beer. Nick warns them, "Not too much," but he doesn't pay attention to how much they are drinking. Nick tells them, "I'm sorry I had to send your mother away. I'm sorry for everything."

By the time they reach the house, the kids are drunk. They keep falling down, dizzily walking in circles. Nick puts them to bed. End of Act Two.

It's six months later. Mabel is coming home. There is a caravan of cars heading to their house: friends, family, Nick's work colleagues. The house is full of people. Nick greets everyone. His mother demands he come to her. She says, "Are you crazy, what is all this? This was supposed to be only the family for Mabel." The wife of the man whose fall Nick caused tells him, "I'm here because I love Mabel. This party is too much. You want to know what I think? You're a shit. You sent her away. You should have picked her up." Nick wanders outside, and some of the party follows. He turns and yells at them, "You can't stand out there. It's a surprise party! Everybody inside!" This is Nick, always trying to take control, and always with an edge (often more than an edge) of anger.

His mother tells him he has to send the people away. He says, "I can't tell them to go, you do it." She makes the announcement. Nick takes over; he thanks everyone for coming and tells them that he will tell her they all came.

As they leave, Mabel arrives. Her parents had picked her up from the hospital.

Mabel is subdued. Nick's mother directs the doctor not to talk about the past, instructs Uncle Adolph what he is allowed to say. We see where Nick gets his bossiness. Mabel quietly asks if she can see the children. It appears that she hasn't been able to see them for the entire time she was away. Nick discourages her; they will start to cry, he says. But his mother contradicts him (we have seen that, too, in how Nick treats Mabel) and says, yes, the children are right over there.

The children tearfully greet her. They tell her they love her; they ask, "Is everything okay?" She greets each of them in turn, but when she asks her daughter if she wants to come to her, Maria says, no, she will just stay where she is. Mabel's face falls. She tells little Angelo, "I'm trying very, very hard not to get excited." She tries not to cry. Soon all the children are hugging her.

She seems shaky, very tentative. The family are staring, smiling at her. Her father says they should leave her alone. Nick insists that her father stay for dinner, and he tells Nick, "I'll only stay if it's not spaghetti. I'm not a spaghetti man." They are in each other's face. Why on earth are they arguing about the meal? Mabel calms them down and sits next to her father. She tells them she is happy to see them all. She asks her father if he thinks she will be okay. He tells her, yes, she'll be fine. She hugs him. He tells her to sit with her mother. She looks deflated.

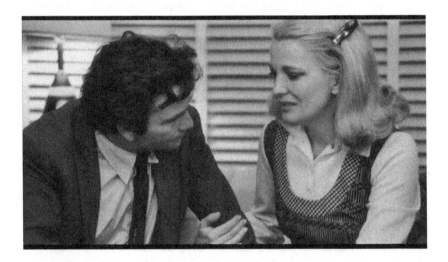

Nick takes her into the next room. "There is nothing you can do wrong. This is your house, to hell with them. Be yourself." This is a much harder demand than it sounds. He imitates her funny noises, "Be happy. Give me a 'beh beh,' no, a real 'beh beh,'" urging her to make her noises like before. She tries, and the family overhears, uncomfortable. They kiss.

Nick announces, "Everyone in the dining room, we are going to have a party. Let's have a little warmth here." Mabel still looks fragile. They greet the children and everyone sits down, Mabel at the head of the table. Nick turns to Mabel and asks what was it like up there; we realize that he never visited her, never saw the place. She smiles. Nick declares something we heard his mother say: "No sense talking about the past. The past is the past, the past is dead. Good times from now on." He is controlling the conversation, dictating what they are allowed to talk about. Mabel winks at him, something that she used to do. Nick is delighted.

Mabel goes to the kitchen and we hear her telling Tina, her cousin, "How did you get so fat?" talking with some of the old energy. She walks back in asking, "Did you see Tina's ass—it's this big!" Tina says, "It's okay, I do have a big ass." Mabel sits with Nick and asks them all to go home, "Nick and I want to go to bed together." Nick's mother says they all came for a party, and Mabel's mom tells her not to talk like that in front of the children. But Mabel is saying what she wants and needs right now.

She says hello around the table, much as she did at the spaghetti breakfast. She turns to Nick, "How am I doing?" Then she repeats her request: "You know we can't talk together while you are still here." They ignore her and urge her to calm down. She starts to tell a joke, complete with voices, "You must pay the rent, the rent. . . ." She starts to cry and presses against Nick for reassurance. Everyone is talking at once and Nick loses it: "That's the end of the jokes; no more jokes, we just talk, hello, how are you, conversation." He is in Mabel's face, telling her what to say, "too hot, too cold, where you been." Mabel starts telling them her hospital routine and tells them about her shock treatments. Nick interrupts her: "Be yourself." Just what version of "herself" does he mean? Mabel looks up and across the table at her father: "Dad, will you stand up for me?" He doesn't understand and begins to get up from his chair. She asks again; he still doesn't know what to do. Her mother gets it. Mabel begins to cry and finally they all decide to go home.

Mabel stands on the couch humming and swaying to *Swan Lake*. The family watches. Nick tells them to get out. He tells her to get off the couch. She runs from him; he chases her. She runs to the bathroom, Nick grabs her as she tries to cut herself, and the children start screaming. They run with her into the living room. She is back on the couch. They ask her, "What's the matter? Don't you hear me, mom?" and when Nick comes closer, the children push him away, protecting her.

Nick tells her if she doesn't get off the couch, he will knock her down. She is in her own world and doesn't respond. So, Nick grabs the children and pulls them all up the stairs into their bedroom. When he lets go, they run back downstairs, calling out for their mom. As they pull at Nick, he slaps Mabel hard, knocking her to the floor. The children rush to her. Nick leans over her, "I'll kill you. I'll kill those sons-of-bitches kids!" They back away. He reassures them that Mabel is all right and, lying there, she tells them that too. Nick drags them upstairs again. They immediately run downstairs again and huddle around her. By now she is standing. Her hand is bleeding.

Mabel takes the children upstairs, with them pushing her from behind. She puts them to bed. She tells Maria she looks just like her father, that she is "daddy's girl." She winks at Nick, and he winks back. It's quiet. In bed, their son Tony tells her he is worried about her. She tells him not to worry, she's a grown-up, she's fine. Angelo asks her to lie down with him and tells her he loves her too. Lots of kisses on the nose. Nick is watching all this. He puts Maria to bed and tucks her in.

Finally, Nick and Mabel are alone. Mabel says to him, "You know, I'm really nuts," and Nick responds, "Tell me about it." Nick begins to care for her hand, rinsing it and putting on a bandage. He is being tender and careful. Mabel asks him, "Do you love me?" He looks at her, nods his head, but the words don't come, "Let's go clean up that crap."

They begin to clear the dining table, working together. Sound-track music returns; it's a jug band. As the end credits begin to roll, we watch Mabel and Nick turn the dining room back into their bedroom. They push the table away and open up the couch, put the pillows on the bed and tighten the sheets. Then Nick pulls the curtain over the doorway and we can see through it that they are getting ready for bed. We watch their return to a normal routine, something they have done thousands of times together. Life goes on.

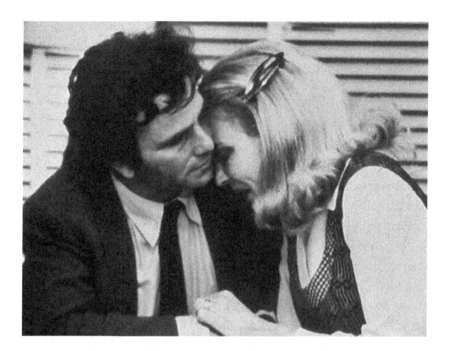

The Madness

There is no question who is supposed to be "mad" in this family, but I hope this walk-through of the film makes it clear that Mabel is not the only one who qualifies. Nick is every bit as emotionally compromised as she is, just in a different way. The extended family and many of their friends are too. Look at Nick's mother or Mabel's father. The *DSM* has little to say about the family issues here, about the many ways Nick contributes to Mabel's strange behavior, even as it defines how he sees her, and himself.

Let's talk about Mabel first. She is constantly checking with Nick, asking him if she is doing what he wants her to do, being the person he wants her to be. The "influence" that Mabel is under is that of Nick, as well as her own need to meet some ideal of the normal housewife and mother.

Mabel knows that she is askew in the world. She often asks her children, "How do you see me? Am I OK? Am I a good mother?" The middle child, Angelo, sensitively tells her she is pretty and smart and nervous. But, of course, he shouldn't have to tell her; she shouldn't need to rely on her children to give her a rating to know who she is or how she is doing. But she does. She asks her children, Nick, almost everyone, except her mother-in-law. She knows what Nick's mother would say and doesn't want to hear it. That is a small sign of strength, knowing and resenting these intrusions into her marriage.

We see how Mabel's moods can turn on a dime, but that there is always an underlying sadness, an uncertainty even when she is broadly smiling.

We are dropped into this family's story in the middle of things. We see Mabel's agitation as she ushers the children out of the house and into their grandmother's care. Mabel is hopping, running back and forth, pressured and micro managing every detail of their short time away, then she misses them terribly as soon as the children are gone. The moment when she returns to the house, silent and dark, and gestures to each corner, is telling; she is alone and suddenly adrift. She has carefully set the table and sits waiting.

Nick can't bring himself to call her and tell her he isn't coming. His hesitation makes a bad situation worse. I think Mabel scares him. He says he doesn't know what she might do, but at the same time insists she is not "crazy." He avoids telling her bad news.

Instead of passively waiting for Nick and perhaps drinking herself to sleep, Mabel goes out, perhaps as a way to get back at Nick for standing her up. She winds up in bed with a stranger, calling him "Nick" and worrying him into thinking she might try to hurt herself.

Nick arrives home with a dozen of his friends in tow, looking to be fed. The friends are a buffer, keeping Nick from having to deal with Mabel's disappointment. He is putting other people between them, something he does again when she returns from the hospital.

Mabel works hard to be the perfect hostess, but it's all a performance. She wants to be friendly and to be appreciated as Nick's wife, but she is insecure and her actions are forced. She tries too hard, misjudges the personal space of people she hardly knows, and most importantly embarrasses Nick, whose temper goes from zero to sixty.

He yells at her to "sit her ass down!" and the party goes silent. After the friends leave and the two are alone, Mabel, quietly sad, asks Nick how he wants her to be: "Tell me . . . I can be that way." It's an admission of a sad dependence on his approval and on his view of how to be in the world, something he can't figure out himself.

They are at cross-purposes later when grandma unexpectedly brings the children home. Mabel urges them off to school and Nick pulls them into bed. When it comes to their comfort being alone together, they are at odds. We see how much Nick cares for Mabel, but he repeatedly shows he is afraid to be alone with her.

Mabel has a nervous energy she can't contain, as we see when she is waiting for the children's school bus. Her behavior is embarrassing. Any child would want to get off at the next stop and find another mother. The way she acts doesn't express joy: it's worry, agitation, impatience, an attempt at control.

The children's party proves to be a disaster. Mabel, in "perfect mother" mode, encourages the children to dance and then to play dress up. The party is chaotic. Mabel seems in her own world; she is the "dying swan" from *Swan Lake*, seems distracted, with quickly changing moods, and makes the father who stayed for the party uncomfortable. When Nick calls, she tells him, "It's working." What does she mean? She is talking about her promise to be what he wants her to be, a "normal" housewife. She is playing a role. But it doesn't feel natural; it has an anxious, desperate quality.

When Nick and his mother arrive, Nick assumes the worst, seeing the man there, and in a rage begins to fight with him. This is one of many times we see his temper out of control. Nick's mother (who has quite a temper, too) screams at Mabel, calling her a terrible mother (the worst thing she could say), and Nick watches Mabel disappear into her own world. She stands on the couch and lists her five "points"; they are all about family and the children. There is no Mabel there, except in relation to them.

Nick, who is always trying to control, to tell people how they should behave, becomes furious and then physically violent when his yelling doesn't control the situation. He tries to persuade Mabel to stop acting "crazy" and, when she can't, he slaps her to the ground. Then we have the grueling scene of the children trying to protect their mother until they are exhausted. We are too, watching.

As we have seen, this family has a problem with boundaries. Nick and Mabel have no privacy in their house—their bedroom is the dining room. The one room where a person can be alone is the bathroom. We discover that Nick tells his mother too much about what happens between him and Mabel, and she flings it back accusingly at Mabel whenever she gets the chance.

A book about family dynamics that I recommend you read is called *Families and How to Survive Them* by Robin Skynner and John Cleese. Yes, *the* John Cleese of Monty Python and *Fawlty Towers*. Skynner was one of the founders of family therapy in the UK. Cleese, a very smart man, was at one time his patient. This book is a conversation between them about how families work, and it is very good. It's meant for a general audience; it even has cartoons. The book talks about how families develop and the importance of boundaries, which change as the family changes.

When you are a child, your world is bounded by you and your parents. As you grow up and develop friendships, you widen your world; your parents are still important but become less central. When you choose a partner, the two of you become a new family and you develop boundaries defining you together as separate from both your parents. There are now things you talk about or decide with your spouse that you no longer discuss with your parents. You are not excluding them; you are just redefining the relationships. As you have children, the boundaries of your family expand to include them, and if your family is an emotionally successful one, your parents assume the role of grandparents, which have different rules. For instance, as grandparents, they need to check with you before making certain decisions about your children. It's when this balance is disturbed or not maintained that things can go wrong.

Things are very wrong in Mabel and Nick's family. Not just across boundaries, but within them too. As we have seen, Nick needs to control Mabel so that she will be "normal."

But we will also see that his definition of normal is that she has to act crazy so that he can feel less crazy. When she returns from the hospital, newly subdued and sad, he misses her energy, her quirky noises and hand gestures. Soon he is telling her to bring them back, even coaching her on how to do them again. He needs her to be crazily anxious and trying too hard. He is troubled by her being quietly in the moment.

At the same time, he complains about how crazy she is to his mother, a violation of the family boundary. It indicates that he hasn't really left the original family system; his mother is still too strong a presence. We also see where he gets his volatile temper. His mother is as full of rage as he is.

Nick is impulsive and not very smart. He has little idea of how to be a father. Declaring "I'm the father!" isn't enough to command respect. While Mabel is in the hospital, he takes the children out of school ("I'm thinking I don't know my own kids"). He barks orders that they have fun, then drags them away if it doesn't match his idea of fun. On the ride home, he lets them get dizzy drunk. Mabel doesn't do anything that crazy.

He is always announcing his version of normal behavior: "[Mabel] cleans the clothes, makes the bed, washes the bathroom, what the hell is crazy about that?" When Mabel comes home from the hospital, he announces, "No more jokes, let's have conversation, hello, talk about the weather, conversation." These are bland clichés of how you are supposed to be, but it is the best he can manage. Nick has a temper, a very short fuse, and he is bossy. He has a limited repertoire of mad behaviors. It's likely that his temper caused the accident at work. He can be violent, easily starting fights and striking Mabel. His work friends seem to ignore it; it's just who he is. Mabel is more creatively diverse in her odd behavior, and he has a hard time with that.

When Nick is trying to talk Mabel down from the couch, he says several times that he loves her. But when she asks him directly, as he is bandaging her hand, he can't say the words. It's too close, too intimate. They have a lovely shorthand of winks and smiles that tells of their long years together, but things can so quickly get out of control. At one moment Mabel's odd hand gestures and noises are just "Mabel being Mabel," and the next moment, usually when they cause Nick embarrassment, he abruptly turns on her.

There is more than one madness in this family.

Mabel certainly seems to have some sort of mood disorder. Do her mood swings justify saying that she is bipolar? I think it unlikely. Her moments of high energy, of euphoria ("It's working!") are too easily deflated. She doesn't show evidence of grandiosity, that she thinks she is terrific or special, with grand plans, nor does she exhibit the irritability of the manic. In fact, just the opposite: she is always asking for reassurance that she is just OK. She can't sit still, is easily distracted, and can't keep up with her feelings and thoughts. Is that mania or mere agitation? Someone with manic symptoms would likely be sleeping less, show pressured speech, talk so fast it's hard to keep up, and spend money they don't have on impulse buys based on grand plans that are often discarded for new ones. A person in a manic state will dominate a room, be alternately charming and domineering, or show impatience with others. The person who is manic is full of themselves, delighted with their own ideas, with their place in the world (though often irritated that others don't recognize just how wonderful they are).

At the extreme, the manic part of bipolar illness can become psychotic. It can be delusional in its excess and in the specifics of the pressured speech and ideas. Odd gestures and noises don't make Mabel psychotic. I see Mabel's odd gestures and noises as not expressions of some psychotic process but as indications of how hard it is for her to express her anger, frustration, and confusion. She never knows what behavior is expected of her, what will please Nick and what will trip an angry outburst. This is quite a tightrope she must walk. It doesn't look manic. It looks more like panic.

Mabel's moments of happiness seem more disinhibited than joyous, sometimes from drinking, but mostly because her moods are so volatile. She certainly appears depressed, sad, empty. She always seems close to tears. The sadness is just below the surface at even the most upbeat moments. In the turmoil of the moment, she tries to cut herself. What is that about? She never expresses a wish to die or a sense of hopelessness. If anything, she seems always hopeful that she will "figure it out," discover a way to satisfy everyone's expectations of her. Is her cutting suicidal or merely desperation in the chaos of the moment? I'm guessing the latter.

So, though this could be a form of bipolar illness, most of the boxes are not ticked for that diagnosis to apply to Mabel. Her madness looks more like an anxious or agitated depression.

This is a form of major depression. Many of the so-called vegetative symptoms of major depression (in contrast to the depression that is not a diagnosis but just another word for "sadness") are less prominent here. Major depression usually presents with sadness and often, but not always, with tears (it is common for those with a more severe depression to report that they are "past" tears, that they feel more empty than tearful). People with depression will show low energy (not getting out of bed, getting dressed, or doing their normal daily routines of hygiene), have insomnia, or sleep for much of the day. They lose interest or pleasure in the activities they used to enjoy: exercise, eating, watching TV, being with friends or family, or engaging in a hobby. They have decreased appetite, decreased interest in sex, problems concentrating, and they withdraw from the world. They often speak softly and hesitantly. They will forget what you asked them or lose track of their thoughts; they don't make eye contact and seem generally lethargic. They will often have suicidal preoccupations. In the next chapter, on *Ordinary People*, we will look at this more closely.

Except for her deep sadness, little of this describes what we see of Mabel. What seems more significant is that she also has excess energy, a jitteriness, and is constantly worrying (about what Nick will think, about whether she is being a good wife and mother). Her restlessness, her inability to sit still, her persistent anxiety with imagined catastrophes regarding her children, with the anxiety being even more prominent than her profound sadness, makes agitated depression seem a better description of her madness.

Of course, real understanding comes not merely from a formal, individual diagnosis but from the dynamics of her relationship with Nick, and with her family. We have been able to see that up close.

In a moment of calm near the end of the movie Mabel says to Nick, "I'm really nuts, aren't I?" and he replies, "I'll say!" I wish he knew enough to say, "Me too," instead.

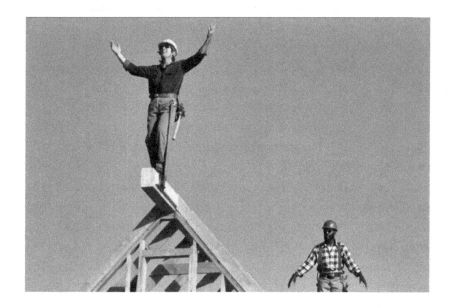

Mr. Jones (1993)

Richard Gere, Lena Olin, Delroy Lindo
Director: Mike Figgis

What recommends this film is Richard Gere's extremely accurate and vivid portrayal of both the manic and depressive parts of the bipolar cycle. The rest is a bit of Hollywood hokum about a therapist falling in love with her patient.

Mr. Jones (Gere) is an architect who, because of his mental illness, has not been able to hold a job. We see him both manic and depressed; we also see him in the hospital and how easy it is for him to avoid treatment. Many people with bipolar illness are addicted to the highs of the manic phase. They crave the energy, the feeling that they are on "top of the world" (to borrow the phrase from *White Heat*, used very differently there). When manic, a person's thoughts are coming a mile a minute, and they all feel like brilliant revelations. It's very hard to give that up, so people can be reluctant to take the medications that might balance their moods, even when the decisions made during a manic phase often backfire, and depression is not far away. There are two moments illustrating the illness that are outstanding here.

Mr. Jones arrives at a symphony concert in a limousine, accompanied by a woman in a ball gown. They are arriving late. He is casually dressed, and hearing the music in the lobby he starts dancing with her. Jones, talking fast, mentions how wonderful his previous girlfriend was: "I think of her all the time. She died, but it's okay." His companion is taken aback.

As they walk toward their seats, Beethoven's Ninth Symphony is reaching its choral climax. Jones is mesmerized, smiling, absorbed in the music. He starts marching down the aisle toward the stage. Then, singing loudly with the music, he climbs onto the stage, waving his arms in front of the conductor and chorus. It's an exhilarating moment—if you know the piece you can understand his enthusiasm (I've sung along and conducted to a recording in the privacy of my living room, so I get it). But taking over a concert is simply not done. Being manic, he does it.

Obviously, there are consequences. He is soon hospitalized.

The other remarkable scene takes place on a construction site. Since he can't get a job as an architect, he gets one as a carpenter, building a house. He is high above the street on the roof, hammering nails. He begins to hammer in rhythm with his new co-worker, Howard, played by Delroy Lindo. A plane flies overhead and Jones goes "whoosh," smiling broadly. He's having a grand time. They talk of Howard's kids, and Jones reaches into his pocket and gives Howard a hundred-dollar bill: "Take the kids out to dinner." Howard demurs: "I can't take your money." Jones tells him he found it on the street, that a voice told him, "give it to Howard . . . I didn't know a Howard, 'til I come here today." It's not likely here that he was hearing voices or that he found the money on the sidewalk; it is more likely that he is making up the story to convince Howard to take the money he is impulsively offering.

Then Jones starts singing James Brown's "I Got You (I Feel Good)" and returns to work. A few moments later he is climbing to the top of the unfinished roof, all lumber and open spaces. He admires the panorama,: "Ever feel like flying, Howard? Just taking off, just fly away." Then he begins walking to the end of the roof beam, commenting on the pitch of the roof (after all, he's an architect), "All we need to do is find the balance, the balance." He starts calculating the wind, arms stretched. Then, saying he could get "lift-off. We are going to fly," he explains how he will swoop down, make a few turns and land on the ground.

Howard knows something crazy is happening, asks for a rope, and works his way toward Jones, who is now standing on one foot, excited about his plans to fly and preparing to jump. At the last minute, Howard grabs him. The scene is incredibly suspenseful. This is mania: euphoric, impulsive, pressured, feeling all-powerful and grandiose to the point of delusion ("I can fly"). The life-threatening behavior is not usually part of the picture—usually the risk is more along the lines of spending all your money or making bad business or personal decisions—but in this film, it works. No wonder the manic high is so hard to give up.

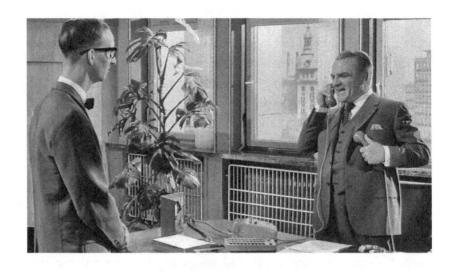

One, Two, Three (1961)

James Cagney
Director: Billy Wilder

Good Morning, Vietnam (1987)

Robin Williams, Forest Whitaker
Director: Barry Levinson

I've put these very different movies together because they both feature defining performances by their leads—James Cagney and Robin Williams—and both portray what being *hypomanic* looks like. Actually, they aren't as different as all that. *One, Two, Three* is a comedy-satire about the Cold War, and *Good Morning, Vietnam* is a comedy-drama about the Vietnam War. In both, we see what might be called manic behaviors, but controlled and modified to the situation, turned on and off, in a way that someone bipolar could not manage.

James Cagney, who was most famous playing gangsters, proves his comedy chops in *One, Two, Three*. He is the manager of a Coca-Cola distribution company in divided Berlin. Coke represents American capitalist excess in contrast to the austerity of East German Communism. The young daughter of Cagney's boss secretly marries an East German Communist, and when Cagney finds out that his boss is on an inspection tour, he has to make the young man presentable, fast. We see Cagney converting him, against his will, into the image of a Capitalist: washed, groomed, wearing socks, fitted in a suit and tie, and with falsified papers proving he is royalty.

Cagney is in full command. Snapping his fingers to punctuate his commands, talking fast and thinking faster, he is managing a dozen decisions with a confidence that is a wonder. It's an acting tour de force, and quite funny. What defines this as hypomanic is how he can stop the pressured speech and decision-making when it's not appropriate and resume it when he is back in work mode. This ability is what defines the success of many presidents of major companies and universities. They often sleep less than most of us, have more energy, make quick decisions, and can dominate a room. This can also make them infuriating, but that's a price they are willing to pay. It's when the manic energy can't be modulated that it becomes a dysfunction, a form of madness.

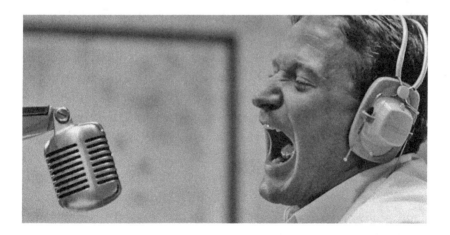

In *Good Morning, Vietnam*, we get to see the closest to a Robin Williams stand-up routine as can be found in his movies. Williams was a phenomenon. He was a brilliant motor-mouth, thinking faster than any of us, doing voices, impressions, and connecting ideas and jokes so rapidly that the speed was part of the fun. But when the "performance" stopped, we could see him tune it all down. He could manage a normally paced conversation, still smart and thoughtful, but at half his performance speed.

Williams was a very good actor and could be persuasive without the hypomanic manner. His performances in *Good Will Hunting*, *Awakenings*, *The Fisher King*, *Dead Poets Society*, and *The World According to Garp* are quiet and sensitive. In many of his movies, that hyper-speed persona is constrained. We can imagine that while filming he kept the crew in stitches with his improvised comments, but those often wound up on the cutting-room floor, sacrificed to the requirements of the story.

In this film, however, being hypomanic is central to his character: a radio disc jockey famous for his wit. It's clear that Williams is improvising most of his radio patter, and it's fast and very funny (even though the "brass" in the story doesn't get it). But you also see him turn off the rapid-fire jokes as soon as the microphone is off. He is in control of this hyperactive thinking in a way someone with a bipolar diagnosis is not.

Ironically, the only other film where that manic energy is let loose is in the Walt Disney cartoon *Aladdin*. Williams is the voice of the Genie and his jokes come fast, tumbling over each other, all focused and clever. It's the best thing in the movie. That's another feature of the hypomanic: even when the pressure is there, it's controlled and goal-directed, unlike the illness of mania, where the distractibility and impulsiveness, added to the cascading thoughts, can lead to confusion and trouble.

I gather that in his personal life Robin Williams wrestled with major depression and anxiety and that he often used drugs. But his depressions do not seem part of a bipolar swing. His performance mode was indeed something he could turn on and off, and it wasn't out of his control, as most manic episodes are. The reports of his suicide suggest that, overwhelmed with the early symptoms of what was later diagnosed as Lewy body dementia (a form of dementia that progresses rapidly and that can cause depression, paranoid delusions, and memory loss, among other devastating symptoms), he was in despair about losing something so central to his identity—his ability to think—and he made a decision to take control of his death. It may have been precipitated by depression and paranoia, or it may have been a rational decision made before he knew he would no longer be able to make rational decisions. Sad, no matter how you look at it. He was a national treasure.

RECOMMENDED READING

Dalio, Paul, and Kay Jamison K. Touched with Fire, Screening Excerpts and Conversation [Video]. YouTube. Available at: https://www.youtube.com/watch?v=UFnuuhnOlNQ. Published April 13, 2019.

Johns Hopkins University, film clips and discussion.

Jamison, Kay. *An Unquiet Mind.* New York: Vintage Press; 1999.

Professor of Psychiatry and a MacArthur Fellow, Dr. Jamison writes vividly of her personal experience of bipolar illness, with severe manic psychosis and suicidal depression.

Jamison, Kay. *An Unquiet Mind* [Video]. YouTube. Available at: https://www.youtube.com/watch?v=eAC6jC4giuo. Published February 10, 2017.

Skynner, Robin, and John Cleese. *Families and How to Survive Them.* London: Oxford University Press; 1984.

Specifically, chapter 3 "Becoming Separate." A dialogue between Robin Skynner, one of the founders of family therapy in England, and his former patient, John Cleese (of *Monty Python*), about families and how they work (and why they often don't).

Vonnegut, Mark. *Like Someone Without Mental Illness, Only More So.* New York: Delacorte Press; 2010.

Following up from his early memoir of "going crazy," The *Eden Express*, Vonnegut, son of the author Kurt, is now a successful pediatrician, despite a history of four psychotic episodes and a diagnosis of bipolar disorder.

▪10▪

"Feelings are scary, and sometimes they are painful. And if you can't feel pain, then you're not gonna feel anything else either."

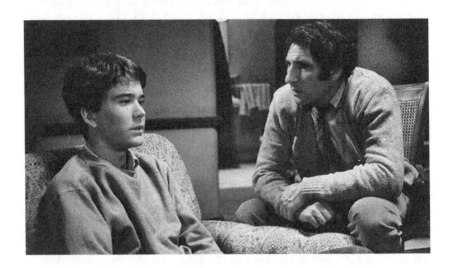

Grief and Depression

Ordinary People (1980)

Timothy Hutton, Mary Tyler Moore, Donald Sutherland,
Judd Hirsch
Director: Robert Redford; Screenplay: Alvin Sargent

I've seen this film dozens of times, and it still makes me cry. It affects me in a way that *A Woman Under the Influence* never does. My students mostly have the same reaction. *Ordinary People* moves them in a way the other film does not. Why is that?

I think one reason is that the parent-child relationship is really what the story is about, a very different focus than the Cassavetes film. I have a son, and I'm a sucker for tender moments of father-son bonding. *Field of Dreams* makes me cry for the same reason. For my Yale students, this family is more like ones they know. And Conrad Jarrett, the troubled son in this family, is close to their age. They can imagine themselves in that world more easily.

Ordinary People allows us to understand more about the Jarrett family's inner lives too, because we get to watch Conrad's therapy with Dr. Berger slowly evolve. We see his father, Calvin, trying to understand what's happening to his family, with help from the doctor. They each talk about their feelings, however hesitantly at first, in a way that never happens with the Longhettis in *A Woman Under the Influence*. It's part cultural, part social class—Mabel and Nick simply don't have the words for their feelings the way that the Jarretts do. Of course, this film is also about not being able to deal with unpleasant emotions like anger or profound sadness.

Mabel and Nick's movie ends in routine: they make up their bedroom as they have done many times before, but there is no sense that anyone has learned anything. In *Ordinary People*, the family seems to be falling apart when Beth, Conrad's mother, leaves, but Conrad and his father are closer to understanding each other and being able to help each other in their grief. Conrad has opened up enough to have a girlfriend, someone who is refreshingly honest about emotions. What brings tears here is that it ends in change, a feeling of hope that things can be different.

This was the first film that the actor Robert Redford directed. It is a remarkably good first effort. It would be remarkably good for an experienced director too. Many years ago, *The New York Times* had a running feature with an actor or director watching a favorite film and talking about it. Denzel Washington was getting ready to direct his first film, *Antwone Fisher*, about a psychiatrist who takes on a difficult patient and transforms his life. He chose *Ordinary People* to watch for the article. He was taken with the level of careful detail in the editing and the set design. The look of the therapist's office, all shades of brown, disordered and messy, contrasted with the Jarrett house, white and uncluttered. The implication was that Dr. Berger doesn't care how things look; Beth Jarrett does. I think the differences are often a bit too emphatic, too pronounced. You want to say, "We get it; she's a neat freak!" Yet, unlike the Cassavetes film, this film is remarkably quiet: it rarely shoves things in your face. Instead, it sneaks up on you. Redford may sometimes be overly careful in his choices, but they work. I guess he didn't want any messes either, in this, his first film as director.

The cast is amazing. This was Timothy Hutton's first movie. He plays Conrad and seems to be living the part. He won the 1981 Academy Award for Best Supporting Actor. Mary Tyler Moore was nominated for Best Actress, and Judd Hirsch was nominated for Best Supporting Actor (competing with Hutton). Redford won Best Director, Alvin Sargent won for Best Screenplay, and the film won Best Picture. Donald Sutherland, who I think is wonderful here, was not nominated.

This was Mary Tyler Moore's first film after a long career on television. She started as the secretary whose face you never saw on the TV series *Richard Diamond, Private Detective*. They only showed her legs as she gave him his messages. From such beginnings, a career is born. She played Dick Van Dyke's wife on his eponymous show, which endeared her to millions. Then, in 1970, came *The Mary Tyler Moore Show*, which ran for seven years and was a top situation comedy during its entire run. Her image was of the girl next door, making it on her own and beloved by all. In the show she was a single girl who worked at a small TV station in Minneapolis; her work colleagues and friends were her family. Shows like *Cheers*, *Taxi*, and *Friends* successfully imitated the formula.

The decision to play Beth, Conrad's mother, was not only a stretch but a risk. Everyone loved Mary Tyler Moore, but it's hard to love Beth. That Moore so quickly made audiences forget her television persona is an acting triumph.

Donald Sutherland has the least dramatic part, one that is hard to play. He is Calvin, the good father, the one struggling with how best to help his son. I think he is very effective. My students used to tell me they loved him as the father here; he seemed an ideal. Sutherland has starred in films such as *M*A*S*H*, *Little Murders*, *Klute* (a thriller with Jane Fonda), *Don't Look Now* (one of the scariest films ever made), *JFK*, *Fellini's Casanova*, *The Great Train Robbery*, *Invasion of the Body Snatchers* (the better remake, directed by Philip Kaufman), and more recently, *The Italian Job*, *Pride and Prejudice*, and *The Hunger Games*. His career is varied and impressive. If he is in a film, he gives it gravitas.

Ordinary People is based on the novel by Judith Guest. Her book and this movie inspired the Yale course that is the basis for this book. When I saw the film at a Yale Film Society screening, with its excellent portrayal of a family trying to cope with grief and depression, and with its sympathetic and realistic scenes of the therapy with Dr. Berger, I wondered if I could find other films that were as powerful in conveying the experience of mental illness. That search led to the creation of the "Madness at the Movies" course. I feel sentimentally grateful to this film that inspired my teaching for so many years.

The Movie

The credits roll in silence and then over a water view we hear the single notes of a piano, tranquil, then a quiet rolling bass; it's the Pachelbel Canon, introducing a chorus of voices accompanied by lovely shots of fallen leaves, woods, and a park empty of people. This is Lake Forest, an upper-class suburb of Chicago. We close in on a school and a choir rehearsing. The camera surveys the young singers, gradually focusing on Conrad (Timothy Hutton). Suddenly we cut to him waking in a sweaty panic from a bad dream. Then we meet his parents watching an amateur theater play. In the car, Beth (Mary Tyler Moore) asks her husband, Calvin (Donald Sutherland), what he was thinking about—he looks preoccupied. At home she walks right past Conrad's bedroom door, but his father stops, noticing the light is on. He knocks, and Con pretends to have been reading. His dad asks if he is having trouble sleeping and reminds him to call the doctor: "We should stick with the plan."

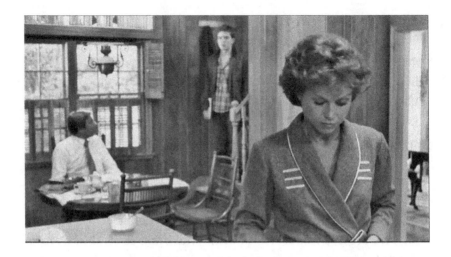

Next morning, Beth is setting up breakfast. Calvin calls for Conrad, who is sitting in his room, upset. When he comes downstairs, Beth offers him "French toast, it's your favorite," and he tells her he isn't really hungry. Calvin starts reminding Conrad that breakfast is the most important meal of the day, but Beth just takes away his plate and dumps it in the disposal. Cal asks Con again if is he okay. When Conrad tells him his friend Lazenby is picking him up for school, his dad says, "That's great," and Con asks why. Calvin says, "I don't see the old gang much anymore, I miss them." Con leaves, and we see Cal begin to eat breakfast, thinking about him as he eats. He suddenly looks up and calls out for his son, who is already outside. It's an interesting director's choice, showing how much Cal is worrying about him.

Conrad's friends pick him up. In their conversation we learn that Conrad lost a year of school. They stop at a railroad crossing and, as he stares at the passing train, Con suddenly remembers rows of gravestones. He looks stunned. In class Conrad stares out the window, distracted. His teacher needs to call his name more than once to get his attention. He sits alone at lunch.

Later he is on the phone, calling Dr. Berger (Judd Hirsch) for the first time. He tells him that his doctor in the hospital had told him to make an appointment.

As the film progresses, we get a taste of Con's days. At swim team practice, he seems very much alone. At dinner, all is quiet, the conversation is trivial ("fish too dry . . . ?"). When Beth asks if Con wants her to sign him up for tennis at the club, he says, "I haven't played in a year," and she says with a smile, "Don't you think it's time to start?" He has no answer. Sleeping, he dreams fleeting images of him and his brother Buck in the water during a storm, clinging to their capsized boat. Some days later, we see Con in the elevator going to Dr. Berger's office, rehearsing what he might say: "I'm fine, couldn't be better, just terrific."

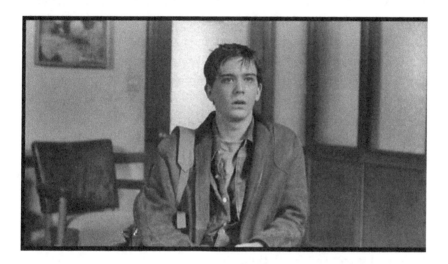

Berger asks him how long he has been out of the hospital. It's been a month and a half. Then he asks, "Are you feeling depressed?" and lights up a cigarette (it's a different time, when smoking was ubiquitous), "Feel on stage? People nervous, treating you like you are a dangerous character?" Conrad, says yes, a little, and Berger asks, "Are you?"

Con was in the hospital four months. Berger asks, "What did you do?" Conrad, irritated, says, "I tried to off myself, isn't it down there" and Dr. Berger tells him it doesn't say how. (This is unlikely. The chart or referring letter would definitely say how and indicate how serious it was.) Conrad answers, "Double-edged, Super Blue"—a razor.

Berger: "So how does it feel being home, everyone glad to see you, friends . . . you're back in school. So, no problems? . . . So, why are you here?" Long pause, and Con tells him, "I'd like to be more in control." Berger asks him, "Why?" Conrad says, "So people can quit worrying about me. My father, mostly." Berger picks up on this: "What about your mother, isn't she worried about you too?" Con interrupts, "I'll be straight with you, I don't like this already," and Berger answers, "Well, as long as you're straight."

They are establishing some rules: Berger asks direct questions and is not put off by Con's hesitations and moments of irritation. He then asks if Con wants to tell him about the boating accident that killed his brother, and there is a long silence. Changing the subject, Berger asks how his work with the doctor in the hospital went, and Con says, "It didn't change anything." Berger asks, "What did you want to change?" and Conrad states again that he wants better control. Berger says: "I'll be straight with you"—mirroring Con's words a moment before—"I'm not big on control, but it's your money—so to speak."

Berger tells him they should meet twice a week: "Control's a tough nut." When Con tells him swim practice would make it impossible; Berger asks him how he wants to solve it, and Con reluctantly agrees that he will have to miss practice twice a week. The session ends with Con again saying he doesn't like being there. This directness, insistence on honesty and openness, makes him very uncomfortable. But it's a good start to their relationship.

The next scene begins with Beth neatly putting napkins rings in a drawer. Con watches his parents talk about not much. Con tells his dad that he went to see the doctor and Calvin is delighted, even though it will cut into swim practice: "It's important." But Beth looks doubtful; she asks where his office is. It's in Highland Park, a lower-class area near Lake Forest. You can see that matters to her.

At swim practice, Conrad's coach notices his lack of interest and energy. He asks him if he is on medication, and Con says he isn't (this is the first we know this). The coach then asks if he had shock treatment. Con says yes (more new information; we are getting some background information that otherwise we would not know), and then the coach makes the insensitive declaration "I would never have let them put electricity to my head."

Conrad has his first conversation with Jeannine (Elizabeth McGovern in her first role, recently seen as Cora Crawley in *Downton Abbey*), a girl in the school chorus who is new in town. She compliments him on his "energy" singing in the choir. End of Act One.

It's Halloween and we see that Beth, being the perfect hostess, has homemade sweets for the trick-or-treaters. She tells Calvin how much she is looking forward to going away to London for Christmas, and he tells her this isn't a good time to be away. She says they have always gone away for the holiday: "Isn't it time we got back to normal?" But Cal doesn't want to interrupt Con's work with his new doctor. He is putting his son first.

Beth comes home a few days later to an empty house. She stops in front of a closed door: it's Buck's old room. She goes in, looking at all his things, still there, untouched. She sits on his bed, lost in her thoughts. When Con comes home from school, he startles her. Their conversation is awkward, out of sync. She asks him about his swimming; he tells her his grade on a trigonometry quiz; she begins to tell him about her experience with math, then changes the subject and walks away.

At a party (we overhear glimpses from a dozen conversations that efficiently define their social world—lawyers, finance folks, people with money), a friend asks Cal how Con is doing, and he tells her he's okay and that he is now seeing a psychiatrist. Driving home, Beth scolds him, says he had been drinking too much, and that talking about the psychiatrist "was in very bad taste . . . a violation of our privacy, the family's privacy."

At the next session with Dr. Berger, Conrad admits to feeling jumpy. Berger tells him that like many psychiatrists he does believe in talking about dreams, but "sometimes I want to know what's happening when you are awake. Something's making you nervous . . . you are making me nervous." Con notices the clock: "You get to tell the time but I can't?" Berger nods his head, yes, that is how it works. Con tells him he doesn't like swimming anymore, and Berger asks if he has thought about quitting. Con asks Berger if he is telling him to quit (that would be too easy, it would be his doctor's fault), and Berger says no, it's up to him. Con says, "It wouldn't look good." Berger comes back with, "Forget about how it looks, about how does it feel?" This will be the theme of much of their work together. Con is angry that Berger won't decide for him: "You're a doctor, I'm supposed to feel better, right?" Wonderfully, Berger replies, "Not necessarily." He asks him about friends, is anything easy? Con says the hospital was "because nobody hid anything there." He remembers that there was one other patient with whom he could talk.

In the next scene, Con is meeting with Karen, his friend from the hospital. She seems upbeat and happy. We see him smile for the first time. They exchange rose-colored versions of their lives now, but they don't really connect. We learn that Karen stopped seeing her doctor and that her dad agreed. She rushes off, wishing him a great year, then urges him to "cheer up."

Con is in the family back yard. Beth joins him, does the mother thing, asking if he wants a sweater. She asks him what he is thinking about. Quietly, we hear the Pachelbel music return. Con is remembering the pigeon that was caught in the garage. Beth remembers too, but Con changes the mood and says, "That is the closest we ever came to having a pet." Beth rightly hears it as a criticism—Buck had

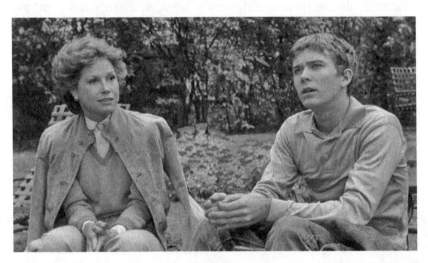

asked her for a pet, a small one—and she starts talking about the unfriendly dog next door. They are talking over each other, and suddenly Con starts barking. She goes into the house.

He follows, and tries to apologize by offering to help her set the table. He wants to be with her, to make peace. Instead, she tells him he can help by tidying up his closet, "because it really is a mess." His look is pleading: talk to me. The phone rings, Beth answers: "No, I'm not doing anything, just getting ready for dinner." Con is forlorn and forgotten, but we see him remembering Buck charming their mom with a story from school. She is smiling and laughing, full of life; Con smiling broadly in admiration of his brother.

Immediately we are back at the doctor's office. The room is bathed in brown; it's dark. Con talks about how he and his mother don't connect. He is bringing to the session what is really happening in his life, what matters, no longer hiding behind "We're doing great." There is a pause and Berger asks what he is thinking. Con tells him, "That I jack off a lot." Berger takes that in stride, asks if it helps. Con admits it does, for a minute. Then he has a memory: his father coming into his room right after Buck died. He sat with him, put his arm around his shoulder, he didn't know what to say. They sat together. "I knew I should have felt something. I didn't know what to feel . . . I didn't feel sad, so much as . . ." Berger pushes: how did he feel? "Don't hold back." End of Act Two.

In the next scene we see Calvin with a work colleague who tells him that Cal is distant, distracted, worried. His friend advises him Con will be gone soon, off to college: "They leave, all that worrying . . . is just wasted energy." On the train home, Calvin remembers Buck as a boy, being chased by his little brother; the boys negotiating over a borrowed sweater; himself banging on Conrad's bedroom door; an ambulance with flashing red lights, the medic commenting, "The cuts are vertical. He really meant business."

Con tells his coach that he wants to quit swimming. The coach warns him, "This is it. Actions have consequences. I'm not taking you back again." His friends ask him what happened, why did he quit? He tells them it was a "bore." He won't talk to them.

Back in therapy, Berger is casually washing his hands, asking Con what his dad said about him quitting swimming. Con hasn't told him, the timing isn't right, he will get more worried. He hasn't told his mother, either. Con reminds Berger that he can't connect with her, then he says, "Look, I'm not going to 'feel anything' today, I'm sorry." Berger scoots his chair over next to Con, very untraditional, but just right: he wants to make a point and being closer helps. "Sorry's out. Remember the contract, control, lack of feeling . . ." He pushes him: "What feelings do you have?" Con says, "I feel things, sometimes, I don't know . . ." Berger says, "I thought you didn't like to fool around, Jarrett. I want you to leave 'I don't know' out there with the magazines!" Pushing him further, he asks if Con is mad. Conrad says "no." Berger pushes harder, "Cut the shit. You're mad as hell. You don't like being pushed, why don't you do something about it. Tell me to 'fuck off.'"

Conrad starts to, but then stops himself. "I can't do it, it takes too much energy to get mad. When I let myself feel, all I feel is lousy!" Finally, he yells back at him and then collapses, exhausted. Berger says: "A little advice about feeling, kiddo. Don't expect it always to tickle."

Here we are reminded about something important in the therapeutic relationship: though it becomes very intimate, it is one-sided. Berger knows more and more about Con, but Con knows little about Berger's personal life. He doesn't even know if he is married or has a family. This is appropriate. The sessions should be about him and not about Berger, though this therapist is untraditional enough that I could imagine him sharing something of his personal life if it would help Conrad better understand himself. Sometimes breaking the rules of therapy is exactly the right thing to do.

Almost too schematically, each scene in *Ordinary People* defines something more about the family. It's done so well that it isn't obvious, but when you have seen the film a lot it becomes clear that there is little in the film and screenplay that is not there for a reason.

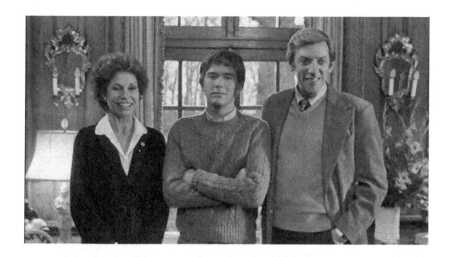

An example is the gathering with Con, his parents, and his mother's parents. They are posing for a family photo. His grandfather tells Conrad to stand between his mother and father. Conrad rushes off after the picture, and Cal says he wants a picture with "Connie and his mother." Beth immediately has a counter-suggestion: she wants "a shot of the three of you men." But Cal has the camera and tells Con to move closer to his mother. He is taking his time to get it right. Beth is clearly uncomfortable standing next to her son. She says, "Give me the camera," but Cal insists he wants this picture. Con watches this exchange, then bursts out, "Give her the god damn camera!" startling himself and everyone into silence.

Beth retreats to the kitchen with her mother, and we hear the sound of a broken dish. As Beth kneels on the floor she says, "I think it can be saved." This is one of the very few too on-point moments in the film, but it gives us a chance to hear what Beth's mother says about Con. As they prepare lunch together, she tells Beth that Con will be all right if she is firm with him. For the first time Beth tells her that Con is seeing a psychiatrist. Her mother says, "I thought we were all finished with that." When Beth says his name, the grandma asks, "Jewish doctor?" and Beth says, "I don't know, maybe just German." Then she holds up the dish, broken in two, and again says it can be fixed, "it's a nice clean break."

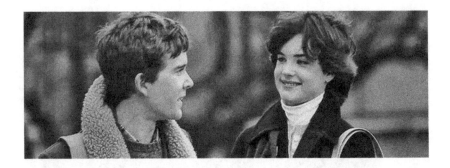

After chorus rehearsal Conrad and Jeannine walk home together. They talk music. Jeannine asks herself why she asks dumb questions and answers, "I'm just showing off." Then she asks why it is so hard when you are first talking to someone. Conrad tells her she makes it look easy. She is honest, straightforward, disarming. She runs to catch her bus and calls out to him, "You really are a terrific tenor." He answers, singing, and walking home he begins singing Handel's "Hallelujah" with great enthusiasm. Then follows a sweet scene where he rehearses a call to Jeannine to ask her for a date. It's perfectly teenage-awkward; a rare comic moment in the film. When he finally calls, she recognizes his stumbling and just says "yes!" making it easy. End of Act Three.

Time passes; it's near Christmas. Cal and Con are setting up the tree. Beth walks in; she is angry. She just found out from her friend that Con had quit swimming weeks before. She more bothered about being socially embarrassed, about not knowing, than by why Con did it. She takes it personally. Cal asks why Con didn't tell them and Con says, "I didn't think it would matter," obviously not his reason. He just doesn't like negative feelings and wanted to avoid a confrontation.

But Beth takes this as an attack, that she wouldn't care. Beth is sure her friends are saying, "Poor Beth, she has no idea what her son is up to, he lies and she believes him." Con explodes: "The only reason she gives a fuck about it is someone else told her first!" Then he accuses her of never visiting him in the hospital, instead traveling in Europe, "Goddamn Spain and Goddamn Portugal!" Beth tells him, "Maybe this is how they talk . . . at the hospital but we are not at the hospital." That moves Con to accuse her that she would have visited the hospital if Buck was there. Beth's reply makes it worse: "Buck never would've been in the hospital!" Con runs upstairs to his room.

Cal pleads with Beth to go to Con with him, but she refuses. When Cal joins him, Conrad tries to apologize. "Tell her I'm sorry—I can't talk to her. It doesn't change the way she looks at me." Cal pleads with him to explain. And Con cries, "She hates me, can't you see that!"

Back in therapy. Berger says you felt great the other day, so what changed, and Conrad says, sarcastically, "You tell me, you're the doctor." Pause, then Berger says, "Don't take refuge in one-liners like 'you're the doctor.' Because that pisses me off," modeling how to be direct and angry. "Everything was fine until you had a fight with your mother and then everything was lousy." Con talks about the "shit" he pulled with her to explain why his mother hates him. Berger says, "I'm talking proportion. What shit?" (Notice how Berger uses Conrad's language when it will advance the moment.) Con talks about how he bled all over the bathroom tiles and she had to re-grout the floor. "I'm never gonna be forgiven for that, never." He adds, "If you think I'm going to forgive, she's going to forgive me . . ." It's a classic Freudian slip. Who needs to forgive whom? Conrad suddenly stops himself; he has had a moment of understanding. This is underlined by the quiet return of the Pachelbel Canon. The music is used sparingly. The film is austere in its quiet; feelings are contained, as they are in the Jarrett household.

They reflect on what he just said. Berger tells him, "That's a hell of a secret you've been keeping from yourself." When Con asks what he does now, Berger suggests he recognize her limitations, that she can't love him enough, or show him her love in a way that connects. Con insists there must be something wrong with him because she showed love to Buck and to his dad. Berger: "Now we're back to the rotten kid routine! She can't love you because you're unlovable. Where does that leave your dad? How come he loves you?" Con says, "Dad loves everybody," and Berger comes back with, "Oh, he loves you, but he's wrong." He is really pushing him.

He tells Con there is someone else he needs to forgive.

Con doesn't know what he means. Berger won't tell him; he needs to find it out for himself, and the time is up. This is a moment when keeping to the time rule matters. Con is frustrated, but this is food for thought.

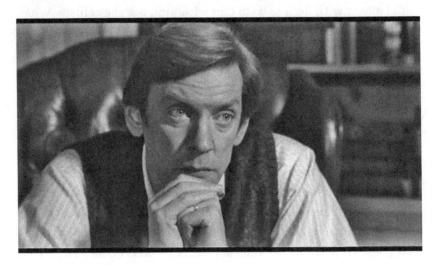

Calvin goes to meet with Berger, who sees him alone. Cal tells Berger he thinks he can shed light on some things. He respects the privacy of therapy and can see that Con is better. Cal feels responsible for Con's suicide attempt, but says it was lucky that he discovered him. Before the accident he used to think he was lucky. Cal sees his son and wife drifting apart; he sees Beth not being able to forgive Con, and that Con is too much like her. "They were the only two who didn't cry at the funeral." Then he says, "I think I know why I came here. I came to talk about myself," and Berger replies, "Okay, why don't we." Berger agreeing to see Cal without Con being present, and agreeing to begin therapy with him alone, are not good practice, but I'll save my discussion on that for later.

When he returns home, Calvin is thoughtful. He asks Beth about Buck's funeral. Why was she concerned then about what shoes he wore, that they didn't match his shirt? Beth tries to walk away and Cal pleads with her to listen: "I just want to talk about something that I have always wondered about." She gives him a hug, but they don't talk.

Later at a shopping mall we see Beth, sad and lost in her thoughts again, easily startled. She meets Cal for lunch and he asks her to join him for a family meeting with Dr. Berger. Beth tells him, "Don't try to change me, Calvin. I don't want any more changes in my life. Let's just hold on to what we've got!" Calvin looks defeated.

Next, we see Con and Jeannine on their first date. They go bowling, then to a burger joint. The conversation starts silly but then gets more serious. Jeannine says she has done things she is ashamed of, and Con says he has too. He looks at his scarred wrists (we see the scars are indeed vertical, the most dangerous kind) and she notices and asks him, "Did it hurt?" Her directness is refreshing. She asks if he is okay talking about it, and he says no one has ever asked. She asks him why he did it, and he begins to describe what happened: "It was like falling into a hole and it keeps getting bigger and bigger, and you can't get out. All of a sudden, it's inside and you are the hole and you're trapped and it's all over. It's not really scary, except it is when you think back on it." He is interrupted by his swim-team friends' noisy arrival, which disrupts the moment and leaves things awkward between them.

They drive home silently. Jeannine invites him to talk some more. She tells him to please call her again.

Beth and Cal fly to Texas to play golf and visit with her brother and his wife. Con goes to watch his swim team. After the meet, Conrad has a confrontation with one of his swim-team friends, and his friend Lazenby sits down to talk to him. "I don't know why you want to be in this alone. You know, I miss him too." That gets Con's attention. "The three of us were best friends." Con tells him, tearfully, "I can't help it. It hurts too much to be around you."

Con returns home. His grandmother is staying at the house while his parents are in Texas. Con phones his hospital friend Karen. Her mother answers, upset. Con learns that Karen is dead; she killed herself. He starts panting and we hear her voice from their last meeting, "Let's have the best year of our whole lives." Con is in the bathroom, crying. He turns on the tap in the sink, the water running, memories of the storm with him and his brother trying to keep the boat upright, his hands now in the water under the faucet, we see the scars of his wrist cutting, then his vivid memory of the boat capsizing and the two of them clinging to the edges of the boat, Buck telling Con, "Don't let go. Everything is going to be okay." Is Con going to cut his wrists again?

Instead, he splashes water on his face, then runs out of the house to call Dr. Berger. The intense memories continue. Buck and Con are holding hands across the boat, then they lose their grip and Buck sinks into the water. Con is crying out his name.

At a phone booth, Con reaches Berger, who says he will meet him at the office.

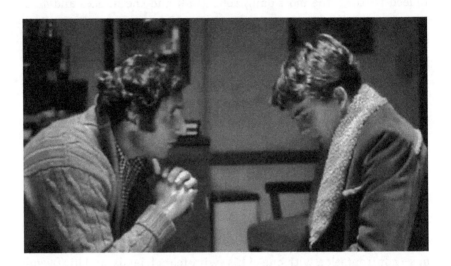

There, Con starts immediately crying, "Something happened, I need . . ." Berger is head to head with him. "I need something, it just keeps coming. I can't make it stop." Berger says, "Don't try." Con continues, "For what I did to him. It's something, it's got to be somebody's fault." Not knowing exactly what he is referring to, but making a good guess, Berger responds, "It happened." Con is still experiencing the storm and the accident: "Bucky, I didn't mean it!" Berger says, speaking as Buck, "I know that. It wasn't your fault." Then Con: "You said get the sail down, I couldn't! It jammed! And you're screwing around, until it's too late to do anything. I'm supposed to take care of it!" Berger, still as Bucky, says, "And that wasn't fair, was it?" Con answers, "No, and then you say, 'Hang on!' and then you let go! Why'd you let go?" And Berger yells, "Because I got tired!" Con yells back, "Screw you, you jerk!" and cries more heavily. Quietly, Berger says, in his own voice, "It hurts being mad at him, doesn't it? Bad things happen even when people are careful."

Berger sits with him. "Okay, so you made a mistake, you should have come in when the storm threatened." Con says again, "Why did he let go?" And Berger says, "Did it ever occur to you that you might have been stronger?. . . How long you gonna punish yourself?" Con says, more calmly, "I'd love to quit. It's not that easy. God, I loved him." Berger tells him, "I know."

What an incredibly powerful and moving scene. Finally, Berger asks him, "You said something happened. What started all this?" and Con tells him about Karen. He starts saying he wishes he could have done something, and Berger challenges him. Con tells him, "I feel really bad about this, just let me feel bad about this!" And Berger tells him he feels bad about it too. They sit quietly for a moment.

Con asks, "Why do things have to happen to people? You just do one wrong thing . . ." Berger asks him, "What was the one wrong thing you did? . . . You know . . ." He encourages him to say the words, and Con says, "I hung on. I stayed with the boat." Berger asks, "Now, you can live with that, can't you?"

Con: "I'm scared."

Berger: "Feelings are scary, and sometimes they are painful. And if you can't feel pain then you're not gonna feel anything else either."

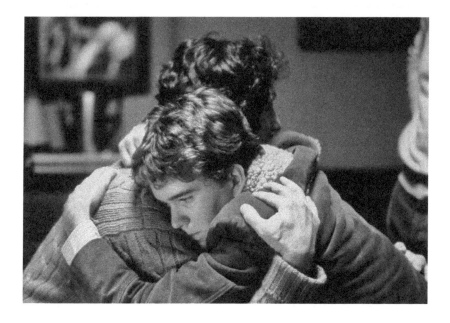

Berger continues, "You're here and you are alive and don't tell me you don't feel that." Con replies, "It doesn't feel good," and Berger says, "It is good, believe me." Con looks at him: "How do you know?" Then Berger offers, "Because I'm your friend." Con asks, "Are you really my friend?" and Berger says, "I am, count on it." Con embraces him, crying.

This is powerful, moving, and sentimental. However, it breaks a rule in therapy that should be respected. I'm not talking about the hug. I'll explain more about this later, but Berger is not his friend. He is not acting like a friend. He is acting like a very good and responsive therapist—and there is a big difference. For one thing, you would not want to burden any friend with the emotionally fraught session they just had. That requires someone with professional distance who can be thinking as well as feeling in the moment. Of course, this wouldn't be the time to explain that to Con. I just wish Berger had not offered it in that way. He was saying it as shorthand to express that he is glad he was there to be able to help Conrad through this crisis, and that he will be there for him as long as he needs him. That's a good and powerful message, but the screenwriter made me cringe when he wrote those lines.

It is particularly true of this movie, but reading my description of therapy moments is not a substitute for experiencing the sensitive, convincing performances. In this movie, you really feel as though you are witnessing something real and important. I do hope you will watch it, if you haven't already.

After the session, Con is standing in front of Jeannine's house. She comes out. They apologize to each other about the awkwardness at the date. "I'd like to try it again," he tells her, and she says yes. He asks her if she is going to school, and she reminds him it's Sunday, then invites him to come inside for breakfast. They walk arm in arm into her house.

Meanwhile, Beth and Cal are on the golf course in Texas with Beth's brother and sister-in-law. They have a quiet argument about whether or not to check on Conrad back at home. It escalates. Cal yells at her to start thinking about what Con needs, instead of how it affects her. This is much more assertive than we have seen him. Beth yells, "I don't know what anyone wants from me anymore!" Her brother and his wife watch the argument and try to intervene, "We want you to be happy." That's the wrong thing to say. Beth replies, tearfully, "Ward, you tell me the definition of happy. But first, you better make sure that your kids are good and safe, that no one's fallen off a horse, or been hit by a car, or drowned in that swimming pool you're so proud of! And then you tell me how to be happy!"

On the plane flying home Cal remembers how they were when they were younger. We see them dancing together, Beth smiling and hugging him. Back at home, Conrad tells them he is glad they are back, and he hugs his mother. Beth doesn't move; she receives the hug but does not hug Con back and instead looks stunned. Cal is watching.

That night she awakens to find Calvin out of bed. Calvin is downstairs sitting alone at the dining table, crying. She quietly asks him to tell her what's wrong. He says, "We would have been all right, if there hadn't been any 'mess.'" He tells her, "I don't know who you are. I don't know what we've been playing at . . . I don't know if I love you anymore, and I don't know what I'm going to do without that."

She says nothing, but quietly turns and goes up the stairs as the Pachelbel returns. She reaches for her suitcase and gasps, shaking, crying. Then she pulls herself together and begins packing.

Conrad wakes up to the sound of a taxi pulling away. He goes downstairs and finds his father standing in the backyard. He asks him what happened, and Cal tells Con that Beth is going away for a while, back to Texas. When Con asks why, Cal says, "I don't know." Con immediately says, "I know why, it's me. Isn't it?" Cal turns on him: "Don't do that to yourself! Things happen in this world; people don't always have the answers for them."

They sit down. Con tells him he should yell at him more often. "Haul my ass a little, get after me. The way you used to, for him." Cal says, "He needed it. You didn't. You were always so hard on yourself I never had the heart. I never worried about you. I just wasn't listening. I should have got a handle on it." Con tells him, "I used to figure you had a handle for everything. I know that wasn't fair but you always made us feel like everything was going to be all right. I really admire

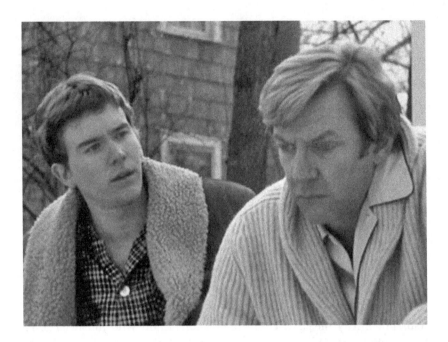

you for it." Cal replies, "Don't admire people too much, they will disappoint you sometimes." Con answers, "I'm not disappointed. I love you." And Cal embraces him, "I love you too."

The camera pulls back and the Pachelbel Canon returns and becomes louder as the credits roll. The End.

The Madness

As I hope this walk-through shows, we need to look at the family as well as Conrad, the identified "patient." They seem a typically successful, upper-middle-class family living in Lake Forest, an upscale neighborhood outside of Chicago. They are a family whose emotional values are defined by Beth, Conrad's mother: *harmony is more important than truth.* What matters is how things look, what other people outside the family think. Private unpleasantness must stay private. Hers is not a house where you drop your coat on a chair. Everything is white, there is no place for a mess, especially the mess of strong emotion.

This may be more familiar to some of us; to others it's quite foreign. But for Beth it has worked . . . until something terrible happens. Her older son Buck dies in a boating accident and her and the family's ability to cope is profoundly challenged.

Though some of my students complained that not much happens in this movie until the catharsis near the end, in fact every scene is filled with powerful emotional beats. The screenplay is eloquent in how much it tells us with small moments. Take the early scene at breakfast. Conrad awakens with a start; he has had a nightmare. When he comes downstairs his hair isn't combed and it's not clear if he has taken a shower or done anything to groom himself for the day. When Beth offers his favorite breakfast, French toast, she is doing what a mother does, feeding her son. It's an expression of care. But for Beth it's something else too: it's her way of saying, "Let's be normal again." He tells her he is not hungry. Calvin, his father, encourages him to eat. He is concerned and trying to gently suggest some healthy behaviors. He also is something of a cheerleader for returning to normality, showing a bit too much delight at hearing that Con is getting together with his old friends for a ride to school. Beth, on the other hand, takes Con's not wanting to eat personally, grabs his plate, and dumps everything into the sink. Her mode is to want things to look normal, for Con to act normal, no matter how he is feeling. He should eat his favorite breakfast because that would mean all was okay, and as it used to be.

More than that, she finds it hard be with him, to find something to say. The rhythm is always off in their communication. The conversation in the backyard is a painful example. When the conversation goes wrong, she goes into the house. Con follows and tries to apologize, offering to help her set the table. He was hoping to share a task with her as a way of being together. But she sends him away to clean up his mess: the mess of his depression, of his suicide attempt. Then, the phone rings and, when asked, she says to the caller, "No, I'm not doing anything important." Beth is relieved to be interrupted by the call, from having to engage with her son.

There are many other examples, like the photo session with the extended family. Beth can't stand next to Con or touch him for more than a moment without becoming uncomfortable. There is another example with Dr. Berger I'll talk about in a moment.

We have seen flashbacks that tell us Beth wasn't always this controlled, this controlling. We see her laughing happily with Buck, dancing with her husband, showing a passionate and joyful nature. But not now. Beth would try to sweep every unpleasant emotion under the rug if she could. Well, that's probably not true since this is not someone who would allow anything messy to stay under a rug; she would want to powerfully vacuum it away. Keeping a pristine house is her version of control, of keeping up appearances.

So, she scolds Calvin for telling friends at the party that Con is seeing a psychiatrist. That is "private," dirty laundry not to be aired. It seems to especially bother her that he is seeing a Jewish psychiatrist. When Calvin tells her later he has met with Dr. Berger and wants Beth to join him, she tells him "Don't change me, Calvin. I don't want to change," and he is deeply disappointed.

Calvin tells Berger, "We would have been okay, if Buck hadn't died." And that may well be true. They might have had the appearance of being "okay." Beth's obsessive need to control, to keep things neat, to look perfect might have continued. But she could not control the loss, though she could control what color shoes her husband wears to the funeral. Calvin doesn't understand that Beth is grieving too. He asks her why she cared about the shoes he wore at the funeral. What he sees, he can't connect with. He has lost sympathy for her. It's what he means when he tells her, "I'm not sure I love you anymore."

When things get upsetting, we all fall back on routine to help us get by. She tries to order her life like the napkin rings in her drawer. She is an extreme example of what happens when that doesn't work. Her coping style gets in the way of her being emotionally available, or of being able to reach out for help. She was a good-enough mother to Buck, maybe more than that because to her he was special, her first child. She allowed him to affect her in ways that her husband and Conrad don't.

If you allow yourself to feel intensely for someone, you leave yourself vulnerable for great hurt if that person leaves you, or if something happens to them. Keeping such feelings under wraps means that you cannot allow yourself to feel great joy, either, or a loving connection. This is a universal dilemma.

After the crisis about Karen's suicide, and the powerful therapy session with Dr. Berger, Conrad seems more relaxed, in a better mood. We see him decorating the Christmas tree when Beth comes home. She is obviously angry. She has just heard that weeks ago Con quit swimming. She takes it personally that she has to find out from a friend, and she is not able to understand any of her son's reasons or emotions. She says to Con, "You always try to hurt me, don't you?" Calvin watches and tries to intervene (his standard role), but the gulf is too wide.

When Conrad first meets Dr. Berger, he tells him he wants to be more in control. Berger tells him, "I'm not big on control. Control's a tough nut." Con is very much like his mother. She too wants to be in better control, to contain things as a way to deal with the devastating sudden loss of Buck. So much of your world you can control, and then the unexpected happens and you reach your limits.

Beth tries harder to keep herself and her diminished family under control, but it's a losing strategy. When Calvin tells her, crying, that he is not sure he loves her anymore, this was the moment for her to sit with him, ask about his pain, and talk about her own grief—but she can't manage it. Instead, she says nothing, goes upstairs, and starts to take down her suitcase. And then, she gasps. For that one moment we see how hard it has been to control the sadness, how alone she must feel. But then she composes herself and starts packing to leave. She makes it hard to feel sympathy for her because she is so unwilling to admit how much she is hurting too.

Calvin is also grieving and depressed, but he shows it differently. His work partner tells him he is distracted, uninvolved, not paying attention at the office, drifting. You don't have to look sad or be crying to be depressed; being distracted, drifting, having trouble concentrating can be depression too.

Calvin tells Dr. Berger he used to think of himself as lucky, but no longer. It was lucky that he found Conrad in time when he tried to kill himself. But you can't feel lucky when your other son dies from drowning. Calvin understands that he needs help too. That it isn't only Conrad who is not coping. He also sees that the work with Berger is helping. Because he sees being supportive as his role, he wants for everyone to get help too.

Conrad's suicide attempt was a cry for "help" for the entire family. We know he wanted to die: it's clear he timed his wrist cutting when he thought that no one would be home. And when we see the scars, we see he cut his wrist vertically, not across, which makes it easier to cut deep and bleed faster. He sees his mother look at him and he imagines she is thinking, why didn't he die instead of Buck, the favored firstborn. He sees that as her wish, and his suicide as fulfilling that wish. But the suicide is also an angry gesture. They had to re-grout her tiles because there was so much blood. He was going to die, but he was going to make a grand mess for her to clean up too.

We see that being angry at someone you love is particularly hard for Con, especially when that someone is Buck who has died. But he is also angry at his mother: for not loving him enough, for so obviously loving Buck more, for not being glad that he is alive. So, his suicide is, as one of my beloved psychiatric mentors, Carl Whitaker, taught me, also a "fuck you" to the person who "made me do it."

Conrad shows the classic symptoms of major depression. His normal grief crossed the line into a self-destructive sadness and inability to function. Remember, we are not seeing him at his worst. Before the events of the film, he was suicidally depressed and tried to kill himself. He was in hospital for four months and had shock therapy. When we meet Conrad, he is supposedly doing better.

We see right away he still sleeps badly, has nightmares, doesn't groom himself (his hair is a mess) or exercise ordinary hygiene. He has little appetite, low energy, is easily distracted (the teacher needs to ask several times to get his attention), and has trouble concentrating. He no longer enjoys the activities and the people that used to mean something to him. He is irritable, tense, tightly wound. He is able to function, but at a low level, barely getting by.

When Lazenby, his swim-team friend, asks why Conrad is avoiding him, he tells Con, "Buck was my friend. I miss him too." Conrad says "it hurts too much" to see Lazenby because it reminds him of who is no longer there. In the therapy sessions we learn that he feels guilty, and over-responsible. He blames himself, but for what we don't at first know—for surviving when Buck did not. We see emptiness more than overt sadness, with anger at himself, at his mother, and, finally, he discovers as we do, at his brother—for letting go, for not "holding on." How can you be angry at someone you love so much, so looked up to, when they are dead?

About Suicide

Central to this story is that Conrad tried to commit suicide by cutting his wrists sometime after the death of his brother. He still has many of the symptoms of depression, even after shock treatment and several months in the hospital. So, he is on the mend, but still depressed when we meet him.

We don't know what precipitated his suicide attempt, what made him decide to do it that day. This is something that his therapist would want to explore in order to judge if there is a risk of it happening again.

A therapist must gauge just how depressed a person is, and more specifically whether the hopelessness that is so often part of depression has led them to consider ending their lives. So, in addition to asking in detail about all the symptoms that Con presents, a trained therapist would ask about thoughts of suicide. We know Conrad has already tried suicide and that he really wanted to die, so his risk is greater. But a therapist will not always know that about the patient at first.

A therapist should stand for life, for staying alive. It is honest to tell anyone who is depressed that, if they survive, they will in time feel different, feel better, and be glad that they are alive. The natural course of even the worst depressions is to cycle toward feeling better. With medication and therapy, the odds of that happening are dramatically improved. When a person feels like they are at the bottom of a black pit with no way out—as Conrad describes to Jeannine—it's hard to believe, or even imagine, that it's possible. Which is how the desperate hopelessness leads to thoughts of "ending it all."

So, the therapist must ask about it, ask them if they have been thinking about life and death and if they have been thinking about wanting to be dead. The therapist looks for signs that they are clearing their world of people and things in anticipation of dying. Are they increasingly isolating themselves from family and friends? Are they giving things away or discarding things that have meant something to them? Have they thought about killing themselves?

By the way, it's dangerous to use euphemisms when discussing this subject. A doctor should not ask, "Have you thought about hurting yourself?" when they mean "Have you thought about *killing* yourself?" Many people will be moved to hurt themselves, to do something that causes physical pain, such as burn themselves with cigarettes or cut their skin with a razor or scissors, to substitute physical pain for emotional pain that feels overwhelming. They don't want to die; they just want to hurt. Often there is a fascination with the process: the scratching is done slowly, drawing blood, and somehow this distracts from feeling so bad.

This is different from wanting to die. On the other hand, many people who do want to die do not want to feel any pain at all. They will take pills and hope the dying is passive and painless.

So, it is important to ask about wanting to be dead in addition to asking about wanting to hurt themselves. These are two different things. Then, if the person acknowledges that he or she has considered dying, they should be asked how they would do it. Risk is gauged by what they say. How close have they come to actually trying? What stopped them? Or if they tried before, how is it that they are still alive? Did they tell someone and ask for help? Was it an accident that the suicide didn't work (they took too few pills, or the gun didn't fire)?

If they say, for instance, that they want to shoot themselves, but they don't own a gun and don't know how to find or use one, the risk of them actually doing it any time soon is low. However, if they tell you that they plan to take a handful of pills, that they have been collecting the pills for weeks, that they know how many they would need to kill them, and that they spend hours staring at the pill bottle waiting for the moment, an alarm should go off. This is dangerous.

Similarly, the person who imagines driving a car into an abutment on the way to work, knows exactly which one they would aim for, and makes a point of noticing it each day, this is also cause for alarm. Certain ways to commit suicide allow for a change of heart. If you take pills, lie back and then suddenly don't want to die, you can try to throw-up the pills or get someone to rush you to the emergency room. But, crashing your car, jumping out a high window, or pulling the trigger—these are irreversible and only luck will keep you alive.

Knowing how someone contemplates suicide is important so a therapist can know how best to respond. If the risk is low and the method leaves room for a change of mind, then a therapist can reinforce wanting the person to stay alive long enough to feel better, arrange to see them more frequently, and suggest they share what they are considering with a loved one or close friend, to encourage their support system, and set up an agreement that, if they feel an increase in the urge to die, they will reach out. As Conrad did with Dr. Berger.

If the risk seems acute and imminent, patients must be advised about the need to protect themselves from their impulses and consider hospitalization. Sometimes their doctor will have to put them in the hospital against their will, to protect them from doing themselves harm. This involuntary commitment is something therapists do reluctantly. We want to help our patients to understand how dangerous their situation is and to accept the help that's needed, but if the person refuses protection, we have no choice but to consider commitment. Eventually, if someone really wants to be dead, they will make it happen. But we want to give them the best chance to learn that it is possible to feel better in the world, and eventually feel good about being alive.

We will talk more about this in the chapter on therapy.

There are different qualities to a suicide. The so-called suicide gesture refers to a usually impulsive act that has not been planned or thought through. Certain personality disorders (such as histrionic and borderline) are particularly vulnerable to this because of a combination of volatile emotionality, poor self-image, and impulsivity. But people simply under stress or feeling overwhelmed are at risk too. Often after an argument or confrontation, or when feeling abandoned or rejected, they will impulsively do something harmful to themselves, something that might kill them; most commonly, taking pills or cutting their wrists. It's not something that has been long contemplated, it's a desperate act of the moment, often (but not always) immediately regretted. So, asking about the circumstances of a suicide is important. Was there a message meant by the action? "You'll be sorry you made me do this," or "Look what you made me do!" or "Please come back, I can't survive without you." These impulsive gestures can be hard to prevent. With some personality disorder diagnoses they may indeed be predictable (it's part of the madness), but not always. The gestures can become a habit even for someone less compromised, a coping style for moments of distress. There will often be a pattern, and over time the patient can be helped to understand the triggering circumstances.

Conrad's suicide was very different. It's likely he was thinking about it for quite a while before he did it, that there was a build-up of grief, guilt, and self-recrimination that brought him to that moment. And that he meant the suicide to succeed; in other words, that he would end up dead.

When someone tells me in therapy that they are contemplating suicide, there are several things I do to hopefully make it less likely that they will actually do it. I want to make it real, because often there is a lot of fantasy involved. I will ask them what they imagine the effect will be on their family and loved ones. Who will react strongly, and who will hardly react at all? And what will the reaction be? This tells you a lot right away about the dynamics of the family. If it's a teenager like Con, I will ask them what they think will happen to their room after they are gone. Will it become a shrine (the way Buck's room is with all his swimming trophies prominently displayed) or will their parents turn the room into a study or TV room, or will they rent it out? What will happen to their clothes? Will the parents keep the closet intact as part of the shrine or just bring their things to Goodwill? A teenager might imagine that the high school yearbook will be dedicated to them (as it too often is, a glorification that can inadvertently encourage copycat suicides), that people will say particularly nice things about them or express the wish that they had treated them better. There is a grandiosity in these fantasies, and built into them is the idea that even though you are dead, you will know about these reactions.

As a therapist, I want to burst these balloons. Remove as many reasons to die as possible. Just raising these questions can make being dead more real, and douse water on any ideas that the suicide will somehow change other people's behavior. A therapist must take a stand on the side of life. Because if you stay alive, there is hope. If you are dead, it's all over.

A Good Therapy

The portrayal of psychotherapy in *Ordinary People* is the best I've found so far in movies. I don't include long-form streaming series, some of which are even better, mostly because they can show more. They have time to show just how long therapy can take before it makes an obvious difference. The show *In Treatment,* which is all about therapy, portrays twelve weeks of sessions with a variety of patients in each season, and the therapy sessions in *The Sopranos* give more of a sense of the longueurs of treatment and how rare the "aha" moments of understanding can be.

The psychotherapy in *Ordinary People* is the gold-standard for a traditional movie. Here we see highlights of some three months of therapy. The highlights seem real, convincing, and emotionally true.

Dr. Berger is presented as a contrast to the Jarrett family. His office is shades of brown, it's disordered, messy, casual. He is relaxed. Conrad first meets him as he is clumsily trying to repair a stereo. He comes across as genuine, not trying to impress or put up a front. All this is in contrast to Beth and to the Jarrett house. If Beth ever came to his office, she would either refuse to enter because it was such a mess or immediately start tidying up.

Unlike Conrad's family, Berger is blunt, to the point. He says what he means. He is a *mensch,* a very useful Yiddish word meaning a real human being: someone of integrity and honor, a person warm yet firm of purpose. It is a high compliment. If Berger sets limits, it is because such limits help the process. In the first session, Conrad tells him that what he wants from the therapy is to learn "control." Berger tells him, "I'm not big on control. Control is a tough nut," and tells him that he needs to come in twice a week. Conrad says he would have to miss swim practice, and Berger lets him squirm a bit before he decides: "Guess I'll have to skip practice." The doctor sets the rules, but the patient has to decide if he will abide by them. If he does, they have a deal. If not, then either they negotiate, or the therapy doesn't happen. Berger honors Con's autonomy. He will not be another parent and tell him what to do. He will treat Conrad like an adult.

The clock faces the doctor, as Con points out. Each session has a time limit that the therapist will monitor, leaving the patient to use the time as best he can. In one session, when Conrad is making some useful connections and needs just a few more minutes to put it into words, Berger calls "time's up" and makes it stick. There are a couple of reasons to do that. One, it compels Conrad to think about the issue outside of therapy, where he is likely to come to the epiphany he is seeking without further coaching. And two, the rules matter. If every time a patient had what's called a "doorway moment"—just coming to understanding, or asking a pertinent question, as they leave with a hand on the doorknob—then every session would go long. It would encourage the patient to look for extra time from their therapist: "If you love me, you will give me more time." Not a useful dynamic. So, the therapist makes it clear that when the clock says it's time to stop, you stop. Soon every patient learns to do the work necessary in the proper time and know that they can continue on their own, or in the next session.

Having said that, when Conrad experiences a crisis and Berger meets with him, they don't set a time limit. This isn't a normal session. This will take as long as it takes, and no one is looking at the clock. So, another rule is that sometimes the rules change with the circumstance: a lesson in life.

Berger is good at his questions. "Do you feel like you are on stage?" and Conrad knows exactly what he means. He feels understood and opens up. Berger rarely gives advice but when he does it's short, sweet, and useful. I like when Conrad complains that he thought you were supposed to feel good after therapy. Berger says, "Not necessarily," and explains that feelings can hurt but that if you try not to feel (which Beth is doing, and Con tries to do) then you can't be open to good feelings when they happen. He is giving Conrad permission to examine unpleasant feelings like anger without actually telling him.

I question a few of Berger's decisions, though. He sees Calvin, Con's father, by himself. This is not a good idea, especially if the primary patient is an adolescent. As Cal acknowledges, therapy is private: the things you talk about with your doctor stay between you. It allows you to think and say things uncensored that you would not want others to hear. Cal doesn't pry. But Con doesn't know that, and once he knows that his father has met with his doctor without him being there, he may worry about what was said, what secret the psychiatrist might have told his father. The solution to this is to never see the parent without the teen being there, or at least giving permission for a separate session and discussing with the doctor what might be off-limits to disclose. We know we can trust Berger to maintain secrecy and respect the boundaries of therapy, but best practices would be for Conrad to be included.

When Cal realizes that he too needs therapy, Berger would do best to refer him to another doctor, or to see Cal and Con together. In my office, I would see them together. They are both grieving, and they both want to change things with Beth. So, ideally, Beth would be part of the family therapy too. Except that she announces firmly she wants no part of it. I would see the men together and hope that, in time, Beth would join us.

It's wonderful how the emergency session unfolds. Berger sees how upset Con is and encourages him as he re-experiences the tragedy on the water. He uses the gestalt therapy technique of role-play, responding to Con in the moment, in the voice of his brother, leading him to understand more about what happened when the boat capsized and Buck let go and drowned. "Why did he let go!?" cries Con, and

Berger says, quietly, "Because I got tired." This is a powerful session, after which they are both exhausted.

That's when there is the "ouch" moment, something I wish they had left out of the screenplay. Berger tells Con, "I'm your friend" and Con asks, "Are you really my friend?" Berger says yes and Conrad hugs him. Berger should not have used that word. If Conrad had asked him the question directly, the proper response would have been, "No, I'm not your friend. I'm your doctor, and I will be there for you when you need me." Your therapist is not your friend. You will not go to the movies together and share a pizza. Your therapist is someone to whom you can tell your most difficult thoughts, who will keep what's said in therapy secret, who will be there for you if you have a crisis, and who will stand by you and help you get better. But your therapist is not your friend. Your therapist is both more and less than that.

Some therapists would also object to the hug Berger gives Con. Berger already breaks some rules of professional distance by his frank questions and informal manner. I think that is a personal choice, in part based on what a particular therapist is comfortable with, and the rules of their brand of therapy. I like that moment. I think sometimes a hug is what's wanted and it can convey more than words: support, concern, caring, reassurance.

We see that Con is getting better. He finds a friend in Jeannine, someone honest and brave enough to ask him about his depression and his suicide, but also someone who is new in town and did not know Buck, so Con has a fresh start with her. He makes efforts to connect with his mom, often clumsy, but he is trying. With Berger's help he begins to forgive her, and Buck, and himself—to lighten up and begin to enjoy life.

After the cathartic role-play, Berger finally asks Con what set him off. Con tells him he just heard about Karen committing suicide. And he says something wonderful, "I feel bad about this. Let me just feel bad about this." Berger understands, and says, "I feel bad about it too." This is not the time to analyze or discuss—right then, being together and being quietly sad is what's needed.

There is a Roz Chast cartoon from *The New Yorker* magazine that I like. A mother and small child are in Central Park in New York. The child has just dropped his ice cream cone onto the ground and is crying. The mother leans over and says, "Do you want to talk about it?"

No, he doesn't. Sometimes you just want another ice cream. And sometimes you just want to feel bad about it.

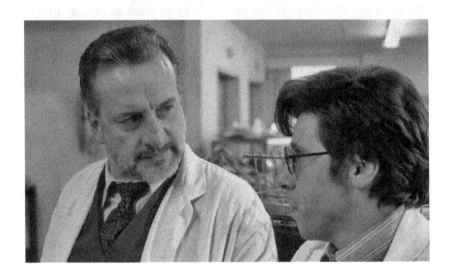

The Hospital (1971)

George C. Scott, Diana Rigg
Director: Arthur Hiller

This very dark comedy by Paddy Chayefsky, the writer of *Network*, which came out a few years later, is an odd mix of absurd, biting satire, and serious drama.

It's a very bad day at a major city hospital, with radicals demonstrating outside against the hospital's slum-clearance project and a madman murdering doctors and patients inside. George C. Scott is Dr. Herbert Bock, the head of medicine, a depressed and exhausted man. It's Dr. Bock's madness that interests us here. The so-called madman roaming the halls killing doctors and switching patients' ID tags so they get the wrong medications is not him.

In an early scene, Bock reluctantly reaches out to a psychiatrist colleague about his depression. Chayefsky's speeches are impassioned and powerful; remember *Network*'s "I'm mad as hell, and I'm not going to take it anymore!" In a brilliant monologue, Bock describes his symptoms and circumstances to the psychiatrist. He left his wife; he is alienated from his "useless" grown-up children and blames himself for their failures. He has lost any enthusiasm for his work as a doctor; he is impotent, drinking heavily, and suicidal. The psychiatrist asks him about his "suicidal speculations" and Bock tells him, "I amuse myself with different ways of killing myself that don't look like suicide" so as not to lose the family's insurance. The psychiatrist replies that digitalis could do it, which encourages Bock to show just how much thought he has given suicide. There is little risk that the psychiatrist's suggestion of digitalis would have added to his suicidal preoccupations. But it does open up the conversation to reveal how angry Bock is and that he has very particular plans.

He is embarrassed and leaves, saying he just needs to pull himself together and get back into his work.

Later that night, in his darkened office, Bock talks with Barbara Drummond (Diana Rigg), an ex-hippie, ex-nurse he has just met who lives with her father on an Indian reservation. He tells her about his impotence; not just sexual, but his loss of "permanent worth," his desire to work, his reason for being. He is depressed, and he is very angry. In a famous rant against his chosen profession, he yells, "We have established the most enormous medical entity ever conceived . . . and people are sicker than ever! We cure nothing! We heal nothing! The whole goddamn rancid world is strangulating in front of our eyes." When she challenges him, he angrily throws her out. She leaves but comes back to find him with a belt tied around his arm, ready to kill himself by injecting potassium. He talked suicide and really meant it.

When she interrupts him just as he is about to put the needle in his arm, he aggressively attacks her, which becomes sexual, his potency restored. Their lovemaking gives him a new sense of purpose. But the film is hardly sentimental. When Barbara suggests he join her on the Indian reservation where he can rediscover his passion for medicine, she says, "If you love me, I don't see what other choice you have." He replies, "I raped you in a suicidal rage. How do we get to love and children all of a sudden?"

This movie is vivid and intellectually powerful. But it doesn't have the emotional heft of *Ordinary People*, in part because the tone of the film switches so often to farce. The acting is extraordinary, however. Chayefsky won an Oscar for Best Screenplay and Scott was nominated for Best Actor. Diana Rigg was not nominated, but she should have been. She is very good. The film is included in the National Film Registry of the Library of Congress.

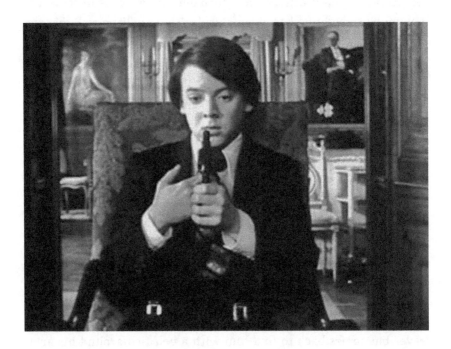

Harold and Maude (1971)

Bud Cort, Ruth Gordon
Director: Hal Ashby

This is one strange movie and a very black comedy. Under the credits we watch Harold (Bud Cort), a young man in his early twenties, carefully prepare to hang himself while Cat Stevens's song "Don't Be Shy" plays. He writes a note and pins it to his jacket, lights two candles, then positions a chair, steps onto it, then off, feet dangling off the floor, a rope around his neck. His mother comes into the room, looks at him, then sits down and picks up the phone. Harold is still hanging. She says to him, "I suppose you think that is very funny, Harold." She cancels her hair appointment. Harold makes choking sounds trying to get her attention. She walks out, pausing to tell him, "Dinner at eight and do try to be a little more vivacious." Later we see her getting dressed and going into her bathroom. Harold is splayed out in the bathtub, covered in blood. This upsets her. In close-up we see the supposedly dead Harold stick out his tongue at her. There will be other "suicides": drowning in his swimming pool, chopping off his hand, setting himself on fire, shooting himself in the head while she fills out a dating questionnaire for him. All fake, and all for the "benefit" of his mother, as he tells the impossibly bad psychiatrist he sees.

When he is asked what he does for fun, Harold replies, "I go to funerals." This is where he meets Maude (Ruth Gordon), seventy-nine years old, who rather than being preoccupied with death embraces life with an enthusiasm that Harold can't resist. He falls in love with her.

These suicide gestures (performances, really) have nothing to do with wanting to die and everything to do with wanting to annoy his mother and resist her plans for him. This is played for comedy but it shows that suicides can happen for many reasons—they can be demanding attention, like here, or a cry for help. Cort plays Harold with a deadpan expressionless monotone that looks very much like the flat affect of low-grade depression. Ruth Gordon's Maude is "lust for life" personified. This is someone who steals whatever she wants and digs up city trees to return them to the forest. There is a cult enthusiasm for this movie, but you either love it for its weirdness or you hate it for the same reason.

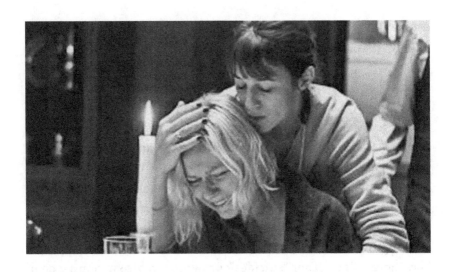

Melancholia (2011)

Kirsten Dunst, Charlotte Gainsbourg, Kiefer Sutherland
Writer and Director: Lars von Trier

This film does something unusual. It not only tells the story of a woman with serious chronic depression but, in every frame, it *is* the experience of depression. I don't find it depressing, though. It's very beautiful and, in the end, it is very sad. How could it not be, since it's about the end of the world?

"Melancholia" is an antique word for serious depression. Here, it's also the name of a large planet that is on a path that will bring it very close to Earth, what's called a "flyby." At least that is what the scientists say; that it will be a spectacular event, a near miss, and nothing to be afraid of.

To the haunting music of Wagner's prelude to *Tristan and Isolde*, the movie opens with dream-like images in slow-motion, so slow that they look like still-life paintings. A woman carrying a young child, whose footsteps sink into the turf of a golf course, a horse sinking to the ground, another woman in a bridal gown, dragging what look like tree roots behind her.

These are the dreams of Justine (Kirsten Dunst). She is the bride at an elaborate and very expensive reception after her wedding. Everyone is asking her if she is happy, and you can see she is trying to be, but she seems pained, distracted, certainly not joyous.

There is family trouble. Her mother's toast at the dinner is to announce she doesn't believe in marriage, especially by members of her family. She is divorced from Justine's father, who seems to be paying more attention to the two women named Betty at his table than to Justine. When Justine tries to talk to her mother, it does not go well. Justine tells her, "I smile, I smile, I smile. But I am frightened. I have trouble walking properly." This is not just the jitters of a new bride, but her mother's response is dismissive. By the end of the evening her groom has left her, and she has had sex with a stranger and she has told off her boss and gotten fired.

Her sister Claire (Gainsbourg) is practical and sympathetic, trying to be supportive but often frustrated and angry at her sister's illness. It's several days later, and Claire is very worried about Melancholia. Her husband (Kiefer Sutherland), an amateur stargazer, tries to reassure her it's safe; the scientists have calculated carefully. Claire wants to believe him, but the internet says otherwise.

Claire is on the phone talking to Justine, who is in real trouble. She is emotionally paralyzed; she seems incapable of getting herself into a taxi to come to her sister. When Justine finally arrives, she is a mess. Disheveled, weak, emaciated, and unable to walk on her own, she immediately goes to bed. The next day Claire wakes her and tries to help her take a bath. It's clear Justine hasn't cleaned herself in days. She can't raise her leg to get into the tub. Is it physical weakness because she has not eaten or is it the extreme lethargy of depression? It is probably a bit of both. She collapses on the floor. When she finally comes downstairs for dinner, Claire has made her favorite meal, meat loaf. But when Justine tries to eat it, she can't: "It tastes like ashes." She is profoundly depressed.

Over the coming days, Claire watches as the planet comes closer and closer to Earth. At the last minute it begins to recede, and she breathes a sigh of relief. But then, the next day, it looms again, slowly filling the sky. Claire's son makes a simple device that shows whether the planet is coming closer, and it is. Justine seems stronger, more calm, less sad, as her sister becomes more and more anxious.

Claire's husband disappears and she finds him dead in the horse barn. He has taken her pills and killed himself, realizing that the scientists were wrong and that the planet will collide with Earth.

In a strange conversation, Justine tells Claire, "I know things. We are alone. There is no afterlife. Life is only on Earth, and not for long." Justine has lived her life depressed, experiencing fear and anguish and emptiness, feeling doomed every day. So, she is oddly better prepared than her sister to confront the real doom of the end of the world.

In a panic for herself and for her son, Claire tries to run, but where can she go?

This is no action picture. There are no scenes of mass hysteria, of scientists trying to solve the crisis, of heroes sent to save the day. This is a quiet film; the dread is real but contained. Finally, it's just two sisters and one little boy, facing the end. Justine tells the boy she can make it safe, because they can build a magic cave. Together they gather sticks and build a small open tent on a meadow near the house. There is something about this small task, being together in nature, that is soothing.

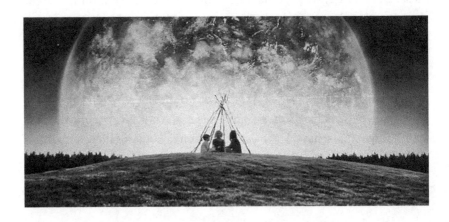

Then, they all sit together inside it, holding hands, their eyes closed. The wind is rising. Justine is calm, Claire is terrified and crying silently, the boy seems content. Melancholia comes closer and closer. There is a powerful light . . . and the world and the movie ends.

RECOMMENDED READING

Agee, James. *A Death in the Family,* Centennial edition. New York: Penguin Classics; 2009.

A remarkable novel, about grief and family.

Barber, Samuel. *Knoxville, Summer of 1915/Essays Nos 1 & 2/Adagio for Strings* [CD]. Cleveland, OH: Telarc audio; 2006.

Knoxville, Summer of 1915 is a haunting vocal work based on the opening words of *A Death in the Family.*

Mack, John, and Holly Hickler. *Vivienne, The Life and Suicide of an Adolescent Girl.* New York: New American Library; 1982.

See "A Clinician's Analysis."

Skynner, Robin, and John Cleese. *Families and How to Survive Them.* London: Methuen; 1983.

Specifically, chapter 2: "Family Structures."

Solomon, Andrew. *The Noonday Demon—An Atlas of Depression.* New York: Scribner; 2001 and 2015.

Describing his own struggles with depression, the author interviews other sufferers, doctors, scientists, policymakers, and philosophers and provides a moving story of depression throughout history.

Styron, William. *Darkness Visible—A Memoir of Madness.* New York: Open Road Integrated Media; 2010.

The author of *The Confessions of Nat Turner* and *Sophie's Choice* eloquently tells the story of his suicidal depression and of his struggles toward recovery.

▪11▪

"You make me want to be a better man."

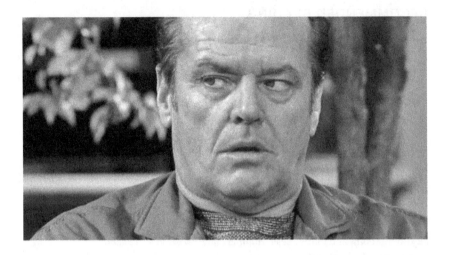

Obsessive-Compulsive Disorder and Other Anxieties

As Good as It Gets (1997)

Jack Nicholson, Helen Hunt, Greg Kinnear
Director: James L. Brooks

We will be exploring several films featuring various forms of anxiety disorder in this chapter. I like to think of this category as "garden variety" madness, because these disorders are much more common than the major madnesses of earlier chapters. They can be every bit as disabling, but what makes them different is that less intense versions are part of everyday living in the way that the psychoses and psychopathic personality disorders are not. Most of us (I might say all of us, it's that universal) have experienced moments of anxiety at times of challenge or stress, but if such anxiety is not something that happens every day, we are able to deal with it, control it, and move on. The characters in these films don't have that luxury. The types of anxiety that they live with are chronic, often overwhelming, and very uncomfortable. But, for reasons I want us to explore, they are often the stuff of comedy.

In these films, the anxiety disorders are sometimes front and center in the story, but more often, they are incidental to the plot. This is quite different from the films we have talked about before. The featured films in those chapters needed to be considered in their entirety to best understand the madness. I don't think that approach works as well here. Therefore, we will be treating the films in this chapter a bit differently. I won't be doing as detailed a walkthrough; instead, I will focus on the moments in each film that best show us what the anxiety is like.

As Good as It Gets is an excellent example. It was nominated for Academy Awards in multiple categories, including Best Screenplay, Best Director, and Best Picture of 1997 (*The English Patient* won). Jack Nicholson won Best Actor and Helen Hunt won Best Actress. Greg Kinnear was nominated for Best Supporting Actor. The film won Best Picture (Musical or Comedy) at the Golden Globes. So, it is a highly lauded film. It is unusual, as a comedy, to get such recognition, but it deserves it.

The Movie

As Good as It Gets is a comedy-drama with real heart and characters of complexity and appeal. Jack Nicholson's Melvin Udall starts out incredibly unlikeable. We first see him trying to entice the neighbor's dog into the elevator so he will pee outside (and clearly hoping he will never be seen again). When that doesn't work, he drops the dog down the trash chute. Then we watch him make fun of his homosexual neighbor, Simon (Greg Kinnear), the dog's owner, and make racist comments about Simon's friend, Frank (Cuba Gooding, Jr.). All of this happens even before the credits begin. Nicholson is a fascinating and original actor, so Melvin comes across as hateful but also oddly charming.

We discover more about him as the credits roll. He enters his apartment and locks and unlocks the door, counting five times, then switches the light on and off five times. In the bathroom, he takes off leather gloves and tosses them in the trash. He opens his medicine cabinet and we see it is filled with dozens of bars of soap, individually wrapped. He takes one, washes his hands under very hot water. We know it's hot because it is steaming, but in an uncharacteristically "actorly" gesture, he mutters, "hot, hot" just to be sure we get it (I don't know who didn't trust the audience to understand—Nicholson or the director—but it's one of the few false notes in the film). He tosses the bar of soap into the trash and picks up another, washing his hands again.

So, we immediately are presented with compulsive behaviors: a number compulsion (needing to do things a set number of times) and a preoccupation with dirt or germs with the ritual of vigorous hand washing.

Melvin is a successful writer of romance novels. Simon interrupts him as he's writing to confront him about the dog, which was found in the basement garbage bin. Melvin attacks Simon for the interruption, asking him if he would like it if he was interrupted when he was "nancing around in your garden." This is a man who is homophobic and proud of it. He demands never to be interrupted again and drives home his point by saying that, even if Simon thought Melvin was dying or dead, or he wanted to celebrate because some "fudge packer" was elected the first "queer president," he should never again knock on his door. Melvin is supercilious, obnoxious, and mean, and completely intimidates Simon.

Later, we see that Melvin, walking to his favorite restaurant, also has a compulsion that does not allow him to step on cracks or to be touched. He must dance his way along the sidewalk, avoiding cracks and contact with people, yelling "don't touch" as he goes. It's an adventure just getting anywhere.

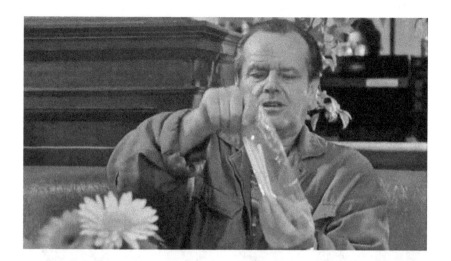

In the restaurant, we meet a waitress, Carol (Helen Hunt). She knows Melvin well; he has a regular table. He complains that there are Jews at his table and insults them until they leave. Carol tells him to "behave," and that the owner says if he ever does that again he will be barred for life. She is neither intimidated by him nor impressed. He brings his own plastic utensils and orders a really big breakfast. Carol jokes that with that diet Melvin is going to die soon, and his comeback is, "It sounds like your son will die soon too" (he knows the boy is frequently ill). She reacts like she was just punched. Silently, she stares at him until he notices. She tells him with quiet intensity if he ever mentions her son again, he will never be able to eat there again. She demands he acknowledge that he understands and calls him "a crazy fuck." He struggles, nods his head, and she gets his order.

Melvin's obnoxious behavior—his racist, homophobic, misanthropic character—has nothing to do with his obsessive-compulsive disorder (OCD). The story will be about his finding a way to be a better human being through his experiences with Carol and Simon. The OCD is a hurdle, making his life that much more difficult, but it's not the reason he comes across as so dismissive of the world and other people. That's who he is when the film starts, and it will take some tough love to help him change.

Simon has a lovely thing to say early on, speaking to a model he is drawing: "If you look at someone long enough, you discover their humanity." That is what this film is doing.

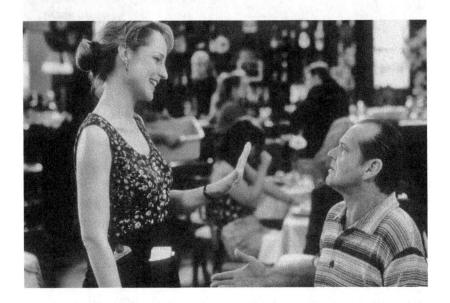

It is another day at the restaurant. We see Melvin trying to get Carol's attention. She asks why he uses his own plastic knives and forks. She suggests he give himself a little pep talk: "Must try other people's clean silverware as part of the fun of dining out." Melvin quietly asks her what's wrong with her son. He even asks his name. It's Spencer. A moment of connection.

Simon's studio is burglarized, and he is badly beaten. He is in the hospital, and Frank demands that Melvin take care of Verdell, Simon's dog. Frank confronted Melvin about his behavior with Simon before, and now has Melvin cowering. This germaphobe with OCD has no choice but to take the dog into the sanctuary that is his home, and Frank has made it clear that he had better make sure no harm comes to him. When Melvin goes to his restaurant, he leaves Verdell leashed outside, and then, worried that someone might take him, changes from his regular booth to keep watch. This small change of routine is a big deal for someone for whom ritual keeps anxiety at bay; that's what the compulsions are all about. But, because he is, in spite of himself, beginning to enjoy the companionship of the dog, he makes the change without realizing it. Carol notices. Later, Melvin takes delight in watching Verdell imitate him and not step on cracks in the sidewalk (very unlikely, but okay . . .). They are bonding.

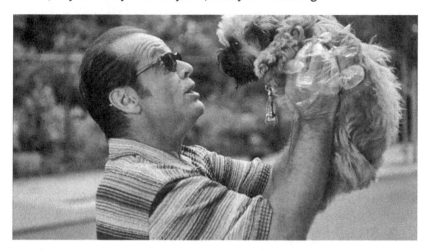

When Melvin is told that Simon is on the mend and will come to pick up his dog the next day, we see him begin to have what looks like a panic attack (breathing faster and starting to cry).

After returning Verdell and finding himself crying again, Melvin does his sidewalk crack-avoiding walk to his therapist's office. Barging in without an appointment, he yells, "Help!" We learn that he hasn't kept his appointments. He asks the doctor if he knows how hard it was for him to come there. The therapist says yes. But when Melvin tries to begin a session, the therapist properly sets a clear boundary and tells him no. Melvin leaves through the waiting room and startles the other patients, saying, "What if this is as good as it gets?"

When he discovers that Carol is not at work and that she may be getting a job closer to home to better take care of her son, he tracks her down. Her building has a foyer with mini-tiles, cracks galore, but he manages to get to her apartment. He asks her to feed him. She says,

"Do you have any control over how creepy you allow yourself to get?" This takes him aback, and, considering, he says, "Yes, I do."

Helen closes the door on him, but her son, who has been chronically ill, has another sudden high fever. She catches Melvin as he is about to get into a taxi and has them drive to the hospital.

Carol comes home from work the next day to find a doctor there. She panics. It turns out that he is the husband of Melvin's publisher and Melvin has asked him to take care of her son (with Melvin paying the bills) because she is "urgently" needed back at work. Melvin is doing a very good deed for a very selfish reason. He wants nothing to interfere with his carefully calibrated routine—a signature of the OCD personality.

As Good as It Gets portrays how problematic medical care in the United States can be for those with inadequate insurance. Simon is now broke because of the hospital costs from his beating. Carol spends much of her time trying to figure out how to pay for her son Spencer's care. But because Melvin has money and connections, a private doctor is not only making a house call, but he has a nurse with him, orders lab tests that will report results that day, and, after reviewing the boy's medical history, finds many steps that were missed because Spencer never had a regular doctor, only emergency room visits.

Carol, frustrated as they are talking about how her insurance didn't support a test the doctor thinks might have been helpful, calls them "fuckin' HMO bastard pieces of shit." The doctor agrees: "Actually, I think that's their technical name." She is astounded when the doctor gives her his home number to call if there are any problems. Another jab at U.S. medicine. The doctor promises that "from now on, your son is going to feel a great deal better."

Later, Melvin agrees to help Simon, who is still recovering from the beating, drive to Baltimore to ask his parents for money. He invites Carol along, and she agrees. When we watch Melvin packing for the overnight trip, we see his obsessive behaviors. He is very organized, everything laid out on the bed. It's the kind of thing that likely makes him more, not less, efficient. Some obsessive habits can be useful. On the other hand, heading toward a restaurant with Carol, he keeps asking whether they sell hard-shell crabs. Getting a yes answer doesn't satisfy; he asks again and again. That's a version of "checking," needing to be reassured over and over that something was done. We will talk about these symptoms more below.

Melvin is charming on this outing until he slips and insults the dress Carol is wearing, hurting her feelings. She demands he pay her a compliment. He asks if they can order first; he does, and then composes his compliment. "I've got this ailment. My doctor told me that pills might help. I hate pills. I'm using the word 'hate' here about pills. My compliment is, that night that you came over, the next morning I started taking the pills. You make me want to be a better man."

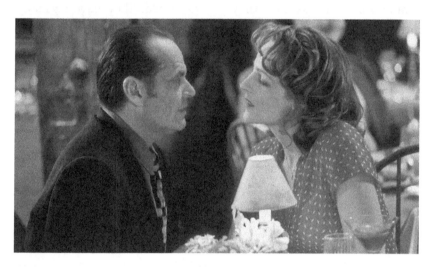

She tells him that's the best compliment of her life. And she kisses him. Then he ruins the moment, once again insulting her. He can't seem to help himself. She gets up and leaves. She wants nothing more to do with him.

Whether it's the pills or love (in real life it would not be love), when Melvin returns home, he forgets to lock the door or to turn the light switch on and off. He's letting go of some of his compulsive behaviors. Melvin does something spontaneous, too, very much against type: urged by Simon, he goes to her home in the middle of the night. As he tries to express his feelings, he can't bring himself to say he loves her.

He says something wonderful to her, then again ruins it. Carol cries out, "Why can't I have a normal boyfriend, who doesn't go nuts on me!?" Her mother, overhearing, replies, "Everybody wants that, dear. It doesn't exist." I love this exchange. Carol invites him in and tells him, "Try not to ruin everything by being you."

It ends happily. That's what comedies do. Melvin even steps on a crack.

The Madness

I find the anxiety disorders fascinating, in part because they are so common but also because they are so varied. They have so many different ways of presenting themselves, of being experienced. It does seem that, at least in Western societies, it is almost universal; some version of anxiety is part of all of our lives. If we are fortunate and relatively healthy emotionally, the anxieties are short-lived and usually tied to an understandable stressful moment: taking an important test, confronting a colleague, giving a speech, worrying about a loved one. Once the moment has passed, or you have survived the worrisome experience (or more commonly, once you actually start doing the thing you were anxious about—the test, the confrontation, the speech; this is called "anticipatory anxiety"), your anxiety level decreases dramatically.

If your anxiety comes and goes as situations and the stresses in your life change, then you are basically living a "life." This anxiety keeps you alive because it helps you to focus on what is important. If your anxiety gets in the way, if you are so anxious you can't focus, or get the job done, then it becomes a dysfunction.

When many people have to perform in public, getting ready to present themselves to an audience, they find their hands shaking, their hearts pounding, or that they are sweating. I've noticed that if you are playing an instrument, normal performance anxiety will often affect what you need to play well—if you are a pianist your hands will sweat (mine always did); if you are a singer, your mouth will go dry. Usually, once you are out there and start to play, anxiety fades and you can do well. This discomfort doesn't necessarily get better with experience. For much of his career, the great English actor Laurence Olivier would throw up from anxiety before every performance—and then be magnificent.

When we see the anxiety in Carol's eyes as she notices the doctor's car in front of her house, thinking her son is in medical crisis, that is a fear that is justified. Her anxiety subsides almost immediately when she finds out why the doctor is there. So, this is not an example of a disorder, when the anxiety would persist despite reassurances, or might always be there. This is a natural and normal response to a situation of worry or stress.

What is anxiety, and how does it differ from fear? Fear is the response to a perceived threat. It generates a "fight-or-flight" response: it gets your full attention and your adrenaline spikes. You sense imminent, external danger and get ready to fight or run. Anxiety, on the other hand, is an apprehension, a sense of worry that has physical manifestations. You tense up and become hypervigilant, but for something you are anticipating, not something facing you in the moment. You will look for ways to avoid what scares you. Most often your sense of threat is exaggerated; that's what makes it a disorder.

For instance, if you are *phobic* (meaning you have a specific fear) of closed spaces—called *claustrophobia* (there is a Greek or Latin name for most anxiety subtypes)—you will do anything to avoid entering an elevator or a crowded classroom or cinema. If you are forced into such a situation your anxiety will peak and you may feel panic (a medical term I will define in a moment). Feeling as though you are trapped, you will look for a way to escape (if you can put yourself near a door, that might help). These fears can really compromise your quality of life.

Those with *acrophobia* have an extreme fear of heights. I must admit to being someone with that disorder. All my life I become anxious in high places and avoid them if I can. I remember going on a hike in the Olympic Peninsula in Washington State, a beautiful rain forest. Halfway through the hike we came to a rickety, wooden suspension bridge over a deep gorge. Very narrow, it was made for one person at a time. I could not bring myself to cross it. I wound up sitting next to the bridge as our friends continued to enjoy their hike on the other side. I waited for them to return and pick me up and head back to the camp site. It was a rather deflating day. When I was viewing the Grand Canyon years ago—magnificent, but you are looking a mile down to the Colorado River—I had to stand far back from the edge. I could too easily imagine the precipice crumbling at my feet, and me falling to the rocks below. It sure interferes with appreciating Nature's grandeur.

One summer while in college, I had a job as the guide for exchange students during their first visit to New York City. I had a new group of students every four days. I loved the job because I love New York City and enjoyed showing people around town. The students were wonderfully enthusiastic. Among other sights, they all wanted to see the Statue of Liberty. In those innocent days visitors could climb to the top and even stand outside on Miss Liberty's torch. The 160-odd steps up to the top of the Statue were an open spiral of cast iron, and at any time you could look down to the bottom. With my fear of heights, ascending the statue felt an impossible ask. The prospect of looking down terrified me. But I had a job to do. I figured out that if I forced myself not to look down, I could manage it. Each time I visited the Statue of Liberty, I had to brace myself and talk myself into it. I had to climb inside that damn Statue some thirty times that summer. I never did manage to get myself outside onto the torch. My students had no trouble with it. I would stand at the doorway to the torch and encourage them to take their time and enjoy it—but not me. The most difficult challenge was climbing down at the end of the visit. Those stairsteps were open, and there was no alternative to looking down during the descent to make sure I didn't miss a step. Looking down enough not to fall, but trying not to see all the way down was hard. I discovered that having to confront those stairs so many times that summer made the task easier and easier. I won't say it cured my phobia, but it sure became less intense.

This was an unplanned version of one of the standard treatments for any phobia—systematic desensitization. The therapist engineers small exposures to the fear-inducing circumstance (like just one step up, then two, then three, for the fear of heights—we will see this in

Vertigo, one of the *Other Visions*), then the therapist teaches the patient how to lessen his or her anxiety (using meditation or relaxation techniques) until it feels under control. The therapist will challenge assumptions, asking what's the worst thing that could happen, discussing how unlikely that is, and brainstorming with the patient about how they could deal with it if that bad thing did happen. Then they try systematic desensitization again, this time with a slightly bigger challenge. Another approach uses "mindfulness" techniques, one of the cognitive behavioral therapies: patients learn to observe their anxieties rather than react to them and can develop a level of control that can significantly ease their symptoms. This technique also can be very effective.

If you have a *social anxiety*, you are made anxious by any encounter with other people, especially if you imagine they might be judging you. Ironically, part of that worry is that your anxiety about being with people will make people see you as anxious and think the worse of you. So, you avoid people. *Agoraphobia* is the fear of being outside your home, in public places and situations. It's different from the specific social anxiety because you avoid places and not just social situations. So, you are avoidant of both open spaces (parking lots, malls, or bridges) and of closed spaces (small shops, theaters, or tunnels when driving). You avoid public transportation, like a bus or train, or any setting where you might be in a crowd of people and be unable to "escape." Anything that draws you out of the comfort of where you live can cause anxiety. Often there is concern that you will panic and draw attention to yourself, making you even more anxious.

Many of these anxiety disorders have in common the added fear that you will have a panic attack and die. The term "panic" in psychiatry has a very specific meaning. It is the physical sensation that you cannot breathe, that you might be having a heart attack. There are symptoms of heart palpitations (your heart pounding in your chest), sweating, trembling and shaking, shortness of breath, tightness in your chest, nausea, dizziness, and numbness in your hands.

You may feel increased derealization or depersonalization—the sensation that the things around you are not real or have somehow changed; or you may feel the sensation that you are watching your-self from outside—that you are separate from yourself, as though you were in a movie, watching what happens. Versions of these symptoms are common in most anxiety disorders (and, we have seen, are often how DID initially presents).

On top of these symptoms, when panicked, you can feel like you are losing control, and that you are dying. It can be terrifying; you will do anything to avoid feeling that way. What causes the sensations that define "panic" is that, as you become more intensely anxious, your breathing changes: you begin to take short breaths and breathe more rapidly. This upsets the balance of carbon dioxide and oxygen in your system, which generates many of the physical symptoms that feel like having a heart attack. The extreme outcome of such panic-breathing is fainting. As soon as you faint (assuming you manage not to hurt yourself when you fall), your breathing normalizes, the oxygen balance returns, and you wake up, perhaps confused and embarrassed, but basically okay. A panic attack is, thus, self-limiting. But you can't tell that to someone in the midst of it. They really do feel like they are about to die.

You may see people subject to frequent panic attacks carrying a small paper bag around with them. This can be an effective treatment for panic. If the person feels an attack coming on, they can put the paper bag tightly over their mouth and nose and hold it there (a challenging thing to do when you feel like you are choking and can't breathe). This causes the person to re-breathe the air they were breathing out too quickly—and the balance of oxygen is promptly restored, stopping the panic sensation before it gets worse. Though it is a hard technique to persuade a patient to try, because it seems counterintuitive ("I'm supposed to breathe into a bag when I feel like I am suffocating?"), I wish other psychiatric crises could be so easily controlled.

When I was treating someone with an anxiety disorder, I would often teach them relaxation techniques. Breathing exercises, medita-tion techniques, and progressive relaxation (mindfully removing the tensions from each body part) can be powerfully helpful. It is difficult to be anxious and "relaxed" at the same time. So, if you can learn to relax, you can begin to control your moments of anxiety. This takes practice, and the exercises take some time, but it can make a world of difference. Learned well, they can even abort a panic attack. My patients used and appreciated this approach but still often carried a small paper bag with them, just in case.

One fairly common version of anxiety is unhelpfully called generalized anxiety disorder. This does not have the specific focus of a phobia, nor the compulsive behaviors of OCD. It describes someone who is chronically worried, apprehensive, restless, on edge, has difficulty concentrating, and often problems with sleep. Many of these are fairly ordinary symptoms and can be connected with other psychiatric diagnoses such as depression or the other anxieties. What leads to this diagnosis is that other symptoms (such as depressed mood, or a specific phobia) are not present, but the anxiety is still disruptive and affects everyday life. Most of Woody Allen's movie characters could fit this diagnosis. Mickey is presented as a hypochondriac in *Hannah and Her Sisters* (discussed below), which is another subtype of anxiety, but outside of his somatic preoccupations, he comes across as chronically and generally anxious too.

I've not yet talked about obsessive-compulsive disorder (OCD). This fits under the umbrella of the anxiety disorders because the behaviors are all an attempt to control and minimize anxiety. But it certainly has its distinctions. *Obsessions* are recurrent or intrusive thoughts, thoughts you can't get rid of, that are disturbing or that drive your behavior. Very often they are of contamination (preoccupations with dirt or germs), of things not being done correctly, consist of violent or bloody images or urges (in your mind's eye, seeing yourself killing or hurting a loved one, or seeing them injured or disfigured), or are religiously or sexually disturbing. These thoughts and images are unwanted and upsetting.

Compulsions are ritualized behaviors that are attempts to manage the disturbing thoughts, to control the anxiety they produce. So, concerns about germs or dirt are coupled with compulsive hand washing (repeated so often that the hands become irritated and even bloodied) and being unwilling to touch a doorknob or water glass that someone else might have touched.

Concerns about safety may lead to compulsive checking—to be sure the gas on the stove is turned off, that the door is properly locked, that everything you want in your briefcase is really there. What makes this a disorder is that this is not the normal checking any of us might do as we leave the house. Once we check the stove, the locks, and the briefcase and see all is well, we can be on our way. But the person with the disorder is never sure they got it right. So they will check, walk away, doubt, then check again, walk away, doubt, and then check again—over and over. Always not quite confident that they got it right.

Very often the compulsions don't have any real connection to the thing being avoided. There is a superstitious quality to them. At least handwashing connects to worries about contamination. Other common compulsions are not so logical; they include needing to do things a set number of times. In *As Good as It Gets*, we see Melvin turning the lock on his door exactly five times before he can move on to something else. Similarly, he turns the light switch on and off five times. That number may differ from person to person, but interestingly it is almost always an odd number—so that after doing the ritual, the lock or switch is indeed moved to the next step (from unlocked to locked, the switch from off to on). If the number was even, the light switch would always stay off (or on).

One patient of mine had to walk around a chair seven times before he could sit down. Another patient was compelled to count the number of leaves on the ficus tree in my office. Have you ever tried to count leaves on a tree? it's impossible! You never can be sure if you aren't counting the same leaf twice. This counting made it impossible for him to pay attention to anything else, like the conversation during his therapy. We solved the problem for the moment by moving into another room without a tree. Other similar compulsions include needing to repeat words or needing to have things placed "just so," often in neat symmetrical configurations. These are all distracting, and often exhausting, for the person compelled to do them.

One of the most common compulsions is avoiding stepping on the crack in a sidewalk or a line on a tile floor. This seemingly superstitious behavior fulfills the need to prevent whatever disaster the obsessive thought implies. There is a feeling that if you can avoid stepping on a crack you will assure that your spouse will not become ill, or that you will not commit violence or a sexual indiscretion, or that the world will not end.

The obsessions are so preoccupying that they make it hard to pay attention to other things. The compulsions can be so time-consuming that they eat up much of your day with activities that have no real useful purpose. It's important to realize that this is not a psychotic illness. Unlike the experience of a psychotic delusion, people with OCD will tell you they know that what they are doing and thinking makes no sense; that it is not true that avoiding a crack on the sidewalk will help avoid illness, or nuclear war, or stop them from dying. They know that, but they can't *not* do it.

Because these rituals have such power and take so much time, people with OCD tend to insist on routine. Every day has to be the same. They have a particularly hard time with unexpected changes—because these changes threaten their ability to complete the compulsive tasks and keep anxiety at bay. So, like Melvin, they will always have their meals at a certain place, a certain table, or a certain time, and they may always order the same meal. Any disruption in their routine can cause increased and sometimes uncontrolled anxiety—a need to undo and return to the rigid routine.

I want to re-emphasize something I mentioned above. Melvin's misanthropic behavior—his rude, mean treatment of everyone around him—has nothing to do with the OCD diagnosis. It is just a conceit of the movie, which is really about how his love for Carol helps him decide to properly deal with his OCD by starting the medications recommended long ago by his doctor, and to begin to treat people with kindness: his decision to try "to be a better man."

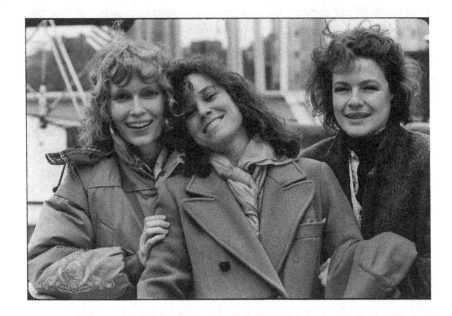

Hannah and Her Sisters (1986)

Michael Caine, Mia Farrow, Dianne Wiest, Barbara Hershey,
Carrie Fisher, Max von Sydow
Writer and Director: Woody Allen

Woody Allen has become a controversial figure: because of questions about his personal behavior, his reputation is in tatters. But there is no controversy about the quality of the films he made in the early years of his career. They are considered iconic; he made some of the funniest comedies of the 1960s, then, in the subsequent decades, brilliant comedy-dramas of increasing depth and seriousness. He has made masterpieces that define their time.

Hannah and Her Sisters is one of Woody Allen's best films. It is a transitional film for him, both funny and serious. His career started in 1950s television as a writer with such comedy giants as Mel Brooks,

Carl Reiner, Neil Simon, and Sid Caesar. Then he moved to performing stand-up comedy. His routines from that period are smart, surreal, and funny; they are classics and defined his style. His first movies were filled with clever jokes and slapstick: *Bananas, Take the Money and Run, Sleeper.* Then there was a leap into greatness with *Annie Hall.*

This was a movie about relationships, romantic yet still funny. Starring Diane Keaton, it was a love letter to her and to Allen's New York, which was the Upper West Side, filled with writers and performers. It was not everyone's New York, but it was the world he knew and could make fun of. *Annie Hall* opens with a joke, told directly to the camera, clearly outside the world of the movie. It's an old joke and not a very good one, but it tells us this movie will be different. And it was. It was a very big hit, winning the Academy Award in 1977 for Best Picture, Screenplay, Director, and Actress (Diane Keaton), and it changed how romantic comedies looked from then on.

The films that followed were in search of a new style. *Manhattan* was a bookend to *Annie Hall,* and very good too. However, Allen's idol had always been Ingmar Bergman, and Allen felt his own films to be trivial compared to the Master. So, he tried to make his own "Bergman" films, austere, serious, and grown-up. *Interiors, September,* and *Celebrity* were all somber attempts, without any humor or wit. They were dull failures. This was not his strength.

Hannah and Her Sisters was his way out. Channeling Chekhov, he created a film about family that was serious and complex. It was lightened with a subplot about Mickey (played by Allen), the ex-husband of Hannah (Mia Farrow), which is conveniently outside the central story. Chekhov would have known how to incorporate humor into the main story, but Allen couldn't yet master it. Instead, he created a new form, and it works beautifully. The film won three Oscars: for Michael Caine and Dianne Wiest as supporting actors, and for Woody Allen's screenplay.

The movie is divided into chapters, each titled with a quote, and with a song from the American Songbook. An innovation of Allen's, the chapters help us keep track of the many narrators. We hear what each of the main players is thinking. The chapter titles and the songs define the moment. A repeated tune is Rodgers and Hart's "Bewitched, Bothered, and Bewildered" from the 1940s show *Pal Joey*. We never hear the lyrics, but the clever title sums up Allen's view of what being in love can do to a person. It's not all hearts and flowers—it's confusing, upsetting, sometimes painful—and wonderful too.

The main story about Hannah and her sisters, Lee and Holly, goes from holiday to holiday, starting and ending with Thanksgiving. Hannah is an actor who has suspended her career to raise a family, with a gaggle of adopted children. (As is often the case with writers, Allen borrows from real life. He was in a relationship with Farrow then, and she indeed had adopted many children. Hannah's apartment in the film is Farrow's actual apartment. The rest of the story is invented.)

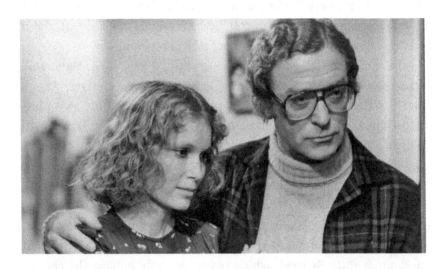

Michael Caine is Elliot, her second husband. He is infatuated with Hannah's sister Lee (Barbara Hershey), who is in a relationship with Frederick, a somber, antisocial artist. Holly (Dianne Wiest) asks to borrow money again from Hannah for her new venture, a catering service, while she is still auditioning for parts in the theater. Allen's screenplay is very efficient in establishing each character. We see in this scene, and in a bravura scene later when the sisters are having lunch together at a restaurant, that Hannah is the support to them all, but that she feels no one is taking care of her. In that later scene, we know that Lee is now having an affair with Elliot, and Holly has given up on acting and wants to become a writer, and that Hannah doesn't know what is behind their moods. As the camera circles around the table during their conversation, there is much unsaid and implied. It's remarkable moviemaking.

But we are here for anxiety. The film up until now has been an earnest exploration of the search for love. Then there is a new chapter, called "The Hypochondriac," and we seem to be in a different movie. It's about Mickey, Hannah's ex-husband, and a showrunner for a television comedy. The scenes telling his story have a new pace and rhythm, filled with nervous energy. We see him hectically dealing with one crisis after another—a sketch that the censors won't allow, a writer complaining about changes in his script, the show running short.

By the way, in the first minute we see a handful of comic actors in their first movie; many have only one line but they have had major careers since. (Allen always had a good eye for spotting talent. See if you can spot Julia Louis-Dreyfus, Lewis Black, and John Turturro.) Mickey is stressed and asks for a Tagamet for his ulcer. Always the drug-of-the-moment.

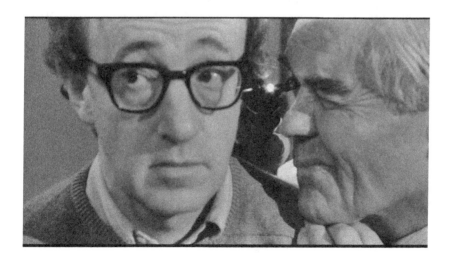

His doctor asks him, "What seems to be the problem, this time?" Mickey is a regular. Mickey says, "This time I really feel I have something." Mickey's father is labeled as the "real hypochondriac," but Mickey is a pretty good example.

He says he feels dizzy and notices hearing loss in one of his ears, but he can't remember which. After some tests, his doctor recommends following up at the hospital. You see in Mickey's reaction that he is expecting the usual report, that it's nothing. He is startled that there might really be something wrong. Like many hypochondriacs, he is quite suggestible. When the doctor asks if he has ringing in his ears, suddenly he has that too.

Next, we see Mickey in a telephone booth calling a doctor friend for advice. He asks what his symptoms might point to and when his friend mentions that worst case, it might be a brain tumor, you see Mickey deflate—immediately assuming that is what he has. At his office, he is very upset. When the phone rings he thinks it's the ringing in his ears. His assistant reminds him that two months before he thought he had a malignant melanoma. He says, "Naturally, with the sudden appearance of a black spot on my back." Her comeback—"It was on your shirt!"—is both funny and telling.

He goes on to insist, "This morning I was happy." She reminds him that everything was going wrong that morning and that he was miserable. He replies, "I was happy, but I didn't realize I was happy." He is someone who enjoys the misery of his job, who is comfortable with the stress, but his health worries are at another level.

The scenes start coming more quickly, brief comic sketches, each ending with a laugh line. There is a montage of hospital tests, and the doctor finds a spot on his brain that requires a closer look. Mickey has a panic attack, and there is a flashback to when he found out he was infertile (consulting with a doctor who has no idea how to talk to worried patients) and he and Hannah ask their friend to donate sperm. It's an awkward situation, made funny by how Mickey tries to make it casual. The friend's wife says to her husband, "We need to discuss this with your analyst, and mine too." A laugh line.

Mickey has a CAT scan. We see him waiting for the doctor to tell him the results. The doctor comes in and tells him, "The news is not good . . . surgery is of no use." The doctor comes in again: "Well, you're just fine. There is absolutely nothing here." We realize the first time was Mickey's pessimistic imagination, running wild.

Now, he is overjoyed—but just long enough to suddenly realize that, yes, this is a reprieve. "Do you realize what a thread we are all hanging by?"; but, that eventually, "I will be in that position—the news will be bad. I will die. It's all meaningless." He is having an existential crisis. Yes, we all, in the back of our minds, know that everyone dies, and that we will too. But we go through life not dwelling on that (except for the occasional dark night when the reality hits), and we find meaning in the moment, in relationships, and in the things we do with our life.

So, Mickey tries to find a sense of purpose, a reason to live. He tries out several religions and questions his own (each sequence ending with a punch line). After consulting with a priest about converting to Catholicism, though he was raised Jewish, Mickey shops for what he imagines every good Catholic would have in his home. He removes from his shopping bag: a crucifix, a catechism, a picture of Jesus, then, a package of Wonder Bread and a jar of mayonnaise. I wonder if you have to be Jewish to get how funny that is? Later, discouraged and depressed, he tries to shoot himself, but shoots a mirror instead (this is funny, too). Then, failing that, he wanders the streets until he stops at a movie house where the Marx Brothers picture *Duck Soup* is playing. This is their most silly, outrageous movie, and Mickey can't help enjoying himself. Suddenly, life seems worth living. These sequences are a masterclass in Jewish humor—staring into the abyss and making it funny.

All of this is interspersed within the larger story of Hannah and her sisters.

Hypochondriasis is one of the anxiety disorders. What is particular about it is the focus on the somatic, on body integrity. Your worries and nervous preoccupations are centered on the possibility, the conviction, that you are ill. Your sense of dread is increased by every imagined or real symptom, and you are convinced that a catastrophic outcome is the only one possible. If you suffer from chronic anxiety, you are under a constant sense of apprehension, always looking for the bad news under any good news, but not necessarily about your health. The anxieties of the person with hypochondria are all about illness and the fear of dying.

Small aches or pains that others might ignore become alarming and threatening. Hypochondriacs are suggestible. When they hear of a symptom, suddenly they have it. You don't have to be a hypochondriac to have this happen to you; the diagnosis only fits if it becomes a way of life. This is something medical students are susceptible to when they are first learning about disease. As you study illness after illness you can easily imagine yourself suffering from that illness. But it doesn't last. You learn how to determine that someone does not have the disease, which is as important as knowing how to make the diagnosis.

A hypochondriac very easily assumes the role of the patient. They will "doctor shop," either looking for someone to confirm their worst fears or for someone to reassure them that, this time, it's okay. But they love putting themselves into the hands of the professional.

The patient role has its comforts. You are relieved of daily responsibilities. You get sympathetic attention. Little is demanded of you while you are in the sick role. Someone will give you medications or do procedures that make you feel cared for. The laying-on of hands is something that hypochondriacs seek—something we all would find comforting, but that most of us would not trade for being seriously ill.

Hypochondria can become a lifestyle; it can lead to having unnecessary surgeries and other procedures or taking strong, unnecessary medications that may cause complications. So, it is not a trivial dysfunction. Sometimes anti-anxiety or anti-depressant medications can be useful. Intensive counselling can help, providing the attention the person seeks in a more constructive way than would other, possibly invasive, medical attentions.

This reminds me of an old joke. The epitaph carved into the gravestone of a well-known hypochondriac: "See, I told you I was sick."

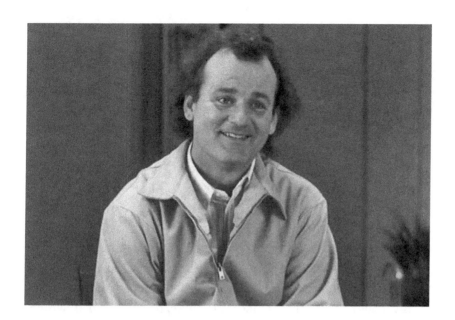

What About Bob? (1991)

Bill Murray, Richard Dreyfuss, Julie Hagerty
Director: Frank Oz

Under the credits we meet Bob Wiley (Bill Murray), chanting a posi-
tivity mantra ("I feel good, I feel great"). We watch his morning routine, including greeting his only friend, a pet fish, Gill. He tells Gill
he has to go to work, then sits down at the desk next to his bed and
punches a time clock. We next see him, a few hours later, pacing in his
apartment, eyeing the door, girding himself to go outside.

In the hallway he does all he can to not touch the walls, then opens
the outside door using a handkerchief. Outside, the loud noises of the
city overwhelm him, knocking him to the ground. The cheery music
tells us we are not to take this too seriously, and Murray, a brilliant
and original comic, conveys Bob's anxieties and strange behaviors
well; he manages to be both funny and real.

At the revolving door to an office building, he enters by pushing with his foot—again, he will do anything not to touch a public object. He is looking for Dr. Marvin (Richard Dreyfuss), his new psychiatrist, whose office, unfortunately, is on the forty-fourth floor. Reluctantly walking toward the elevator, Bob notices a janitor washing the floors. Suddenly he is walking very slowly, exaggeratedly dragging his feet to avoid the catastrophe of slipping. His world is full of everyday dangers.

Worse is to come—he can't bring himself to stay in the elevator. Murray's exquisitely tortured body language as he tries but can't bring himself to get into the elevator is something to see. So he climbs the stairs instead—to the forty-fourth floor.

The next scene is really quite wonderful, funny and strange and well played by both actors. Bob shakes Dr. Marvin's hand holding a tissue so as not to touch him, then, noticing a picture of the doctor's family, tries to guess their names. Of course, he gets them all wrong, but when Dr. Marvin corrects him, the names are telling—and funny. His son is named Sigmund and his daughter is Anna (two Freuds).

Bob's description of his problems: "I worry about diseases, so I have trouble touching things . . . I have a real big problem . . . moving. In my apartment, I'm okay. But when I want to go out, I get . . . weird." Dr. Marvin replies, "Talk about 'weird,'" a standard and clichéd therapy response. Bob says, "I get dizzy spells, nausea, cold sweats, hot sweats . . . difficulty breathing and swallowing, blurred vision, involuntary trembling, dead hands . . . pelvic discomfort." Melvin asks him a better question, "What are you truly afraid of?" and Bob says, "What if my heart stops beating? What if I'm looking for a bathroom and my bladder explodes?" He suddenly bursts out shouting obscenities, and quietly explains that if he does that on purpose it proves to him he doesn't have Tourette syndrome (a neurological illness with motor tics, head shakes, and uncontrolled and often obscene outbursts).

Then Bob mimes a heart attack—it's the same bizarre logic: if he fakes it, then he doesn't have it. Dr. Marvin is unfazed by all this, and as Bob is lying on the floor after his fake heart attack, asks him if he is married. Bob tells him he is divorced, and that he left his wife because she liked the singer Neil Diamond. Dr. Marvin points out that

Bob is the one with problems and that maybe he didn't leave his wife over a singer, but instead she left him. This hits Bob hard: it's a revelation. (What did he do with all the other psychiatrists he has been seeing? This is not a profound observation.) He announces that he is convinced the new doctor can help him: "For the first time in my life I feel there's hope. I feel I can be somebody." Then Dr. Marvin gets up—he has been sitting behind his desk, not a good choice for therapy (which we will talk about in the next chapter), and tells him about a "ground-breaking new book that is just out." He surveys his bookcase as though looking for it. The entire bottom shelf is filled with copies—it's *his* book. It's called *Baby Steps* and it is actually a good title for a good idea, a version of the systematic desensitization I described earlier. Initially, Dr. Marvin comes across as pleasant, but pompous and full of himself, leaning on a bust of Freud as he explains that "baby steps" means setting small goals, one day at a time, each step getting you closer to being able to deal with your problem.

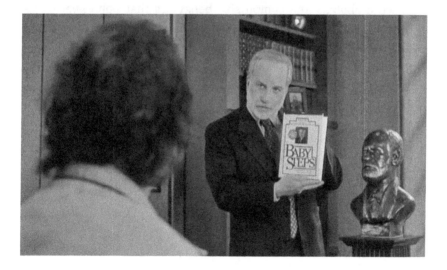

Bob takes it literally, walking with little steps around the office with increased confidence, until the doctor tells him he is about to go on his annual August vacation, a tradition among psychoanalytic therapists. Bob is dismayed—what will he do without him for a full month? He has become instantly dependent on his doctor.

The rest of the film follows from this setup. Bob pursues the doctor to his vacation home in New Hampshire. He has a great need for family connection, and his eccentricities, seen as charming, ingratiate him with the doctor's family. Dr. Marvin can't stand it: yes, being valued by family could help Bob, just not the doctor's family!

For its first two Acts this is a perfect comedy, introducing its two main characters, Bob and Dr. Marvin—with Bob's array of anxieties, phobias, and compulsions, and the doctor's irritability and self-importance—then throwing them together. Unfortunately, the last Act becomes chaotic, as the doctor goes to increasingly unhinged lengths to remove Bob from his life. That's not a reason to avoid the film—the beginning sequences are priceless. But don't expect a satisfying conclusion; though, this being a comedy, it does end happily, at least for Bob.

No single person in real life would have Bob's full collection of anxieties. As too often happens in mainstream films, his symptoms are a grab bag of madness, mostly there to drive the plot. Though the array of specific phobias and compulsive behaviors that Bob experiences doesn't fit reality, the way he describes each of them is pretty much on target. He not only displays a comic expression of the tensions of phobic avoidance in scene after scene but also explains well how he thinks about them. This is why I find this film valuable. And watching Bill Murray is always a treat.

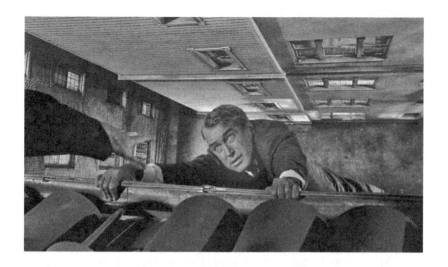

Vertigo (1958)

James Stewart, Kim Novak, Barbara Bel Geddes
Director: Alfred Hitchcock
Score: Bernard Herrmann

Entire books have been written analyzing this film, one of Hitchcock's most intriguing and complicated. The story is unexpected and strange. Its use of color, Jimmy Stewart's performance (and Kim Novak's too), and the insinuating music of Bernard Herrmann leave a haunting effect. It is on many lists of the greatest films ever made.

Vertigo is a story of obsession and deceit. In this case, "obsession" does not refer to the obsessive thoughts that someone with OCD experiences; those thoughts are unwanted and unpleasant and are coupled with compulsive rituals to ward off the intrusive images and ideas and make them go away. The obsession here is our hero's intense preoccupation with Madeleine, a woman he hardly knows, but whom he has fallen in love with. This obsession takes over his every moment and seems to give meaning to his life. But it blinds him to what is really going on with her, and with him.

As interesting as this is, I want to focus on a different aspect of the film—its portrayal of acrophobia.

Vertigo starts with a chase. James Stewart plays Scottie Ferguson, a police detective chasing someone on the roof of a high building in San Francisco. The person being chased jumps from one rooftop to another, and Scottie and another policeman make the jumps, too. Scottie slips and grabs a gutter to stop himself from falling. He is dangling high above the street. Frozen there, he looks down, terrified. The policeman turns back to help; as he reaches for Scottie, he loses his balance and falls to his death, with Scottie watching helplessly.

In the next scene Scottie is talking with Midge (Barbara Bel Geddes), a good friend who is quietly in love with him. He tells her he quit the police force because of his fear of heights, his acrophobia. He blames himself for the policeman's death and has nightmares about it. The acrophobia gives him vertigo, a form of extreme paralyzing dizziness. As they talk about how disabling the fear of heights can be, he starts with a ridiculous example, looking down to pick a pencil off the floor. Of course, that doesn't trigger the vertigo. But it gives him an idea. He says, "I have a theory. I think if I can get used to heights, just a little bit at time, progressively . . . ," and he demonstrates, standing on the lowest step of a step stool.

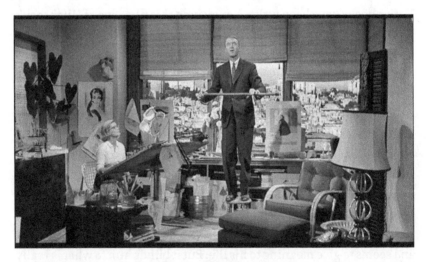

"I look up, I look down . . . there's nothing to it!" But, when he stands on the top step and looks down, he has a flashback of the view from that rooftop and falls in a faint. This is a failed attempt at systematic desensitization. It fails because it is not guided by a therapist, who would be careful to choose the gradual exposures likely to be tolerated at the start and what each new exposure should look like; and would have taught him techniques to reduce anxiety during the desensitization trials. Scottie tries to be his own therapist and too quickly and too directly challenges his phobia. The best lesson for him to take from this failure of a good idea would be to find an expert to guide him.

What I find interesting here is that this experiment speaks more of post-traumatic stress disorder (PTSD) than acrophobia. The shock of watching that man fall has given him nightmares, and standing on the stool he doesn't just get vertigo but has a vivid flashback to the rooftop. He may well have acrophobia (which he first experienced on that rooftop), but his vertigo here, on the step stool, which causes him to break out into a sweat and become tremulous and faint, seems triggered by the flashback from that traumatic event; more a symptom of PTSD, an anxiety disorder brought on by a stressful, traumatic experience which is relived as though it is happening now, than simple acrophobia.

Scottie is hired by Gavin Elster, an old college buddy, to follow Madeleine (Novak), Gavin's wife. He is worried about her. She seems to believe she is possessed by Carlotta, her great-grandmother, who died of suicide. Is Madeleine unbalanced and at risk? Scottie begins to follow her for Gavin, first intrigued and then in love. He follows her to a museum where she spends hours staring at a portrait of her grandmother.

When he sees her jump into the waters of San Francisco Bay, he rescues her. Now he is part of her life and they spend time together. She says she loves him, but is clearly troubled.

At a Spanish mission she runs into the church, insisting Scottie stay behind, and then climbs the stairs of the bell tower. Scottie runs after her, close behind, but he becomes frozen near the top of the stairs, his acrophobia causing vertigo when he looks down. This is visualized with a camera movement invented for this film—a zoom-out/track-in that is dizzying.

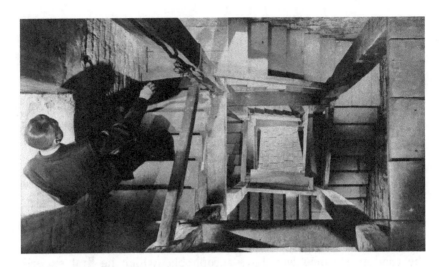

Clutching the railing, in a cold sweat, he watches her reach the top, and seconds later fall to her death.

Scottie becomes profoundly depressed and is in the hospital for months. When released he is obsessed by her memory, going back to all the places he saw her, and having recurrent nightmares. This doesn't quite fit with

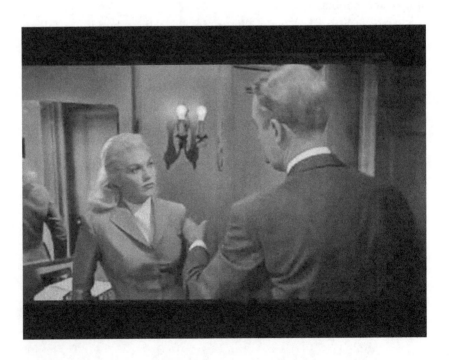

PTSD; the nightmares do, but typically the person with PTSD will do anything to avoid whatever reminds him of the initial traumatic experience. Instead, Scottie is immersing himself in those moments.

And then he sees Judy (also Novak), a woman who looks like Madeleine.

Scottie single mindedly tries to make her over to become the image of the woman he lost, not knowing that they are the same person. Judy was part of a deception and regrets it. (Unexpectedly, now Hitchcock shows us what really happened in that bell tower, something that, in another movie, would have been saved for the very end. It's a bold choice.)

Judy resists the attempted transformation. In love with him, she wants Scottie to appreciate her for herself, not because she reminds him of another woman. Having insisted that Judy wear the same dress and shoes as Madeleine and dye her hair blonde like Madeleine, he finally tells her to put her hair up like Madeleine's. Judy reluctantly complies. When she walks out of the bathroom, the image of her doppelgänger, she seems to be standing in a green mist, a ghostly presence. A famous moment in the history of film, the effect is magical.

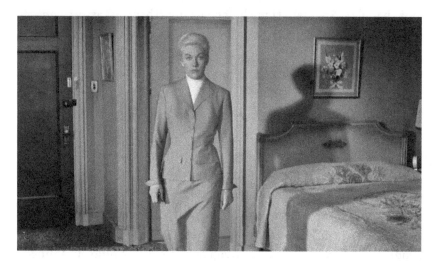

They embrace, the music swells, and the camera swirls around them—you can feel the passion. However, Judy has not admitted her deception. There will be one more time at the bell tower and another experience of vertigo; it does not end well for either of them.

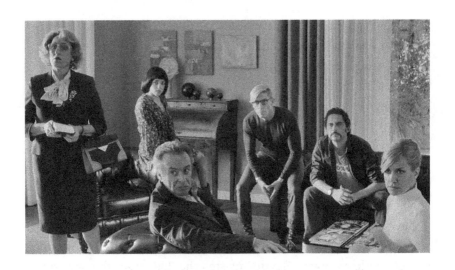

Toc Toc (2017)

Oscar Martinez, Alexandra Jiménez, Paco Léon
Writer and Director: Vicente Villanueva

This popular Spanish comedy brings together an assortment of patients waiting for their first appointment with a famous psychiatrist, a specialist in OCD (TOC in Spanish), who has been delayed. Because of a computer glitch, they are told they were accidentally all scheduled for the same time.

We meet them in turn as they introduce themselves to each other—a taxi driver who has counting rituals; a woman who works in a lab and, obsessed with dirt and germs, cannot stop cleaning; a religious woman who cannot stop checking and checking; a young man who can't step on a crack in the pavement; and a young woman, a personal trainer, who has echolalia, compulsively repeating words and phrases that others say. An older man in the group tells them he has Tourette syndrome, which is not an OCD diagnosis, but is also quite disabling—forcing him to shout obscenities.

The film is very funny and treats the characters in the story with respect, mostly accurately showing how their OCD syndromes complicate their lives.

Occasionally, a portrayal goes wrong. For instance, the taxi driver looking for number coincidences shares them loudly with his passengers, often driving them to leave his cab in annoyance; most people with his sort of compulsion would try to hide it, finding it socially embarrassing. He also is a calculating whiz, something more often associated with people in the autism spectrum. Most of the other characters are portrayed more realistically, even if they are broadened for comic effect.

By sharing their experiences, the patients wind up feeling better about themselves, and look forward to meeting again. The film ends with an unexpected and very gratifying surprise. It's worth seeking out.

The comedies here, and others like them, give us exaggerated versions of the everyday frustrations most of us experience. That is why, I think, we find them funny. We can identify with them in a way that we can't with someone psychotic or bipolar. We are familiar with being anxious before a date or an important meeting, we might be rather obsessive about our daily schedule, or compulsive in arranging our room or a closet just so. We are likely to be phobic of something; maybe not germs, but perhaps snakes or spiders or clowns, or closed spaces, or in my case, heights. Most of us are able to get past these phobias, but we can appreciate what it would be like to not be able to.

What makes it funny in a movie is not only that it is familiar but that it is happening to somebody else. If bad or uncomfortable things happen to other people, and their life seems complicated, knowing it's pretend, we can laugh. The laughter brings relief and delight because we know how it feels, and because it's not happening to us.

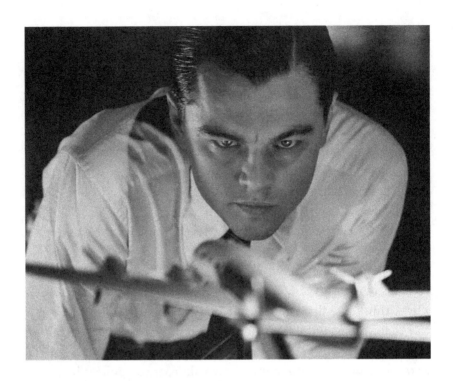

The Aviator (2004)

Leonardo DiCaprio, Cate Blanchett
Director: Martin Scorsese

The Aviator is an evocative biopic about Howard Hughes, the richest man of his day. Hughes was born into money and used it to underwrite his passions. He was a brilliant engineer who loved airplanes. He also made movies. His first, *Hell's Angels* (1930), had convincing and exciting airplane battles, still remarkable today. He invented the technology to film them. The story in *Hell's Angels* is not much, but those battles set the standard. He was a pilot and broke air speed records in planes he designed, including the fastest time flying around the world solo. He also built the largest flying boat in history, made from wood because aluminum was in short supply during World War II. Using his engineering expertise, he designed a brassiere to increase the cleavage of the already well-endowed Jane Russell for his movie, *The Outlaw* (1943).

His careful, obsessive attention to detail was remarked upon and served him well for years. He made planes (and brassieres) that worked.

He also dated the most glamorous film stars of the day, including Katharine Hepburn, Jean Harlow, and Ava Gardner. The first part of this film glories in his successes, and in the excesses of Hollywood in the 1930s and 1940s. But all that time Hughes is fighting demons (severe anxiety, OCD, and then paranoia) and gradually they overwhelm him, and the story.

Oftentimes, obsessive attention to detail and insistence on getting things right gets the work done and done well. But, if the obsessive preoccupations become extreme, develop a life of their own, and become the reason for what a person does instead of making them more thorough and effective, then it edges into madness. That's what happened to Hughes, and this film documents it well.

He had the need for order that one finds in most people with OCD. At lunch with Hepburn at the Coconut Grove (the in-place for Hollywood in the 1930s) he is a regular, and the chef knows his preferences. He is served a steak with exactly twelve peas, arrayed on the plate in a precise grid.

The actor Errol Flynn stops at his table uninvited and takes one pea from his plate. Hughes pushes the plate away—someone has touched it, the grid has been violated; he can no longer eat. Hepburn notices how uncomfortable he is; she will be his most devoted friend.

Hughes was profoundly germ-phobic. Several scenes illustrate this with clinical precision. He is in a restaurant bathroom. He takes a small case out of his pocket: it's his private bar of soap. Carefully he picks up the soap and begins to wash his hands.

A toilet flushes, and he winces—there is someone there. The man is on crutches and walks with difficulty toward the sinks. He asks Hughes to hand him a towel. There is a long pause, "Sorry, I really can't do that." That would require touching. As the man laboriously does it himself, Hughes turns his back on him to avoid contact.

The second bathroom scene, in another restaurant, is even more awkward. We see him vigorously wash his hands, so much so that they bleed. He reaches for a towel to stop the bleeding. Then he notices a spot on his shirt, pulls out the shirttail and tries to wash it, rubbing hard. He grabs a towel to dry the shirt and his soap-case, discards the towel and walks to the door. But he can't touch the doorknob without a towel. When he looks back, he sees the soiled towels in the waste basket, and the empty towel tray. He is paralyzed, unable to leave. Anguished, he stands by the door, waiting for someone to come in, so he can dash out.

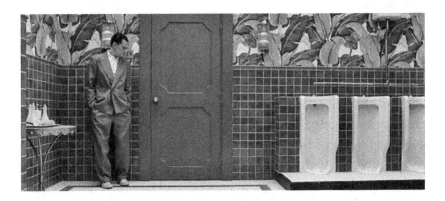

It gets worse. He is at his factory where they are building the Spruce Goose, the largest airplane made at the time. Studying the blueprints, he makes a quick decision that the rudder plans are okay. But then he tells his partner, Otis, "We need to look at the [steering] wheels." His partner says, "We have looked at a dozen wheels, choose one, please!" Holding one wheel, Hughes tells him, "This one is pretty close." Moments before he was quickly decisive. Now, he can't decide.

Making a decision is hard for someone with obsessive tendencies. They are often on the fence, balancing their choices, "on the one hand, on the other hand," unable to commit. If they do decide, they are frequently immediately overwhelmed with doubt—was that the right decision? And so they are right back where they started—unable to be sure, unable to decide.

It is the same sense of doubt that drives repeated "checking" compulsions. "Did I really turn off the stove? Did I lock the door properly?" So, you check again and again, unsure each time as you try to walk away.

Hughes suddenly focuses on a janitor slowly sweeping the floor: "Why is that guy looking at me?" With paranoid intensity he demands that he be fired.

This raises an interesting point. We will see that Hughes eventually becomes profoundly paranoid, locking himself away in a room for years. But his suspicious look at that janitor was not without reason because people really were "out to get him" (the classic paranoid concern); soon he would be accused of profiteering from the war. It is possible to have the madness of paranoid delusions, and to discover that people really do want to harm you. Separating the reality from the fantasy is often difficult for the therapist, and even more difficult for the patient, but it's very important.

When I was in training at the VA Hospital, I began working with a patient who claimed he was head of a major movie company. I assumed that was a paranoid delusion: he had been labeled as suffering from schizophrenia and he had other crazy ideas, too, like insisting he hadn't taken a breath in ten years. When I did some research, I discovered that he was telling the truth: before he became ill, he had indeed been an executive in Hollywood. That didn't make him any less mad; it's just that what his madness consisted of was different from what we had first been led to believe. And that made a difference in how we understood him and how we thought about his treatment.

As Hughes continues to work on plans for his airplane, he asks to look at the blueprints again. He starts muttering over and over, "Show me all the blueprints." He begins to walk away, repeating it, "Show me all the blueprints," grimacing with anxiety. He can't stop saying it over and over. Once alone, in a panic, he tries to hold his breath and then, slowly spelling "quarantine" letter by letter (a mindfulness technique), he begins to calm down.

Much later, he is under more stress; a senator is investigating him for defrauding the government during the war. His symptoms are getting worse. He is pacing in his screening room, bare-chested, muttering, "I sleep in this room, in the dark, I have a place, I have a chair." He is running *The Outlaw*, the Western film he made with Jane Russell, a highlight of his movie career. Looking at the image on screen, he says, "I like the desert. It's hot but it's clean." He can't sleep.

There are bottles of milk carefully lined up on the floor. Staring at the milk bottles, he says, "Wait a minute—that milk is sour, that milk is bad, I shouldn't pick up the bottle of milk in my right hand and I shouldn't take the top off with my left hand." He says it over and over. Again, he can't stop himself.

Hepburn is worried about him. She tries to persuade him to open the door and talk to her. He sends her away.

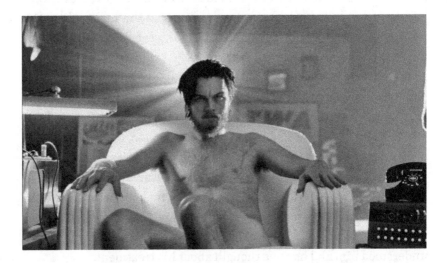

Later, we see that he is not eating. He is sitting naked, unshaved, saying "Come in with the milk" over and over; then, he gives instructions into a microphone, "He needs to open the bag with his right hand, hold the bag out to me at a forty-five-degree angle so I may reach into the bag, without touching the paper . . . Repeat it from the beginning, repeat it from the beginning."

There is a line of milk bottles on the floor—this time holding his urine. The bottles are uncountable; he spells out "quarantine" again and again.

This is no longer just OCD or anxiety. This is paranoid psychosis. He retains many OCD symptoms; they are an attempt to calm himself and manage from moment to moment. He is the richest man in the world and he is urinating into milk bottles, unable to leave his room.

RECOMMENDED READING

Barlow, David H. *Anxiety and Its Disorders; the Nature and Treatment of Anxiety and Panic.* 2nd edition. New York: Guilford Press; 2002.

Germer, Christopher, and Ronald Siegel and Paul Fulton. *Mindfulness and Psychotherapy.* 2nd edition. New York: Guilford Press; 2016.

▪12▪

"Well, it seems that our time is up for today."

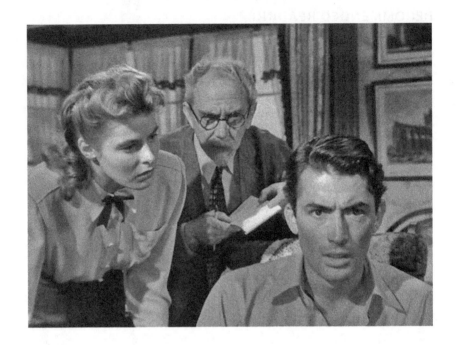

Hollywood Healers

PSYCHOTHERAPY ESSENTIALS

Over the years, as I looked for movies that portray different forms of madness, I noticed that many of them make an effort to show how psychotherapy works. Some are earnest in the attempt; some are antagonistic, either suggesting it doesn't help or that it is trying to impose something on the patient; and, not uncommonly, many just make fun of the therapist (not a difficult task—therapists can be pretty full of themselves, very much worthy of being parodied).

I found myself asking: What is this process we call therapy? There are many different models for psychotherapy, "the talking therapies" (I won't be dealing with medication treatments here). Some work better than others for specific types of madness: psychosis, or mood disorders, or the anxieties. Is there a common element that makes these treatments therapeutic, that allows us to call them "therapy"? Are there elements that make them less likely to be helpful? How can you tell good psychotherapy from bad? How can you tell a good therapist from a bad one—a different question?

I'd like to see if we can come up with answers, looking at an array of films we haven't talked about before, as well as a few that we have.

First let's look at Alfred Hitchcock's *Spellbound* (1945). There is a good reason to start here, because in the 1940s being in therapy, which meant psychoanalysis back then, became the thing to do among the Hollywood elite. Despite the stigma of admitting to emotional difficulties, a cult developed around this form of therapy, in part because it smacked more of trying to "understand" yourself better than admitting to a diagnosable madness. It was new, a boldly different way of looking at mental illness and treatment, and exotic, since many of the therapists were German and Austrian Jews seeking refuge from Nazis. *Spellbound* traded on the interest that Freudian psychoanalysis aroused and was the first of many films to glorify and explain it to the masses.

Spellbound is second-shelf Hitchcock. It's heavy-handed and dated, especially in its portrayal of women. The story is contrived, the characters mostly clichéd. But it has its moments, and its explanation of psychoanalysis is rather good. Gregory Peck plays J.B., who presents himself as Dr. Edwards, the new head of a psychiatric hospital. It is soon apparent that he is an imposter, that he suffers from amnesia and may have killed the real Edwards. Ingrid Bergman is Constance, a psychoanalyst colleague at the hospital who falls in love with him and tries to treat him to prove he is not a murderer. We know Constance is a doctor because she wears glasses and her hair is in a bun (in another dated stereotype—she lets her hair down once she is in love).

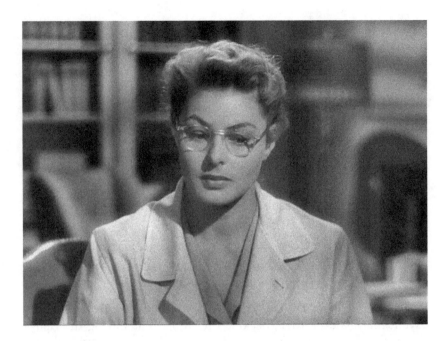

She brings him to the home of her mentor, Dr. Brulov, played wonderfully by Michael Chekhov (coming from the Moscow Art Theater, Chekhov was a celebrated acting coach to the stars, including Peck and Bergman). Brulov tells Constance that "women make the best doctors, and when they fall in love, the best patients." (Ouch.)

In a very Hitchcockian scene, J.B. goes into a sort of trance while starting to shave after staring at the white porcelain sink and then the lines on the bedspread where Constance is sleeping. He is holding a straight razor, which the camera focuses on as he walks past her and down the stairs. It is quite suspenseful—will he do something violent with that razor? Brulov is at his desk and offers J.B. a glass of milk to help him sleep (but also to make sure about that razor). He hands J.B. the glass and J.B. drinks it—as he does, we see Brulov, distorted, from inside the glass. The scene fades to the next morning. J.B. is sleeping on a couch.

Brulov had put bromide, a sleeping medication, into his milk. He shakes J.B. awake (a moment of humor as a gentle shake becomes a gesture to hit him) and Brulov tells J.B. that he wants to use analysis to help with his amnesia and to find out who he is. Brulov explains the therapy, a shorthand version of something that usually takes years.

"Don't fight me, I'm going to help you if I can. I'm going to be your father-image, I want you to look on me like your father. Trust me, lean on me."

J.B. says, "Go ahead, I'm leaning," and Brulov says, "Maybe you have something you want to tell me, a single thought. Words in the corner of your head, whatever comes into your head, just say what it is . . . Maybe you dreamt something? What did you dream?" J.B. says, "I don't believe in dreams. That Freud stuff is a lot of hooey." Brulov, offended, tells him, "You are a fine one to talk. You've got amnesia, you've got a guilt complex, you don't know if you are coming or going, but 'Freud is hooey,' this you know . . . wise guy!" Brulov goes on to explain about dreams: "The secrets of who you are and what has made you run away from yourself . . . are buried in your brain. But you don't want to look at them. The human being often doesn't want to know the truth about himself because he thinks it will make him sick. He makes himself sicker, trying to forget!"

So Brulov has given a simple but clear definition of transference ("treat me like your father") and free association ("tell me whatever comes into your head, maybe you dreamt something"), basics to the psychoanalytic process.

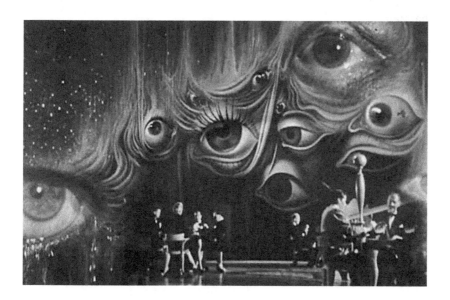

This brings us to the most famous part of this film—the dream sequence and its interpretation. The dream was designed by Salvador Dalí and is filled with his iconic eyes, melted watches, distorted wheels, and bizarre landscapes. Brulov explains, "Dreams tell you what you are trying to hide but they tell it all mixed up . . . the problem of the analyst is to examine this puzzle and put the pieces together in the right place and find out what the devil you are trying to say to yourself."

This is where the film begins to go wrong in trying to portray this new therapy. Brulov and Constance listen to details of the dream, and they tell J.B. what *their* associations are to its images instead of asking what they mean to him. They treat the dream as though they are detectives looking for clues to a crime, rather than therapists helping the patient understand himself. This is a real distortion of how this sort of therapy is supposed to work. For instance, in the dream a winged shadow chases J.B. down a hillside. Brulov says, "That shadow is Constance. If Constance grew wings, she would be an angel." That is very much Brulov's association, not J.B.'s. But then Constance runs with it—and wonders if the location of the dream is Angel Valley. That jogs J.B. memory and he says, no, it's Gabriel Valley. The therapist's interpretation led him there, but it's a distortion of how it might really happen.

In classic psychoanalysis, the therapist would repeatedly ask the patient what his associations are to the dream. One way of getting a better understanding is to have the patient retell the dream again and again, with the idea that new details will emerge that might help "solve the puzzle." The therapist would never impose her own association on the patient, though if she thought the patient was missing something she might gently make a suggestion in hopes the patient will then see it for himself.

The objective is not the "aha" moment too often seen in films (which must hurry the process to keep it interesting), but the patient's gradual new understanding, not just of the dream but of himself. This is one of the common elements in all therapies—not only the ones based on Freudian and other analytic ideas.

The therapist helps the patient develop a story about how he got into the situation that is troubling him, and then the therapist works with him to figure out how to get out of it. When Brulov says the therapist's job is to "put the pieces of the puzzle in the right place" he is describing a certainty, a sense of authority, that gives therapy (and, too often, those therapies based on psychoanalysis) a bad name. There is rarely a single "right" answer to what something means, or what happened in someone's childhood that might still haunt them. There is only the most convincing story you can manage to discover together with your therapist that allows you to move past whatever is holding you back from feeling good about yourself.

It really may not matter if the explanation is valid (most psychoanalysts would dispute this), but it has to be one you can agree on with your therapist, so you have a common language to better work together. This takes a while. Real therapy usually takes a while.

Spellbound and the presumptions of psychoanalysis are parodied to very good effect in Mel Brooks's *High Anxiety* (1977), a film that teases a raft of Hitchcock movies, from *North by Northwest* to *Vertigo* to *Psycho*.

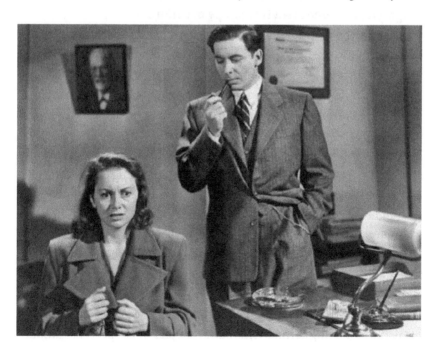

I started with *Spellbound* because it is a first attempt to feature psychoanalysis as central to the story. Just a few years later, Olivia de Havilland won an Oscar for her portrayal of a patient in *The Snake Pit* (1948). By this time, portrayals of psychoanalysis were hagiographic, placed on a pedestal as the gold standard of therapies. When Leo Genn, playing her therapist, explains to de Havilland why she is no longer feeling depressed, he tells her she doesn't need to understand why, as long as she can "feel it." He then proceeds to tell her exactly what happened in her childhood that got her there. This is condescending, paternalistic, and misleading about the nature of therapy, but was common in many films of the 1940s and 1950s.

Throughout this scene, a photo of Sigmund Freud is benignly looking down and approving just over the therapist's shoulder. This sort of thing was meant in earnest, but, in later years, it is played for laughs. In *What About Bob?*, as the therapist Dr. Marvin explains his "baby steps" theory, he leans on a bust of Freud, like they are buddies. When Bob tries to guess the names of his children, the doctor corrects him—they are named Sigmund and Anna (Anna Freud, Sigmund's daughter, pioneered analytic therapy of children).

Most of the therapies that followed psychoanalysis were either inspired by it or in opposition to it. Classic psychoanalysis is rarely practiced today because therapeutic change, if it happens at all, develops very slowly and at an enormous expense in time and money.

There have been many schisms in the psychoanalytic world over the years, and as many schools of thought, sometimes defined by something as seemingly simple as whether the analyst should answer a personal question ("Do you know anything about golf?" for instance). However, there are still many areas of agreement within the field.

During classic psychoanalysis, the patient would lie on a couch with the therapist sitting out of sight, usually behind him. Freud invented this structure to make it easier for the patient to free associate without responding to body-language signals from the therapist. He also admitted that he preferred this setup because he did not like his patients looking at him. Whether to lessen Freud's personal anxiety or to make it easier for the patient to be uncensored and open, this became a standard analytic rule. In order for the therapist using the psychoanalytic model to wear the mask of significant others, like a father or mother (encouraging transference, as Brulov explained in *Spellbound*), he must try to be anonymous, passive, and unrevealing about his personal life. Another rule was that sessions occur four or five days a week at a set time, for the classic fifty-minute hour. This is quite a commitment. The only interruption allowed was for several weeks, usually in August, when the therapist took a vacation. Though it is rarely required now, in the heydays of psychoanalysis all major decisions were supposed to be postponed until the therapy ended, or until the therapist had a chance to examine them closely with the patient and approve. A powerful dependence on the therapist is still encouraged and central to the work. Psychoanalysis can be interminable and run for years.

Freud himself had a sense of the limits of his technique. He understood that it was not recommended for anyone psychotic, for instance: the open invitation toward free association could worsen their disconnection from reality. He famously described his therapy as having the goal of "transforming neurotic misery into ordinary unhappiness." Not a high bar, though perhaps a realistic one. Even with that low expectation, classic psychoanalysis is quite inefficient as therapy, though it remains fascinating as theory and is often useful to academics when analyzing literature.

To address some of these concerns, a modified form of the therapy developed in the 1950s called psychodynamic psychotherapy. It uses many of the concepts of classic psychoanalysis, but in a way that changes the dynamic between the therapist and patient. First, the therapist and patient sit facing each other. This puts the concept of transference in the back seat: it's harder to do when you see each other. The therapist asks the patient to take responsibility for bringing concerns to the therapy and may be more active in asking for clarification and offering interpretations. The more conservative therapists will still ask the patient to free-associate, which sets up the therapy to be open-ended, while other therapists will ask the patient to settle on a goal for the work that can happen in a limited and agreed-upon amount of time.

Though my initial training as a child psychiatrist taught me psychodynamic principles and traditional play therapy, I was fortunate to find mentors, Carl Fellner and Carl Whitaker (the two "Carls"), who were pioneers in developing family therapy as an alternative way of helping children.

There are many schools of family therapy; most use some aspects of systems theory (emphasizing here-and-now interactions and looking for family rules that make it difficult for family members to change) and focus on communication and the emotional experience of being part of the family as well, without looking for causes or exploring history.

Both Carls started their careers as psychoanalysts but found that limiting and looked for something that might provide more immediate relief for their patients. Their analytic intuition, coupled with the immediacy of working with families as a system, proved incredibly powerful and exciting. The idea is that though a child (or adult) might be the "identified patient," the one whose behaviors brought them to the doctor, it is likely that if you can see the family together, learn how they function from day to day, see in your office the habitual patterns they fall into that can either exacerbate or worsen the diagnosed madness, you can engage them actively and help them change those patterns. This process can be a revelation for the family, not only pulling the focus away from the child (which relieves a great deal of stress) but also helping the family to see each other anew.

This work requires active engagement from the therapist and sometimes is best done with two therapists in the room, working together. Carl Whitaker used to joke, "Never let them outnumber you," to acknowledge how helpful it can be to have the second therapist there, to model how to argue or defuse a confrontation, or to simply demonstrate that there is more than one way to see a problem or find a solution.

In individual therapy sessions, I've never been good at just listening, though I like to think I am a good listener. I have a hard time not talking (shades of Sean, whom we will see in *Good Will Hunting*), so being an active participant with a family works for me. When, as part of my training, I was able to be the second therapist working with a master like Carl Whitaker, it was exhilarating. I learned so much about how to be with patients, families, and individuals.

The families in *Through a Glass Darkly*, *A Woman Under the Influence*, and *Ordinary People* might have really benefited from this model. Think about it: in each of these families we discover that the person labelled "mad" is not the only one who is troubled and may not even be the one who is the most disturbed. In *Through a Glass Darkly*, Karin has schizophrenia, but her father is depressed and overwhelmed with guilt. In *A Woman Under the Influence*, Mabel is depressed and may appear bipolar, but Nick is impulsive and has a violent temper. In *Ordinary People*, Conrad is depressed and suicidal, but his mother Beth's emotional coldness and pathological grieving tears the family apart. Seeing them together as a "system" might well have encouraged each family toward a better life together.

Let's talk about some therapy ground rules. When beginning therapy, the therapist needs to make clear to a potential patient what the rules and expectations are if they are going to be able to work together. Many rules are explained explicitly, and many are simply conveyed by what happens in the early interactions between the patient and therapist. Based on the therapist's training and preferences, which she should discuss early on, she will specify how often they should meet, who should participate in the therapy (is this going to be individual, couples, or family work), how long each session will be, and what the goals are. If it's not clear what the goals are, because the patient is not sure or doesn't know what is possible, then the first goal is to figure that out.

I always also made a point of emphasizing that I will make every effort to start each session on time, and that sessions will end on time as well. The fifty-minute hour is common (it allows the therapist time between patients to make notes, return a call or go to the bathroom), but some therapists prefer forty-five minutes and some seventy-five minutes. If you are working with a family, the longer amount of time is more likely to be productive. But for individual patients, fifty minutes seems close to the ideal time that both therapist and patient can maintain focus together. If the patient's or therapist's schedule does not allow weekly sessions or if the therapist doesn't think the problem needs such frequent meetings, the therapist should say so and plan accordingly. In the United States, unfortunately, questions of insurance and payment must also be sorted out. It's best to avoid any rude surprises later about money.

The next level of discussion is about the nature of the relationship. A psychodynamic therapist pledges to make the patient's issues central to the work. He will pay attention, not be judgmental, and help the patient stay focused. The therapist doesn't need to say all this; demonstrating it in the first sessions will make the point.

Carl Whitaker, practicing family therapy, would start the work before even seeing the patient. When arranging a first appointment he would ask whoever called to tell him who was in the family, and then insist that all the members of the family come to the first session. If the person calling objected, declaring this is only about my son who is depressed, or my husband is too busy with work, or my daughter has music lessons that make it impossible for her to be there, he would say that he would not see them unless they were all there, and give the person calling the task of making sure that happened.

This immediately tests the system. Is this a family that can come together about a problem? Can they talk to each other well enough to adjust to what is demanded? If they manage it, they will have already begun the therapy and perhaps even begun to change. If they couldn't manage it, Carl might relent and agree to only see the parents and the identified patient child, but would use those first sessions to help find a way to bring the others in.

To be effective, any therapy requires that patients feel that their privacy is honored and that they are assured of confidentiality. This is a big and important subject that I will try to summarize here.

What is said in the office stays there. However, there is an exception: when a therapist becomes concerned for the patient's safety, that they might be suicidal or want to do violence to someone else. In that circumstance I always tell my patients of my concern and then try to evaluate what needs to be done to keep them safe. If the patient can make an honest agreement with the therapist to contact him if the suicidal or violent preoccupations become more intense, then it might be okay to send him home. The therapist makes sure the patient knows how to reach him at any time of day or night.

If the patient isn't able to make that commitment, the therapist would then explain that a parent, spouse, or friend needs to be brought into the session to see if they are able to protect the patient from acting dangerously. If that is too much a burden for family or the trusted friend (and it is a lot to ask), and if the therapist thinks the risk is immediate, then the patient will need to be hospitalized.

If this is explained, most patients are accepting of this violation of confidentiality, knowing it is the best way to keep them safe. If they refuse to cooperate with the plan, then the doctor may have to commit them—which means legally requiring them to go into the hospital to be evaluated and treated until they are deemed to be safe.

This circumstance can be difficult. Psychiatrists are sometimes bad at evaluating risk. There are no absolute measures. That's why it is always a good idea to consult with a colleague to ensure that the situation is being read correctly. To protect confidentiality, a therapist will usually not identify the patient to the person they are consulting with, but will only describe the thoughts and behaviors that make them concerned for the patient's safety.

I had a patient once whom I was seeing for his agitated depression. He was convinced that the obstetrician who delivered his new baby had caused her injury. As his agitation worsened, he began to make violent threats in our sessions about killing the doctor, finally telling me his plan to go to the doctor's house and shoot him when he answered the door, and then turning the gun on himself. I became convinced that this was no fantasy, that he really intended to do it. We talked about what the consequences would be; that he would be responsible for someone's death and would either be dead himself or be arrested and kept away from his wife and child. But he could not shake this obsession.

I decided that for his protection and to protect the obstetrician, I had to commit him. He was not able then to agree to going to the hospital on his own. Taking this step was difficult for me. It is not easy to take away someone's freedom, even to protect them from themselves. Committing him required that I sign a formal declaration, then call an ambulance to take him to the hospital and a policeman to be sure he got there. Fortunately, he went without a fuss.

There is a legal "duty to warn" that overrides confidentiality in many states, including where I live. So, I called the obstetrician, whom I did not know, and told him what was happening. He thanked me profusely and was relieved to know my patient was in the hospital. A few weeks later, the patient returned to me, no longer suicidal or obsessed with revenge, and we were able to continue working together. Sometimes that can't happen if the patient harbors anger at the therapist for forcing hospitalization. The therapist can only encourage him to find another counselor to work with. In this case, though, he thanked me. The doctor he had threatened did too; he brought me a potted plant.

Another version of this exception to confidentiality is when the therapist is seeing young children or adolescents alone.

For teens especially, telling them that the details of their therapy will not be reported to their parents is essential to gain their trust. If a parent asks what was discussed, the answer must be that what was discussed is confidential. If teens want to tell their parents about the session, that's fine. But, without express permission, a therapist will not disclose this information to them.

Patients must be told, however, that there is an exception: if the teen expresses something that makes the therapist fear for their safety—suicidal or dangerous behavior, cutting, severe eating issues, or the like—then, after discussing the specific concern, the therapist will call a parent in to include them in the work.

In *Ordinary People*, which I think of as a particularly good example of how therapy is done, none of this was made explicit. But it is clear that Conrad understands how it works—after all, he had been in therapy at the hospital for months.

My own most common mode of therapy with children and teens is family therapy, including parents, other children, and often grandparents if they live nearby. If that is the only mode of therapy I'm using, the bubble of confidentiality includes the whole family. I often will see teens separately as well, giving them the opportunity to talk about things with me that might be hard to say in front of mom or dad. Those sessions will be confidential. Under those circumstances, if I think it will help, I might encourage the teen to talk with their parents in a family meeting about a particularly difficult issue. If there is agreement, we can rehearse how to talk about it, with me offering to be backup in case the parents respond badly.

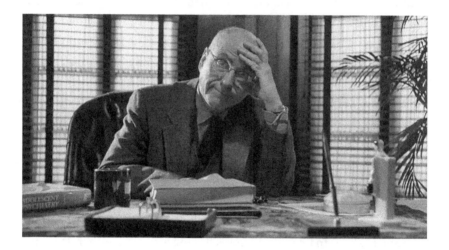

Grosse Pointe Blank (1997) is a romantic comedy with Alan Arkin as Dr. Oatman, a psychiatrist, and John Cusack as Martin Blank, a hitman who returns home for his high school reunion. There are several funny and real examples of challenges to the rules of therapy.

Martin's latest job brings him near his hometown. He's been depressed and on edge, so he finds a psychiatrist who has written a book about killers. Martin is tempted to go to his high school reunion, "But I don't know how much I have in common with those people anymore. They all have husbands and wives and can talk about what they do and what am I going to say, 'I killed the President of Paraguay with a fork, how have you been?'"

Alan Arkin (another actor who I think is a national treasure—warm, quirky, and funny) is his very reluctant therapist. After their fourth session, in which Martin first discloses his occupation, Dr. Oatman tells him, "I'm not your doctor. I'm emotionally involved with you, I'm afraid of you . . . It would be unethical for me to work with you." The doctor tells Martin that he doesn't want to work with him, "and yet you come back every week at the same time. If you are thinking of committing a crime, I have to tell the authorities." Martin says he knows that, but he is serious about wanting to get help, "and I know where you live." That not-so-veiled threat doesn't go down well. Martin insists he was joking, but Oatman says it didn't sound like a joke, and he is intimidated and feels like he has to be really interesting or Martin will "blow my brains out. You are holding me hostage here."

Throughout this conversation, Dr. Oatman is sitting behind his desk. If he were actually intent on doing therapy with Martin, he would have moved to a nearby chair. He puts the desk between him and Martin as a defense, non-verbally saying, this is not happening.

Therapy requires an openness on the part of the patient and the full attention of the therapist. A desk gets in the way. Not only does it make it hard for the therapist to see and read the patient's body language, but it feels to the patient like a barrier to honest connection. Therapists shouldn't be taking notes during a session, either. If something needs to be written down, either for the patient's records or to remember details of the session for next time, it should be done after the session ends, during that ten- or fifteen-minute break between patients. If the therapist is writing during the session, they are not paying full attention to what is happening in the room.

Martin, frustrated, asks what they should talk about, and asks if he should talk about his dreams. Dr. Oatman says, "It's your nickel," and Martin relates one of several dreams about his old girlfriend from high school (Minnie Driver) whom he is anxious about meeting at the reunion. This dream is about the "battery bunny" in television commercials and he, Martin, is that bunny.

Dr. Oatman says that sounds like a depressing dream and explains, "It [the bunny] has no brain, no blood, no anima! It just keeps going and going." Then he tells him, "Time's up," even though it's only been twenty minutes. He wants Martin gone. Martin says, "At least give me some advice," and asks if he should go to the reunion. The doctor says, "Sure, get out of town! Go see some old friends . . . Don't kill anybody for a few days, see what it feels like." Martin says, "I'll give it a shot," and the doctor replies, "No, no, don't shoot anything." After Martin leaves, the doctor leans on the wall and groans.

I like this very much; it's funny and oh so wrong. The first boundary violated is that Martin refuses to accept that his therapist, in being afraid of him, can't work with him. That should have ended the relationship. Part of the expectation for a relationship to be therapeutic is the development of trust. Usually, it's the patient who must learn to trust his new doctor, which takes time. In this case, the doctor can't trust Martin, who waited four sessions to admit to what he did for a living and then refuses to let the doctor off the hook.

Dr. Oatman's agenda for this whole session is to get it over with as quickly as possible without making his patient angry and possibly killing him. That's probably why, if we take the moment seriously for learning purposes (instead of allowing it to be the comic exaggeration it is), he reacts to Martin's dream by telling him what it means instead of asking him. His interpretation is his reaction to the battery bunny in the dream and may not be Martin's at all. But we will never know, and neither will Martin because as soon as a therapist leaps in to interpret that way, he closes off the possibility of the patient venturing his own ideas. It takes a lot of self-confidence to contradict your therapist, and most patients starting therapy are anything but self-confident. When Martin asks for advice, under normal circumstances most therapists would be reluctant to give it, at least directly. If they give advice, they would want it to be part of a longer conversation with the goal of the patient discovering the best advice himself. Dr. Oatman gives Martin what he asks for to appease him and to get him to leave. "Don't kill anybody for a few days" includes him too.

A word about "firing" a patient: it doesn't happen often, but it requires honesty. If the issue the patient needs to work on is one that either makes the therapist too uncomfortable or is a problem that the therapist is not adept at treating, it is okay for the therapist to tell them that and refer them to someone else, preferably someone who specializes in their problem. For me, that would be people who abuse alcohol: I'm just not good working with them, but I know people who are. If that is a patient's central problem, better they should work with someone more expert and more comfortable with it than I am.

A person doesn't always declare up front what all their problems are: they might not even know what all their problems are, and it may take a few sessions to discover them. If what the therapist discovers tells him this is not someone he can help as he would want, referring them to someone better equipped to be helpful makes sense and is appropriate. It's important that in doing so the therapist doesn't label the person as bad or burdened with an impossible problem; just that the fit is bad. The patient might come to the same conclusion, which is why some doctor shopping is a good idea. It should be contained, but it's okay for patients to want to be sure they feel comfortable with the manner and therapeutic model of their therapist. A good way to deal with this is to suggest the patient try, say, six sessions and then decide. This is useful in general: it's not a bad idea to pause after a certain number of sessions and ask, "How are we doing?"

Admittedly, being afraid of your professional-killer patient is not a normal therapy situation. More typical is the situation we see in the film *Klute* (1971).

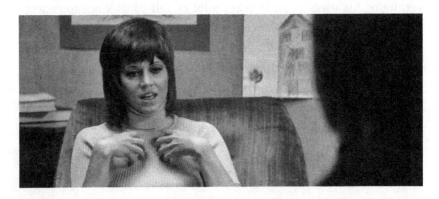

Jane Fonda, who won an Oscar as Best Actress for this film, is Bree, a high-priced call girl who wants to stop scoring tricks. We first see her complaining to her therapist that she has been seeing her for a long time, yet she still feels compelled to trick. Her doctor, a woman who sits opposite her in profile (an unusual position since most therapists would sit directly facing their patient) first reminds her that she doesn't have a magic potion to make her conflicts go away, and then asks her what she likes about being a call girl.

Bree talks about liking the sense of control, knowing that she is good at it, "for an hour I am the best actress in the world, the best fuck . . . You just lead them in the direction they think they want to go; you control it, and you call the shots and I always feel great right afterwards." But, she says, she never enjoys it physically. In another session, she talks about the detective (Donald Sutherland) who is investigating the disappearance of a businessman. Initially distrusting each other, they have recently begun an affair and Bree has unexpected feelings for him. "I enjoy making love with him, which is a baffling thing for me, I've never felt that way before . . . All the time I feel the need to destroy it, to break it off, to go back to the comfort of being numb again." Bree talks freely. Her therapist says very little. She is just a very good and sympathetic listener. This is the portrait of a therapy that is well established, that has been going on for a while. There is trust and an understanding of what to do from session to session—mostly, for Bree to think out loud, not only to express her fears and uncertainties but to hear herself putting them into words and begin to think about them differently. The therapist poses the occasional question, but Bree is doing most of the work. Which is as it should be. If the therapist is working harder than the patient, then something is very wrong. Here, we only see brief moments of therapy (we don't actually see the work), but we see that Bree is changing, and we can believe in that magic potion.

Paul Mazursky is the writer and director of several films that were very popular in the 1970s. These were serious, comedic dramas about relationships among upper-middle-class New Yorkers who routinely brought their troubles to therapy. Mazursky is rather forgotten today but he was very good, and these are films worth watching.

An Unmarried Woman (1978) stars Jill Clayburgh as Erica, whose husband suddenly leaves her for a younger woman. She is wrestling with defining herself outside of marriage, outside of a relationship with a man. Mazursky had a habit of using real therapists in his films. The therapy sessions are interesting, and were mostly improvised.

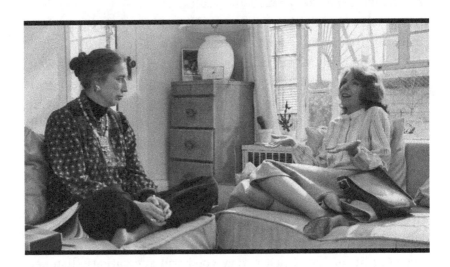

In *An Unmarried Woman*, Erica sees Tanya. They are both sitting cross-legged, shoes off, on low cushions. Tanya directs Erica away from talking about her childhood and asks what is happening now. She repeats what Erica has just said, but in slightly different words. This is a way of telling her patient that she is listening carefully and confirming that Erica's experiences are not unique—that she understands, and that Erica's confusion will clear up in time. Then she recommends that Erica come twice a week for a while and then move to once a week, "because it's a lot more important what you do out there than what you do in here." This is a very different message from that of classic psychoanalysis. She is setting the boundaries for the work—how often they will meet, for how long, and what kind of responses Erica can expect from the doctor. But we also see that one of her standard replies will be to predict that things will get better.

At another session Erica is in tears. She can't help noticing all the affectionate couples and feels jealous and lonely. Then Tanya does something unexpected and, frankly, unprofessional. She tells Erica that she, too, was lonely when she got divorced. Erica didn't know she was divorced. Tanya then begins a litany of telling her it's okay to feel lonely, that you are supposed to: "It's really okay to feel anything, anger, jealousy, depression . . . it's okay to feel." Erica then says she feels guilty, and Tanya switches gears and suddenly announces that feeling guilty is not okay and that "it's something I get livid about, it's sort of a man-made emotion" (whatever that means). Tanya then gives her an assignment: Stop feeling guilty for one week. "And don't feel guilty about feeling guilty," she says. This is bonkers.

First, Tanya gives her too much information, telling Erica that she has been divorced, an observation that probably is meant to convey that she understands what Erica is going through. Of course, she can't really understand unless she asks more about it, which she doesn't. She tells Erica she can't talk about "guilt" because it makes Tanya upset and angry, which closes off any discussion of why Erica feels guilty or what she feels guilty about. Then she tells Erica to stop feeling guilty, as though that is easy, or even a good idea. One bad intervention after another. What is interesting, though, is that with all these mistakes, Erica seems to value the relationship and her sessions. She finds, in Tanya, a sympathetic person, someone she can talk to who helps assuage her loneliness. And for her, that seems to be enough. But it's not good therapy.

In *Bob and Carol and Ted and Alice* (1969), also co-written and directed by Mazursky, the psychiatrist is Dr. Donald Muhich, who was Mazursky's personal analyst. He is a very strange man, with an oddly passive manner that I find quite off-putting. One wonders what prompted Mazursky to use him, what conversations they had to decide that it was professionally okay for Muhich to do it. It certainly would complicate the nature of their relationship. My fantasy is that this is Mazursky's revenge on his doctor, putting him on display for all to judge.

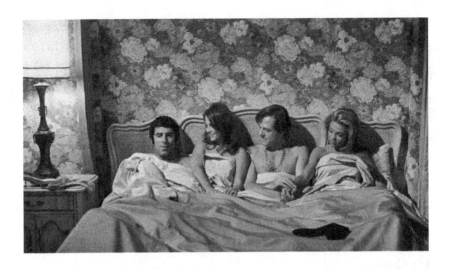

Bob and Carol and Ted and Alice is very much of its time with an extended sequence showing a marathon "gestalt encounter group" experience. The four title characters are two couples, longtime friends, looking for enlightenment and sexual adventure together. The encounter group has rules: you commit to the full day or weekend, and one of the rules is that "there are no rules." But of course, there are. "No rules" is a rule. Also, there is a rule that there must be no physical violence, that you will work to be in touch with your feelings, and that you will express it in the exercises the leader sets up. There are trust exercises, like falling backwards and trusting that a stranger from the group will catch you; looking deeply into another person's eyes and trying to communicate without words; and getting out your angry feelings by physicalizing it, for instance by punching a pillow.

All this can be exhilarating—letting your guard down and seeing others do the same. But, the effect usually doesn't last, in part because there is no narrative, no story that helps you figure out what to do next, outside of the group. Many of these techniques were developed by Fritz and Laura Perls, creating ways to encourage you to think less and be more in the moment. They have much in common with psychodrama, where you act out feelings and relationships rather than talk about them. Gestalt therapy groups' popularity was very much a response to the failings of psychoanalysis. As the leader says in the movie, "Perhaps this marathon will open up some doors." Doors that psychoanalysis did not seem able to open.

In *Ordinary People* (1980), we see the technique of psychodrama during the emergency session with Berger after Conrad has heard that his friend from the hospital has killed herself. This is clearly not something Berger does routinely with his patients. But, when he sees Conrad so upset, intensely reliving the moment when his brother drowned, he goes with it. Conrad cries out to him, "Why did you let go?" and Berger responds in the voice of the brother, "Because I got tired." Notice, that he uses "I"—in that moment he is *being* the brother for Conrad, allowing him to yell back, "Well, screw you, you jerk!" and then collapse in tears. The drama is over, and quietly Berger says, "It hurts being mad at him, doesn't it?" This opens up a new and healing conversation; a different narrative toward understanding.

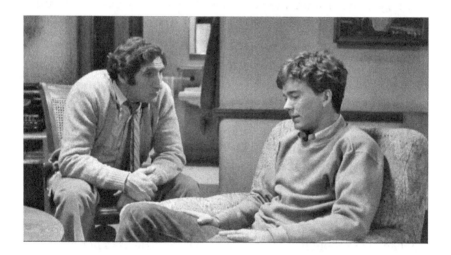

What I want to emphasize here is how Berger's human connection with Conrad allowed this to happen. Berger is good about keeping the focus of their work on Conrad. When Con is mad at him in an earlier session, he yells something about Berger going home to his "fat wife." We realize that neither Conrad nor we in the audience know anything about Berger's personal life—is he married, does he have a family, where is he from? This is good. Conrad doesn't need to know for his connection with Berger to be real and meaningful. All this is not to say that Berger is the perfect therapist—he makes mistakes too. As I mentioned earlier, I cringe when he tells Conrad he is his "friend." He is both more and very different from a "friend," and that distinction is worth holding onto.

In general, another boundary rule is no hugs, no touching. The therapeutic relationship is an unbalanced one; the patient is usually emotionally vulnerable and dependent. It is not a relationship of equals, and it can be too easily misunderstood or abused. But sometimes that human connection is necessary, and even appropriate. It needs to be carefully considered, not something a therapist does impulsively. Though I think declaring himself Conrad's friend was the wrong message, I think the hug was just fine. They have been through an intensely felt and important moment, with Conrad finally able to be angry at his brother and face the fact that he survived the boating accident because he was stronger. A hug that conveys support and understanding and acknowledges this shared moment says a lot that needs to be said. In this, and most of the decisions we see him make, Dr. Berger shows himself to be a mensch, a person with compassion and good character. If I could choose a movie therapist as my doctor, it would be him.

Back to *Bob and Carol and Ted and Alice*: In addition to the gestalt group experience, all the characters are in traditional therapy, and their therapist is Dr. Muhich. The session with Alice is particularly revealing. She is uncomfortable telling the doctor that she has lost interest in having sex with her husband; she doesn't want to be touched, even though she is a "happy person." He asks her what she means. She tells him "I like my husband, I love my child, I love my friends," and he points out she said she likes her husband, but she loves her friends. A good point and one worth examining. So far Muhich is doing well. Alice is taken aback; did she really say that? Several of the close-ups of the doctor show him staring, unresponsive; you could read anything into his expression, which I guess is the point. And then there is a half-smile that looks more like a smirk. He comes across to me as cold and unsympathetic and maybe enjoying her discomfort.

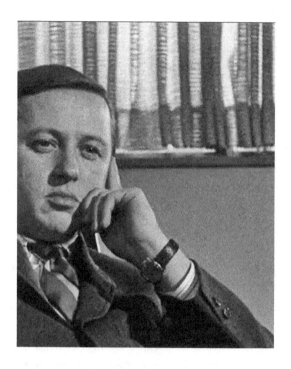

When she makes a "Freudian slip" and says their friend Bob's name (instead of Ted, her husband) when talking about having sex, we see that odd half-smile again. Then he tells her that their time is up, and he gets up to walk her to the door. But Alice is still in mid-thought: she is beginning to wonder if she doesn't trust Ted. Is she suspicious that he is interested in her best friend, Carol, and is that why she was short with her the other day? She is trying to figure something out, something important. But Muhich keeps repeating, "Let's continue Thursday, we can discuss it then." This is a classic "door knob moment," something that happens often in therapy. Something may be difficult or embarrassing to face; the patient delays talking about it until the last moment of the session and then presents it on the way out the door. The temptation is to be glad this is finally being talked about and explore it—but if the therapist allows it, it can become a habit. All the difficult subjects will be saved for the last minute, not only because the time running out increases the pressure to finally blurt out the worry or thought that you have been sitting on all session but also because it is gratifying to be given extra time; it feels like a gift and makes the patient feel special. But there are better ways to hold to the time limit than Muhich's method. He comes across a bit like Dr. Oatman's "battery bunny": He has no anima, he doesn't show a human connection with his patient. He just repeats himself, pointing to the time boundary rule and to the door.

We see a much better example of how to do this in *Ordinary People* when Dr. Berger sets the same limit with Conrad. Berger's manner is very different from that of Muhich. He is in conversation with Conrad, asking challenging questions, questioning Conrad's assumptions, but in a way that encourages a response, and encourages him to think differently about what he just said.

They are talking about how Conrad's mother has a difficult time showing that she loves him, Berger challenging Conrad's conviction that this proves that he is unlovable. Finally, Berger says to Conrad, "There is someone besides her you have to forgive," and he lets that sink in, looking intently at Conrad, in silence. Conrad is taken aback, asks him what he means. All Berger offers is, "Why not give yourself a break" and then tells him, "Time's up!" This is not one of those intentionally delayed "doorknob" moments; they have just run out of time. Conrad tries to get him to answer, and Berger says, "Come on, Con, you know the rules. You think about it." Conrad isn't happy, but even if he hasn't been given extra time, he has been given something to contemplate until they next meet.

Muhich offers nothing like that to Alice. As I have pointed out before, if the therapist can help patients come to the understanding on their own, with whatever coaching is required, they will more easily own the new understanding and be able to use it. The general rule is that if you tell your patient the answer to an important question, they either won't get it or can too easily dismiss it. It's always best for them to figure it out for themselves. A therapist can lead them there, but for it to carry emotional weight, for it to mean something, they have to discover the final bit of ground themselves. And, sometimes having to wait until the next session to explore the answers is the best way to find them.

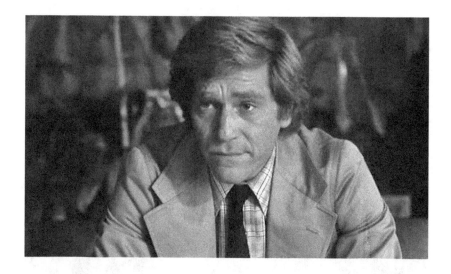

Another very good Mazursky film is *Blume in Love* (1973), starring George Segal as a lawyer, distraught because he is still in love with his ex-wife. In a therapy session with the ever-present Dr. Muhich, Blume is reporting that whenever he hears mention of his ex-wife's name, he becomes impotent with the woman he has been seeing. Blume talks freely; he is used to therapy. Muhich asks if it has happened with anyone else, and Blume says there isn't anyone else right now, then asks if Muhich is suggesting he should go to bed with another woman. Muhich's response is, "I wasn't telling you to do anything" (making clear he will not give advice), and then he says, "but, sometimes after people get divorced, they go through a period of 'sport fucking.'" This is not only an odd phrase but it sure sounds like a suggestion, and Blume takes it that way. In a later session, Blume tells Muhich that he thinks he wants to stop therapy. He tells him, "Sometimes I think this is a waste of time, that it doesn't do any good." The doctor replies, "Sometimes it doesn't." Blume asks him why he does it. As the camera pulls in on his face, Muhich replies, "Because, sometimes it does. And until we find something better, what else is there to do?" Poignant and dispiriting words about your life's work.

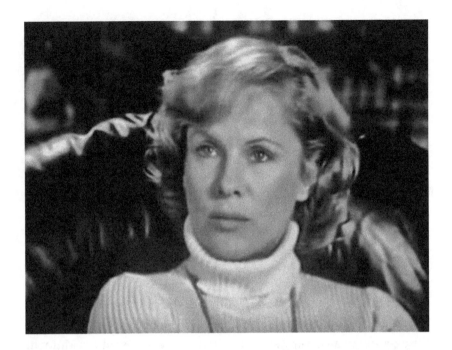

In *I Never Promised You a Rose Garden* (1977), Deborah (Kathleen Quinlan) is in therapy with Dr. Fried (Bibi Andersson). She has symptoms of schizophrenia with intensely vivid psychotic hallucinations. Dr. Fried uses the model of psychodynamic psychotherapy to explore why Deborah feels so guilty and suicidal. They sit opposite each other, and the doctor asks her about her latest suicide attempt—she has cut her arm badly. She asks Deborah to remove the bandage and tells her she wants Deborah to see it, to see the scar. She then asks her why she did it. The therapist is determining the direction of the therapy, telling the patient what she needs to work on. Because Deborah is psychotic, suicidal, and in the hospital, this level of guidance seems right.

Deborah says she is poison, that everyone she touches gets hurt. And then she tells Dr. Fried that many years ago she tried to kill her baby sister. As Deborah describes what happened, the doctor asks questions about it and points out that what Deborah remembers could not have happened the way she remembers it. Then she provides an interpretation: that Deborah was angry at her little sister and wished her dead. She asks her to imagine the event again, to remember more, and suddenly Deborah does, realizing that this was a false memory. But then she becomes panicked and the psychotic images return. She begins to talk about her unreal world, Yr, and the doctor asks Deborah to tell her more about it. She is accepting and open, and as Deborah hesitates, the doctor asks her to trust, saying, "I won't betray you."

Telling Deborah she needs time to prove her trust, she defines what is special about therapy and is hard for films to convey: therapy is a process that is slow, hesitant, with many setbacks, and which takes time to make a difference. Later, as the therapist learns more about Deborah's delusional world, she tells her that the god of her world is too punishing. Deborah is receptive enough now to say, "not always." She is allowing the doctor to look at this world and comment on it, something she would not allow earlier. Later conversations about her father encourage Deborah to see him as a man with flaws, who, wanting to protect her, simply said the wrong things. This makes Deborah cry for the first time, and Dr. Fried encourages her to hold onto the feeling even if it hurts or is scary, that it is part of the human condition (very much the same message Berger gives Conrad). She also gives her permission to return to her delusional world if she chooses—"I can be crazy if I want to . . . bats?"—a movie conceit you see rather too often. This is simply not something one has control over. But a version of this message is worth giving—that the patient can either work toward change or choose not to. Deborah's use of the word "bats" opens a nice exchange when Dr. Fried, whose mild accent betrays her not speaking English as her first language, asks her what it means. Deborah explains the phrase "bats in the belfry," and then reaches out to touch the doctor's face, inviting a gentle touch in return. It's a lovely moment.

Contrast this scene with the time Deborah must see a substitute doctor because Dr. Fried is away. This doctor responds to hearing about Deborah's delusional world language by pulling out dictionaries to try to find a source. Deborah is being treated as an object of interest, not a person needing help. In a sign of progress, she forcefully calls him on it.

When patients of mine tell me they are depressed, I don't leave it at that. I ask them what they mean, what experiences they have that they would call "depression." I may help them if they are struggling by telling what other people experience when they are depressed, asking if they, too, have these symptoms. But first, I want to hear them describe it; I want to learn their language, their meaning. Do they mean that they are simply sad? Does it mean they cry a lot, or not at all? Do they not feel sad, but have low energy, poor concentration, and no longer enjoy their favorite activities? That can be depression too. Novice therapists will often bring their own assumptions about meaning into the relationship and not give the patient a chance to explain. That can cause misunderstandings that can lead them astray—simply because they didn't ask.

"My dog just died," says the patient. It would be easy to assume that this is sad, to almost insist on it. Patients want to please the therapist, to be liked. They want this process to go well, so they may let the therapist persuade them to agree. But maybe they are not sad, but relieved, because their dog was very old and in pain, or maybe it was a nasty animal, or maybe it was too much trouble to take care of. These are all different scenarios for which "how sad" is not an appropriate response. It is important to give the patient a blank page to fill in and the time to do it. In movies, the "essay question" too often becomes "fill in the blank" because the film doesn't have time to show the normal back and forth of therapy.

One of the benefits of long-form serial television is that it has time to show this progression. Our focus in this book is on the stand-alone two-hour movie, so we won't be discussing these shows here. But they deserve attention too. For portraits of therapy, long-form series such as *The Sopranos*, *In Treatment*, and the recent *Mare of Easttown* are definitely worth a look.

Empathy is a necessary element in any successful therapy, even in the more mechanistic therapies like cognitive behavioral therapy, which is much more focused on the left brain and encourages the patient to think through alternative narratives rather than trying to uncover repressed feelings. This is a therapy that is structured more like a tutorial; you are given homework assignments and things to practice, such as meditation and desensitization techniques. It is focused, particular, and usually time-limited, with no room for dreams or free association. But still, even a therapist utilizing this model needs to be able to connect with the patient and establish a working relationship. In all therapies, the therapist needs to convey that they are giving their full attention, something we rarely experience in the course of our day, and that the therapist will be nonjudgmental and open to explore what the patient brings to the work.

A therapist may have some strong ideas on what is important, but they need to start where the patient is. When Conrad tells Berger that he wants to work on "control," Berger says "Okay, it's your money," even though he thinks that is not what is needed. But he will start there, and even make it a reason for Conrad to come twice a week, "Control's a tough nut." Berger has confidence that as they tell their stories to each other (first Conrad's version, then Berger's different take) they are likely to change the nature of the quest.

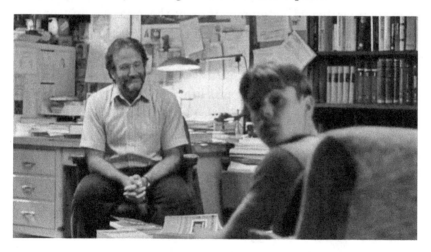

Good Will Hunting (1997) is a study of everything a therapist could do wrong and still help his patient. That can only happen when you do some important things right. Robin Williams is Sean, the psychologist assigned to Will Hunting (Matt Damon, who wrote the script with his friend Ben Affleck), a preternaturally brilliant young man from South

Boston, the wrong side of the tracks. Will has blown off several other therapists' attempts to engage him.

It tells us something that we never know Sean's last name. He is not the traditional therapist who will insist on being called "doctor." His office is institutional, papers scattered and piled high, books everywhere. Knowing that Will is not there voluntarily, Sean tries to connect with him by finding things they may have in common. Will makes a condescending joke, asking if the books came as part of a "shrink kit," and Sean turns it around to ask Will if he likes books. Will says curtly, "Yeah," trying to shut down the conversation. Sean pushes it, pointing to his books and asking if Will has read any of them. So, in trying a "joining" maneuver he is also beginning to challenge Will, asking him what he thinks of the ones he's read. Will fires back, "I'm not here for a fuckin' book report. They're your books, why don't *you* read them?" Sean says, "I did. I had to." It's like a boxing match, punch for punch; so far, it's a draw. But he has gotten Will talking.

Will starts smoking and pacing around the office. Sean tells him, "You know you would be better off shoving that cigarette up your ass," matching Will's casually vulgar language, and Will comes back with a sarcastic, "Yeah, I know, it really gets in the way of my yoga." This allows another joining topic as Sean asks if Will works out. Sean says he does, free weights, and Will asks him what he benches. Sean tells him, 285 pounds, then asks him what he lifts—and Will, who obviously can't top Sean in weight lifting, abruptly changes the subject.

Will sees a watercolor of a boat in the ocean and asks about it. Again, Sean initially sees it as an opening and asks if Will likes art, does he draw or like music? Will begins to criticize the drawing, and then to read it as reflecting Sean's state of mind, "I think you are about one step away from cutting your fuckin' ear off!" Then he pushes too far, "Maybe you are in the middle of a storm . . . maybe [that's why] you became a psychologist . . . maybe you married the wrong woman." Sean replies, "Maybe you should watch your mouth," but Will pushes further, "What happened, did she leave you, was she banging some other guy?" Sean takes off his glasses and throttles Will by the throat,

"If you ever disrespect my wife again, I will end you!" Will, when he can get his breath, says "Time's up," and walks out.

So, the joining goes wrong, and Sean violates a major rule: you don't touch, and (to state the obvious) no matter how provoked, you don't attack your patient.

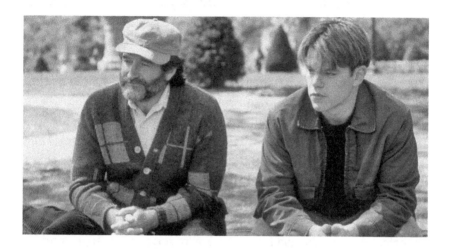

Later they meet on a bench by a lake. Neutral territory. Sean tells Will that being smart intellectually does not make you smart emotionally. He knows Will's family life has been chaotic and hard and that he doesn't have experience of love or lasting relationships. Sean calls Will on his arrogance to think that because he is smart, he can figure it all out. He then talks about his marriage and the painful time dealing with his wife's cancer and with her death, all to make the point that Will knows little about life with another person who really matters. Sean is being much more open about himself than most therapists would choose to be. (Contrast this with therapist Tanya's casual mention of her divorce, a revelation that is a joining maneuver, but which doesn't go anywhere.)

In so many words, Sean is telling Will that Will can decide he doesn't want to work with him in therapy, but if he does decide to, he must commit to do the work and not be a smart-ass. This overlong, artificial, and sentimental movie moment brings Will back to therapy. And they do bond.

Will returns to Sean's office. He tells him he went out on a date, and when he is asked whether he is going out again, Will says he hasn't called her, even though she is beautiful, she's smart, she's fun, and different from most of the girls he's been with. Sean says, "So call her up, Romeo," and Will says, "Why? So I can realize she's not that smart . . . this girl is fuckin' perfect right now, I don't want to ruin that." Sean's response is very good: "Maybe you're perfect right now, and you don't want to ruin that . . . a super philosophy. That way you can go through your entire life without really getting to know anybody."

Sean shares an anecdote about his wife farting in bed (this was an improvisation by Robin Williams that they decided to keep). They laugh together. Sean tells Will, "She's been dead two years and that's the shit I remember. Wonderful stuff. Those are the things I miss the most, those little idiosyncrasies that only I knew about. That's what made her my wife. And she had the goods on me too . . . These imperfections are the good stuff . . . You're not perfect, sport, and let me save you the suspense, this girl you met, she isn't perfect either. But the queston is whether or not you are perfect for each other. That's the whole deal, that's what intimacy is all about." Will smiles and says, "You fuckin' talk more than any shrink I ever seen in my life," and Sean replies, "I teach this shit. I didn't say I knew how to do it."

It's true, there is way too much talking *at* Will: lecturing him about life, about what he doesn't know, and what Sean's superior wisdom could teach him. But the way Sean works to find common ground with Will, the way he doesn't give up on him, the way he models openness about feelings, all this is "the good stuff" even if it strays far from how actual therapy works.

Let's end with a couple of funny therapists. Psychiatry, and therapists in general, are easily made fun of. We often take ourselves too seriously, are too earnest, and too many of us think we understand more than we do. We are ripe to be taken down a peg or two. And, of course, to the extent that we represent authority, we are ripe for satire.

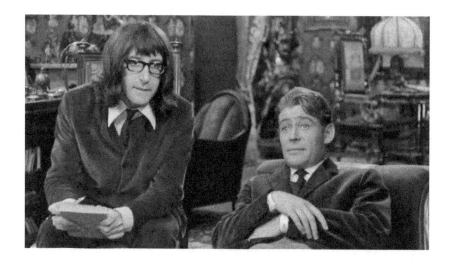

In *What's New Pussycat* (1965), Peter Sellers is Fritz Fassbender, dressed in red velvet, with a Beatles haircut, an obvious quack. We first see him being chased by his wife for being a "lascivious adulterer" ("Don't you dare call me that again until I have looked it up!"). Then in the midst of his temper tantrum, lying on the floor and pounding it, a new patient arrives. It's Peter O'Toole, essentially playing himself. He was Lawrence of Arabia, and he is very handsome. He lies on the couch and tells the "doctor" he has a problem with women; they chase him, and he can't say no. Between slugs of whisky, Fassbender asks, "So, what is your problem?" Peter wants to be true to his girlfriend, Carole.

As they continue, O'Toole gets up and Fassbender lies down on the couch. Fassbender leans in and whispers, "Why don't you marry her and cheat?" Then Fassbender volunteers, "I like thighs. Do you like thighs?" Then, "I can't take more than fifteen minutes of your sex life at one time!" and he ends the hour. Fassbender invites O'Toole to group sessions. "You'll like this. It's a real freak show. If it gets dull, we sing songs." Turned on by all this talk of sex, Fassbender gets on the phone with his mistress: "Hello my little laxative. This is baby Fritzie here." O'Toole's reaction is, "He must be a genius!" There is nothing right about any of this, but it is very funny.

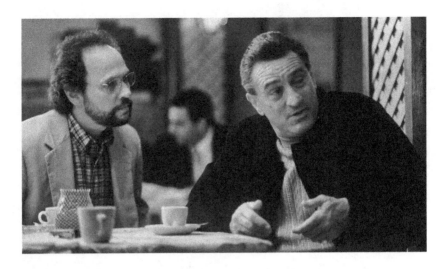

Analyze This (1999) is less anarchic but also very funny. Billy Crystal is psychologist Dr. Ben Sobel, and the first post-credits scene is priceless. He is in session with his patient, Caroline (Molly Shannon), who is in the middle of spouting clichés about "getting in touch with my uniqueness" and is crying. She can't believe that her marriage is over; maybe there is still hope. Dr. Sobel responds, "Well, he did take out a restraining order against you, and I have to be honest, that's usually not a good sign." She whines, "What should I do?" and he stands up and shouts at her, "You are a tragedy queen, 'Steve doesn't like me!' Who gives a shit. Get a fuckin' life!" Then we see him sitting quietly and we realize that was a fantasy, what he wished he could say. Instead, he now tells her what she was saying was very interesting and he wants her to think about it until after his vacation. She tells him he is just like her husband, wanting to throw her away. He responds, "That's not true, I'm gonna see you next week, whereas Steve never wants to see you again," and then he winces at what he just said out loud.

This is funny because it suggests something real. There are many times I have wished I could allow myself to say what I was really thinking instead of a carefully measured response. I've had mentors who have modeled doing just that, and it is liberating; a family therapy teacher of mine once stood up on a chair and shouted at an arguing married couple to "shut up!" It got their attention. You need a lot of confidence to pull that off.

A complicated series of incidents has gotten Paul, a Mafia boss with anxiety issues played by Robert De Niro, to rely on Ben Sobel to help him with his panic attacks. Ben asks Paul about his relationship with his father, who died suddenly years ago. Paul relates that his father slapped him around because as a kid he was hanging around with a bad crowd. Ben wonders if Paul was angry with his dad at the time he died and gives a solid explanation of the Oedipal conflict. Paul takes it literally. When he hears that Oedipus killed his father to marry his mother, he goes, "Fuckin' Greeks," and then asks, "Have you seen my mother? Are you out of your fuckin' mind?"

Later, in a smart and funny scene, Paul is angry and upset. Ben suggests he hit a pillow to get his anger out (a gestalt technique). Crossed meanings: gangster Paul pulls out his gun and shoots the pillow to smithereens. Ben nervously asks, "Feel better?" And Paul admits, "Yeah, I do."

+ + +

When I was in college, I had an English professor named Kenneth Koch. He was a highly regarded poet and a wonderful teacher. His course was called "The Comic in Modern Literature." He told us this story on himself.

Koch had been in classic Freudian psychoanalysis for years, when one day his therapist suggested that they should begin to consider when to end the therapy. Koch says he sat straight up on the couch and protested, "We can't stop now! I still get anxious before I give a talk. I get really depressed when a poem I'm writing isn't working!"

There was a long silence.

Then, his analyst, offering the grace of perspective, said to him, gently, "And you are going to die someday too."

This is what passes for psychiatric humor. It's both profound and funny, very much like life.

RECOMMENDED READING

Gabbard, Glen, and Krin Gabbard. *Psychiatry and the Cinema*. 2nd edition. Washington, D.C.: American Psychiatric Press, Inc.; 1999.

> This is more about how psychiatry is portrayed in films than about madness or therapy.

Lindner, Robert. *The Fifty-Minute Hour*. New York: Other Press; 1999.

> A classic of the 1950s, these psychoanalytic therapy sessions read like short stories, revealing the inner world of the therapist as much as of the patient.

Minuchin, Sal. *Families and Family Therapy*. 2nd edition. London: Routledge; 2012.

> A founding text on family therapy.

Napier, August, and Carl Whitaker. *The Family Crucible: The Intense Experience of Family Therapy*. New York: Harper and Row; 2017.

> As someone who had the privilege of working with Whitaker, I can vouch for the accuracy of the moment-by-moment examples of Carl's work with different families.

Yalom Irvin. *Love's Executioner: And Other Tales of Psychotherapy*. 2nd edition. New York: Basic Books; 2012.

> Tales of psychotherapy, from an unconventional therapist.

I would have never written this without the support and patient persistence of my son, Noah Charney. Noah is an established author, an expert on art crime, with some twenty books to his credit. Knowing my passion for the course I taught for so many years at Yale, he encouraged my wish to try to capture the experience in a book, and offered to guide me through the process of finding a publisher. His faith in my project, his practical advice, and his loving wish to help me fulfill a dream, were invaluable.

My wife, Diane, was my number-one cheerleader for this project. A retired Yale professor of French and Writing, she tirelessly read every chapter and gave me detailed edits—catching grammar mistakes and inconsistencies, as well as making sure my thoughts and sentences were clear. Her enthusiasm and encouragement, chapter by chapter, really made a difference. She would want you to know that any unnecessary semicolons are my own (I can't help it–I like semicolons).

Urška Charney, my daughter-in-law, is my perfect reader: intelligent, curious, and thoughtful. Her queries and suggestions were always spot-on, helping me clarify my ideas and my explanations. The book is infinitely better because of her efforts. An excellent copy editor, she meticulously helped me prepare the manuscript, frequently and patiently rescuing me from the computer wilderness, making Word do what we needed it to do. On top of all that she is a gifted photographer. I was so pleased when she offered her work as my author photo. Urška is talented, warm, and wise. How lucky I feel to have her in our family!

I want to thank several friends and family members who read individual chapters and took the time to give me their reactions and suggestions: Robert Horwitz, Frank Corcoran, Chris Livesay, Erika

Bizzari, Bobbie and Peter Bartucca, Susan Miller, and my sister, Nancy Hayes.

I am thankful to colleagues whose suggestions helped me shape my discussions, including Vincent Casaregola, former Director of the Film Studies Program at Saint Louis University, whom I met when he did a peer review for Johns Hopkins. His advocacy for how well my book could serve in courses in abnormal psychology and film studies, and his appreciation for my choice of movies, were especially valuable. Nathan Dunne, a world expert on Tarkovsky, also wrote a much-appreciated review supporting the use of *Madness at the Movies* in academic settings. Clinical and Research Psychologist Diane Sholomskas pointed out some confusions in my discussion of DID and its treatments, which I was glad to correct.

Of course, any errors of fact or judgment are mine alone.

Dudley Andrew, R. Seldon Rose Professor Emeritus of Comparative Literature and of Film Studies at Yale; Peter Salovey, current President of Yale, and Chair of the Psychology Department at Yale when I was teaching my "Madness at the Movies" course; and Jeffrey Brenzel, former Dean of Admissions for Yale, Lecturer in Humanities and Philosophy, and former Master of Timothy Dwight College, also cheered me on with this project.

I must express my gratitude to the students of my "Madness at the Movies" course at Yale College, The American University of Rome, Arcadia University in Rome, and at the University of Ljubljana, Slovenia. Their insightful questions and their enthusiasm for the subject made teaching a real joy.

This is my first book and everything about the process of publication was new to me. I want to especially thank a group of friends who called themselves "Team Madness"—Lyndsey Posner, Ian Morley, Andrew Fitchie, and Annie Loui. We had animated discussions throughout the negotiations with Johns Hopkins University Press during which they generously gave me the benefit of their experience.

I want to thank Joe Rusko, my editor at Johns Hopkins University Press, who championed the project from the start and shepherded me and the book through the tall grass and brambles of what seemed to me a byzantine vetting process.

I am grateful to the folks at Newgen, Production Manager Rashmi Bhate, Production Editor Alan Bradshaw, and Copy Editor Erin Ivy, for their enthusiasm and thoughtfully detailed suggestions. They managed the feat of keeping the book very much my own but helping me say what I meant with greater clarity and economy. Our discussions made this stage of the book-making a joy.

I wrote *Madness at the Movies* to honor my students, and to have a written record of a teaching experience that was the academic highlight of my life.

And I wrote it for my beloved, wonderful granddaughters, Eleonora and Izabella, so when they grow up they will be able to know me, their "Greppen," a little better.

Chapter 1: *One Flew Over the Cuckoo's Nest,* United Artists, 1975

Chapter 2: *Through a Glass Darkly,* Janus Films, 1961; *Benny and Joon,* Metro-Goldwyn-Mayer, 1993; *Network,* United Artists, 1976; *I Never Promised You a Rose Garden,* New World Pictures, 1977

Chapter 3: *Repulsion,* Compton Films, 1965; *Spider,* Odeon Films, 2002; *A Beautiful Mind,* Universal Pictures, 2001; *Saint Maud,* Escape Plan Productions, 2019; *The Shining,* Warner Bros., 1980

Chapter 4: *Taxi Driver,* Columbia Pictures, 1976; *The Treasure of the Sierra Madre,* Warner Bros.–First National, 1948; *Dr. Strangelove or: How I Learned to Stop Worrying and Love the Bomb,* Hawk Films, 1964

Chapter 5: *The Night of the Hunter,* United Artists, 1955; *White Heat,* Warner Bros., 1949; *American Psycho,* Lions Gate Films, 2000; *Joker,* Warner Bros., 2019

Chapter 6: *Strangers on a Train,* Warner Bros., 1951; *Cape Fear,* Melville-Talbot Productions, 1962; *Cape Fear,* Amblin Entertainment, 1991; *The Talented Mr. Ripley,* Miramax, 1999

Chapter 7: *Psycho,* Paramount Pictures, 1960; *The Three Faces of Eve,* 20th Century Fox, 1957; *Dead of Night,* Ealing Studios, 1945; *Primal Fear,* Paramount Pictures, 1996

Chapter 8: *Peeping Tom,* Michael Powell, 1960; *Blue Velvet,* De Laurentiis Entertainment Group, 1986; *Reservoir Dogs,* Live Entertainment, 1992

Chapter 9: *A Woman Under the Influence,* Faces International Films, 1974; *Mr. Jones,* Rastar Productions, 1993; *One, Two, Three,* Bavaria Film, 1961; *Good Morning, Vietnam,* Touchstone Pictures, 1987

Chapter 10: *Ordinary People,* Paramount Pictures, 1980; *The Hospital,* Simcha Productions, 1971; *Harold and Maude,* Mildred Lewis and Colin Higgins Productions, 1971; *Melancholia,* Zentropa Entertainments, 2011

Chapter 11: *As Good As It Gets,* TriStar Pictures, 1997; *Hannah and Her Sisters,* Orion Pictures, 1986; *What About Bob?,* Touchstone Pictures, 1991; *Vertigo,* Paramount Pictures, 1958; *Toc Toc,* Âtresmédia Ciné, 2017; *The Aviator,* Forward Pass, 2004

Chapter 12: *Spellbound,* Selznick International Pictures, 1945; *The Snake Pit,* 20th Century Fox, 1948; *Grosse Pointe Blank,* Hollywood Pictures, 1997; *Klute,* Warner Bros., 1971; *An Unmarried Woman,* 20th Century Fox, 1978; *Bob and Carol and Ted and Alice,* Columbia Pictures, 1969; *Ordinary People,* Paramount Pictures, 1980; *Blume in Love,* Warner Bros., 1973; *I Never Promised You a Rose Garden,* New World Pictures, 1977; *Good Will Hunting,* Miramax Films, 1997; *What's New, Pussycat?,* Famous Artists Productions, 1965; *Analyze This,* Village Roadshow Pictures, 1999

obsessive-compulsive disorder (OCD), 11, 125, 336; in *As Good as It Gets*, 335-36, 347; in *The Aviator*, 366-71; defined, 345-47; medications for, 347; symptoms, 338, 345-46; in *Toc Toc*, 264-65; *See also* compulsions; obsessions

Oedipus complex, 212, 407

One Flew Over the Cuckoo's Nest (1975), 17-22; awards, 19; filming location, 19-20; group therapy session in, 21; Kesey's novel and, 17-18, 19, 20; narrative change for film, 19; paranoia in, 18, 19, 21; screenplay, 19; *Through a Glass Darkly* compared with, 24

One Flew Over the Cuckoo's Nest (novel, Kesey), 17-18, 20

One Flew Over the Cuckoo's Nest (play), 17-18

One, Two, Three (1961), 286-89; bipolar illness versus hypomania in, 286-87

Ordinary People (1980), xviii, 37, 281, 290-93; act structure of, 297, 299, 302; awards, 292; cast, 292-94; diagnostic commentary, 310-23; grief and depression in, 291-93, 311-14, 318; influence of, 291; opening scene, 293; screenplay, 292, 300, 311, 322; suicide in, 304, 311, 314-23; walk-through description, 293-310

Ordinary People (Guest), xviii, 293

Ormonde, Czenzi, 163

O'Toole, Peter, 143, 405

Oz, Frank. See *What About Bob?* (1991)

Ozu, Yasujiro, 89

Page, Anthony. See *I Never Promised You a Rose Garden* (1977)

panic attacks, 337, 343-45, 352, 407

Pantoliano, Joe, xx

paranoia: conspiracy, 75-76, 116, 118-20; defined, 106-7; delusions, 10, 39, 75, 83, 105-12, 117, 289, 369; in *Dr. Strangelove or: How I Learned to Stop Worrying and Love the Bomb*, 118-20; grandiosity, 39-40, 54-56, 75-76, 111, 116-17, 280, 285, 319; projection, 106, 116; in *Taxi Driver*, 105-17; in *The Treasure of the Sierra Madre*, 115-17

paranoid schizophrenia, 40, 81-83, 143, 153

parent-child relationships, 290-91. *See also* father-daughter relationships;

father-son relationships; mother-daughter relationships; mother-son relationships

Passgård, Lars, 26

pathognomonic, definition of, 112

Peck, Gregory, 182, 183, 373, 374

Peeping Tom (1960), 6, 11, 67, 225-32; act structure of, 235, 239; delusions in, 244, 248; diagnostic commentary, 241-50; movie conceits about psychopaths in, 244-50; obsession in, 238, 247-48; opening scene, 225-26, 242; restoration, 232; screenplay, 227; voyeurism in, 231; walk-through description, 232-41

Perkins, Anthony, 193, 200, 231, 232

personality disorders: antisocial personality disorder, 112, 125, 140, 159-60, 177-78; borderline personality disorder, 125, 212, 213, 317; defined, 123; *DSM-5* on, 124-25; dependent personalities, 125, 212; depressive personality disorder, 124; medications for, 125; narcissistic personality disorder, 125, 141; types of, 125. *See also* psychopaths

Phillips, Todd. See *Joker* (2019)

phobias, 341-45, 358, 365; acrophobia, 341-42, 359-63; agoraphobia, 343; claustrophobia, 206, 259, 341; germaphobia, 336, 345, 364, 367; treatments for, 342-43; in *Vertigo*, 359-63

Phoenix, Joaquin, 154, 161

Picasso, Pablo, 14

Polanski, Roman: *Chinatown*, 8, 60; as controversial director, 14; *Knife in the Water*, 60; *The Pianist*, 60; *Rosemary's Baby* (1968), 260; *The Tenant*, 60. See also *Repulsion* (1965)

post-traumatic stress disorder (PTSD); in *Taxi Driver*, 104-5; in *Vertigo*, 361, 362-63

Powell, Michael, 226-32, 233, 235, 241, 243, 246, 247, 250. See also *Peeping Tom* (1960)

Pressburger, Emeric, 227, 231

Primal Fear (1996), 222-23; dissociative identity disorder in, 223

projection, 106, 116

psychiatrists, xxi, 2, 8, 9; in *Bob and Carol and Ted and Alice*, 391; in *Dead of Night*, 220; in *Grosse Pointe Blank*, 385-86; in *Harold and Maude*, 327; in *The Hospital*,

von Sydow, Max, 25
von Trier, Lars. See *Melancholia* (2011)
voyeur: male gaze, 243; movie watchers as, 67, 198, 226, 233–42, 246–47; as murderers, 231, 241–50; in *Peeping Tom*, 231, 242, 246; reviewers as, 246; therapists as, 239–40. See also *Blue Velvet* (1986); *Peeping Tom* (1960)

Walker, Robert, 181
Wallace, George, 89, 108
Walsh, Raoul. See *White Heat* (1949)
Washington, Denzel, 291
Wayne, John, xiv–xv, 89
Welles, Orson: *Citizen Kane* (1941), xi; *The Magnificent Ambersons* (1942), 127; *Touch of Evil* (1958), 193
What About Bob? (1991), 355–58; anxiety disorders in, 355–58
What's New Pussycat (1965), therapy in, 405
Whitaker, Carl, 314, 380, 381, 382
White Heat (1949), 147–49, 283; psychopath in, 147–49
Whitman, Walt, 14

Wilder, Billy, 4; *Witness for the Prosecution* (1957), 127. See also *One, Two, Three* (1961)
Wilder, Thornton, 163
Williams, Robin: in *Good Morning, Vietnam*, 286, 287–89, 401, 404; in *Good Will Hunting*, 288, 401, 404; suicide of, 288–89
Winters, Shelley, 129
Wolff, Tobias, 14–15
Woman Under the Influence, A (1974), 257–61, 381; act structure of, 270, 271; anxiety in, 268, 281; awards, 260; bipolar diagnosis and, 280–81, 381; diagnostic commentary, 275–82; major depression in, 280–82; opening scene, 261; screenplay, 260–61; walk-through description, 261–74
women: stereotypes, 9, 181, 373; violence against, 64–65, 69–75, 211, 231, 249. *See also* mother-daughter relationships; mothers; mother-son relationships
Woodward, Joanne, 213, 218, 219

James Charney is a clinical professor of Psychiatry and Child Study at the Yale School of Medicine, where he teaches psychiatric interviewing and diagnosis to medical students and residents. He recently retired from a thirty-five-year practice of child and family psychiatry in New Haven, Connecticut. For twenty-five years he was the psychiatric consultant to the Choate-Rosemary Hall school in Wallingford, Connecticut, a private, boarding high school whose alumni range from John F. Kennedy to Jamie Lee Curtis. For thirteen years he taught Madness at the Movies, a popular senior seminar at Yale College, and the inspiration for this book. Since retiring from private practice, he continues to teach at the School of Medicine and consult at a private high school in Rome. He has taught a version of Madness at the Movies at Arcadia University of Rome, at The American University in Rome, and at the University of Ljubljana in Slovenia.